The
Framework of
Systemic
Organization

The Framework of Systemic Organization

A Conceptual Approach to Families and Nursing

Marie-Luise Friedemann

SAGE Publications
International Educational and Professional Publisher
Thousand Oaks London New Delhi

For information address:

SAGE Publications, Inc.
2455 Teller Road
Thousand Oaks, California 91320
E-mail: order@sagepub.com

SAGE Publications Ltd.
6 Bonhill Street
London EC2A 4PU
United Kingdom

SAGE Publications India Pvt. Ltd.
M-32 Market
Greater Kailash I
New Delhi 110 048 India

Printed in the United States of America

Library of Congress Cataloging-in-Publication Data

Friedemann, Marie-Luise.
   The framework of systemic organization: A conceptual approach to families and nursing / Marie-Luise Friedemann.
        p.   cm.
   Includes bibliographical references and index.
   ISBN 0-8039-4913-8 (alk. paper). — ISBN 0-8039-4914-6 (pbk. : alk. paper).
      1. Family nursing.   2. Family nursing—Philosophy.   I. Title.
   RT120.F34F76   1995
   610.73—dc20   95-21327

This book is printed on acid-free paper.

95   96   97   98   99   10   9   8   7   6   5   4   3   2   1

Sage Production Editor: Diane S. Foster
Sage Copy Editor: Gillian Dickens
Sage Typesetter: Christina M. Hill

Contents

Foreword

When I began my doctoral dissertation on family development processes in the mid-1970s, I approached the task with great anticipation. As a member of a new doctoral program in nursing, my mood went from anxiety, to nonbelief, to anger when I could not find linkages between existing nursing theory and family theory—most of which was developed external to nursing. The nursing perspective on family, including values and assumptions of the discipline transmitted across time, was virtually nonexistent. I believed then, as now, that nursing could use family theory external to nursing but that this theory *must* be reformed for our purposes. Because each discipline has its own societal mandate and perspective, theories external to nursing were not adequate to the task unless they were reformulated. Moreover, I believed then, as I do now, that nursing could and should not just reform existing theory external to nursing but should also develop its own family theory.

It became clear to me that this could be accomplished in a variety of ways; for example, one might reform family theory external to nursing by using nursing conceptual models. In an equally plausible method, one might reform this theory using existing middle-range theory in nursing and/or practice theory. Likewise, one might develop a theory using some hypothetical deductive and/or inductive means.

All of these efforts need to be examined in terms of theoretic criteria, such as internal consistency, as well as in multiple studies; the scrutiny of the marketplace would thus be brought to bear on these products. The good news today is that nursing scholars have accepted that challenge that lay before nursing more than 20 years ago. Nursing has labored long and hard to develop the nursing knowledge base needed to serve families. Today there are "family schools of thought" within nursing, excellent programs of research focused on testing family theory for nursing, and scholars such as Dr. Friedemann who have published textbooks designed to guide nursing practice, education, and research. I believe Dr. Friedemann's continuing family development within nursing might be seen as falling within the "crises" school of thought. With the indelible mark of an experienced nurse, Dr. Friedemann is concerned about how nurses might address assessment of families' diagnoses of problems, intervene to assist families with these problems, and evaluate the practice outcomes. This textbook is a welcome addition to family knowledge within nursing. Dr. Friedemann has developed family theory for nursing by using a variety of methods. The chapters are rich not only in practice implications but also in suggestions for research.

Today there are threats to developing family theory in and for nursing. One of these is a nihilistic view within nursing that sees all theory as useless. Far from this view of 20 years ago, which in essence assumed that all nursing must develop theory-based family practice, these reactionaries would return to atheoretical practice, education, and even research. As bizarre as this sounds and as nondefensible this position is, good will come from this struggle internal to nursing. Because of this challenge, whole family schools of thought within nursing will become more tightly integrated with corollary programs of research, and we will have had the scholarly debates within nursing that will show us just how far nursing has progressed. Textbooks such as Dr. Friedemann's will be viewed 20 years from now as an excellent contribution to our struggle to develop family nursing science. But for now, let us revel in the breadth and depth of Dr. Friedemann's discussions of family from a perspective that is undeniably of nursing.

Ann L. Whall
Ann Arbor, Michigan

Introduction

The family has been a central theme throughout the history of modern nursing. A focus on the family was already evident in 1876, when Nightingale wrote instructions for district nurses and home missioners (Miller Ham & Chamings, 1983). On the basis of a review of historical literature, Whall and Fawcett (1991) found that much had been written about the family over the years, but the development of formal midrange family theory that is useful in practice has started only recently and still needs much work. Since the 1980s, several nursing leaders have attempted to formulate family theories based on existing conceptual models or have adapted theories from other disciplines to nursing (Clements & Roberts, 1983; Fawcett, 1975; Whall, 1986). Even though definitions of nursing have become holistic and include family and community (Murphy, 1986), the theoretical formulations are not specific enough to serve as practice guidelines and models for family research and the formation of hypotheses.

The framework of systemic organization is presented here as both a grand and a midrange theory. The theory originated from Wayne State University and was published initially in 1989 (Friedemann, 1989a). It includes philosophical underpinnings and propositions that form the basis of processes described at the midrange level. The nursing metaparadigm—environment-person-health nursing—has been expanded to include the dynamic concepts of family and family health to guide the explanation of systemic functioning of individuals, social and environmental systems, and interactions between them. These processes at the midrange level can then be made specific to various clinical situations and built into the nursing process. Furthermore, processes at the midrange level lend themselves to theory testing through research. In short, this framework bridges the various levels of theoretical abstraction and closes the gap between theory and nursing practice.

As all viable conceptual frameworks, the framework of systemic organization has evolved through a process of both inductive and deductive thinking processes. It represents a synthesis of my life and professional experiences, my worldview and personality, and is enriched by insights from scientific literature and research. Consequently, bits and pieces of the writing of scientists and practitioners in nursing, such as Rogers (1980), King (1981), and Newman (1979, 1983), and family specialists and researchers, including Kantor and Lehr (1975), Minuchin (1974), Haley (1976), and Beavers (Beavers, 1981; Lewis, Beavers, Gossett, & Phillips, 1976), have been reformulated and become part of my universe of discourse. Today, the evolutionary process is by no means complete. The framework continues to experience growth and change through discussions with groups of professionals, students, and colleagues and through the findings of theory-based research.

The framework of systemic organization is being taught to undergraduate, graduate, and doctoral nursing students at Wayne State University, numerous universities across the United States, and in German-speaking Europe. Likewise, a practice model derived from the framework (Friedemann, 1989b) is being used and tested in a variety of settings with families of acutely, chronically, and mentally ill clients; substance abusers; and families who have problems with parenting or coping with stress. Readers are asked to absorb and critically examine the thoughts and reasoning presented in this book, and if the truths about persons, families, and the role of the nurse correspond with their own, they may want to use this framework in their own creative way to grow as nurses and as people.

This book is organized into five parts. Part 1 constitutes the theoretical presentation of the framework and discusses the major concepts and their relationships to each other. In Chapter 1, the metaparadigm constructs of environment, person, and health—supplemented with family and family health—are discussed in depth. The presentation of the construct of nursing—a complex process that involves the inter-action of the nurse with the client(s) in need, the family, and their environment—is reserved for Chapter 2.

Part 2 includes three chapters that explain the interaction of modi-fying factors with the family process. A fourth chapter is added to sum-marize issues concerning the function, process, and use of family research. Family structure (Chapter 3), family life span considerations (Chapter 4), and the influence of culture (Chapter 5) contribute to the many variations of families. The focus is on family health and healthy adaptation to changes. Chapter 6 addresses tenets of positivist-empiricist science and their influence on theoretical debates, the challenges of the operationalization of midrange theory, the confrontation of the quantitative and qualitative paradigms, and the use of triangu-lation.

Problems nurses often encounter with families in crisis are described in the remainder of the book. Family processes related to all topics are presented theoretically with the help of clinical examples. Findings from existing researchers and theoretical discussions in the literature will be cited to validate the theoretical propositions and process descriptions.

Part 3 focuses on crises from within the family system. The frame-work is applied here for the support of families struggling to find health in their own specific way. Chapter 7 discusses crises arising from developmental transitions and concentrates on possible difficulties families encounter as individuals reach various stages in their lives. Chapter 8 focuses on structural changes in the family. Crises resulting from family dissolution, adjustment to losses and structural change, and the merging of individuals and families in the formation of a new system are also addressed. Chapter 9 presents a broad view of addic-tions as they arise from and severely impair the family process. Crises with substance abuse, violence, and other addictions are explained as cyclical interpersonal processes encouraged and maintained by the family process as a whole and each individual's personal attempt to meet needs. Chapter 10 addresses methods of research and their use-fulness and limitations in theory testing with families in crisis.

Part 4 applies to crises with illness. Chapter 11 discusses the inter-action of families and the acute care system and focuses on the nurse's role in addressing crises quickly and effectively. The focus of Chapter 12 is terminal illness and the preparation of the family for death. Chapter 13 discusses crises that can occur as families give care to chronically ill members, with special emphasis on the transition from home care to institutionalization. Chapter 14 deals with issues around caring for members with developmental disabilities, mental illnesses, and dementias and their devastating effects on families. Nurses are shown ways to assist families as they experience severe losses in their relationships with the afflicted individuals and how growth can be promoted within the process of caring. Chapter 15 relates to issues of research and measurement within the topic of families and illness.

Part 5 addresses crises from the environment. Family reactions to external assaults or adverse conditions, such as violent crimes, prob-lems with work, unemployment, poverty, and homelessness, form the content of this part. Chapter 20, the final chapter, focuses on research implications. The readers are also offered suggestions for the conduct of their own studies with the families in discussion.

In absorbing the content of this book, the reader is guided toward a concept of nursing that unifies theory, clinical expertise, and research and pursues the one important aim of supporting the process of seek-ing health and well-being unique to each individual and family.

Acknowledgments

The development of a theoretical framework is an ongoing growth process. Without the critical thinking and excellent feedback of many nurses and students engaged in practice, teaching, and research at universities, health care institutions, and social service agencies locally, across the nation, and overseas, this book could not have been written. I wish to thank all the people who have applied this framework to real-life situations and reported the encouraging outcomes that nourished my enthusiasm and maintained my belief in the reality of a nursing process that truly reaches out to families and their members. I deeply appreciate the efforts of all teachers and researchers who use my publications to enhance the growth of their students and guide them in exploring the depths of the family process. These people have convinced me of the need for this book to explain and tie the various pieces together into a unified whole.

Specifically, I extend my sincere thanks to my associates and students who have contributed their time to the refinement of the framework, treatment model, and assessment instruments: Dr. Rhonda Montgomery, Director of the Gerontology Center, University of Kansas, and longtime mentor and research associate; Dr. Adele Webb, faculty member at the University of Akron and research associate; Clementine Rice, Rosanna DeMarco, and Ann Smith, PhD candidates at Wayne State University who are involved in research with this framework; and Olivia Washington and Margie Miller, both faculty members at Wayne State University, College of Nursing, and instrumental in launching my treatment model in the community. Finally, very special appreciation goes to my husband, Heinrich, for his endless patience and hours of proofreading and critiquing the manuscript.

PART
1

The Framework
of Systemic Organization

1

The Framework and Its Propositions

The major concepts of the framework of systemic organization explained in this chapter are environment, person, family, health, and family health. Each is presented with its underlying propositions and the theoretically deduced dynamic processes that define its relationships to the other concepts.

Environment

Propositions
1. All existing things are organized as open systems of energy and matter in movement.
2. The basic order of the universe is ruled by conditions largely unknown to humans. It is timeless and limitless, and its power is awesome. Under universal order all existing systems are connected and congruent in pattern and rhythm.
3. The organization of systems on Earth follows an order secondary to and dependent on the order of the universe: the laws of the earthly conditions of time, space, energy, and matter.

All matter and energy are organized into systems. Systems are defined by rhythms and spacial patterns. Rhythm involves the time of revolutions of matter and energy around the system's center of gravitation, whereas the spacial pattern describes the system's use of space. The state of systems being attuned to each other in their rhythms and patterns in a way that energy can flow freely within and between systems is called *congruence.*

Examples of systems include microsystems, such as atoms, molecules, and cells; inorganic systems as in rocks, metals, water, or air; biological systems of plants and animals; ecological systems; nature as a whole; the terrestrial system; the solar system; and finally the universe. The terrestrial system, subordinate to the universal system, is specific to Earth and depends on the earthly conditions of time, space, energy, and matter.

Open systems theory is applicable here (Weinberg, 1975). This view of living systems is global in that it looks at phenomena in their totality. It does not reduce the whole to simpler parts but instead explains the parts by the function they perform as a contribution to the operation of the total system (Constantine, 1986). Open systems view is *organismic,* meaning that each living system has a specified internal mechanism for maintenance and development that determines the interaction process of the parts and makes the prediction of outcomes difficult (Ackoff, 1974). The system therefore has properties of its own that are different from the sum of its parts (von Bertalanffy, 1968). Furthermore, all living systems exchange matter, energy, and information and are interrelated and interdependent.

Human organizations are social systems of differing size and complexity in which the individual person always functions as the smallest subsystem (von Bertalanffy, 1968). Social systems are institutions such as families, schools, workplaces, recreational organizations, communities, governments, and economic systems. They differ from biological systems in that their human subsystems have the capability of directing internal systems operations through a decision-making process. Furthermore, humans simultaneously carry assigned roles and function as subsystems in numerous other social systems. Consequently, they help to shape these systems by exchanging information, energy, and material with them and, in turn, their own personal system experiences growth and an ongoing process of change and evolution.

The concept of environment comprises all things outside the system in the focus of nursing (e.g., a person, a family, a hospital system). The environment is therefore the inescapable dynamic context in which each focal system evolves.

Person

Propositions

1. Human perception is limited by the structure and function of the human body.
2. Persons have the ability to realize their dependency on natural forces and foresee death. This threat to their systemic existence has the potential to evoke a disturbance of system processes and incongruence. All incongruence is experienced as anxiety.
3. Humans have attempted to decrease their vulnerability by creating an artificial environment or civil system within which they maintain a sense of control.
4. Persons have the capacity for transcendence through which they can re-establish congruence with systems of their environment and with the order of the universe.
5. Culture is the total of human life patterns. Culture is everchanging through the integration of new knowledge in the human way of life, leading to new patterns while forgetting old ones and transmitting the new patterns to the next generation.

Because forces that move electrons around the nucleus of an atom also move planets around their suns, human system organization is a universal organization, and consequently, humans are intrinsically one with their environment and the universe and therefore congruent in rhythm and pattern. However, only if humans fully accept their connectedness and live without a pretense of vain power can they sense their congruence and be free of anxiety (Jung, 1953). For centuries, the purpose of human life has been the major theme of philosophy and the striving of humans to find that purpose to live accordingly has been viewed as a distinguishing feature between humans and other living organisms. Humans who want to live purposefully have to base their actions on a certain undisputed set of values assumed to be central to existence and true. These values serve as the underpinning that allows the emergence of intellectual and emotional experiences or the processes called individuation, which will be explained later. Individuation, however, can occur only in a state of relatively low anxiety. Therefore, the most basic human processes, the system dynamics described in the following paragraphs, curb anxiety.

According to the interpersonal theory of Sullivan (1953), people who do not find themselves supported or approved of by others sense anxiety in the form of tension and energy that they will transform into action to reduce the anxiety. Similarly expressed, in terms of the theory of systemic organization, anxiety arises through systemic tension resulting from system incongruence. From the perspective of human perception, a state of congruence among people and social systems on Earth is a Utopia. Although all systems are involved in a struggle to attain congruence, their rhythms and patterns are often attuned to sharply opposed forces and contradictory ideologies, beliefs, or principles. Humans involved with systems that fail to reflect their own values and beliefs experience incongruence. If the horizontal flow of energy through their own system and the vertical flow through the systems network are blocked, humans will respond with anxiety and will activate system processes in the attempt to reestablish congruence and the flow of energy.

The basic organization of human system processes to buffer anxiety and attempt congruence is shown in Figure 1.1. It is identical to the processes of all social systems in that it involves the four targets of stability, growth, control, and spirituality. Each person or social system emphasizes these targets in a unique way and uses processes learned and acquired over time. The pursuit and balancing of the targets occur on an abstract level through subconsciously determined behaviors. These behaviors are triggered by a value and belief system acquired from the older generations or the environment, most of which has never been consciously examined and challenged. Nevertheless, actual behaviors or actions used to meet the targets are observable and can be assessed within the nursing process. These concrete strategies can be categorized into the four process dimensions of system mainte-

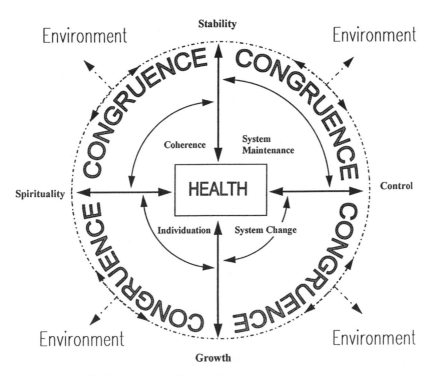

Figure 1.1. Life Process of the Human System

nance, system change, coherence, and individuation, which are indicated as quadrants of different sizes in Figure 1.1.

The System Targets

The four targets of control, spirituality, stability, and growth are shown in Figure 1.1 as they interact with each other along the system periphery to form a dynamic equilibrium through which the healthy system continuously adjusts to find congruence between its own order and that of its environment.

Control. The target of control serves the purpose of reducing anxiety evoked by a sense of vulnerability and helplessness. Through control, humans maintain the system unchanged or regulate and channel knowledge and information to produce desirable changes.

Since the beginning of human civilization, great strides have been made to control external forces that threaten human existence. Protective systems that originally consisted of little more than caves and fires to keep warm have been expanded into elaborate arrangements, such as economies for the supply of goods, political systems to enforce and control leadership and subordination, and social systems to ensure cooperation and division of labor. As a result, modern humans have achieved considerable control over their dependency on nature through a superimposed civil system and a sense of power that have made it possible to deny the awesome power of the universe during most of their lifetime.

Humans in industrialized countries have attuned their own system to their superimposed civil system. They work according to prescribed job descriptions and schedules, use transportation, buy goods to stimulate the economy, and produce and educate offspring for the purpose of survival within the civil system. Values are imposed by media pressure and many people fail to recognize that their personal freedom has been lost to daily routines and a blind pursuit of material commodities. Civil systems originally thought to protect mankind have become increasingly complex and difficult to control. An individual's contribution to the total system has become insignificant and the sense of power it originally granted is eroding.

Humans invariably experience moments of universal truth as they become aware of their vulnerability and unavoidable end. They are reminded of it by reports of wars and epidemics as well as by pictures of natural catastrophes and loved ones who have become victims of tragedy, illness, or crime. Furthermore, many circumstances in their personal lives cannot be handled by regular means of control.

Spirituality. Humans who live in primitive conditions target spirituality as their major defense against helplessness. In today's world, spirituality is becoming increasingly important again in that it leads the alienated person back to experiencing connectedness and the order of the universe. Spirituality does not signify resignation but is an active pursuit that employs the intellect and the emotions. Instead of willfully controlling and modifying environmental influences, through spirituality humans adjust their own rhythm and pattern to render them congruent with chosen systems of contact: a person, an organization, nature, or the universe. Healthy spirituality results in congruence or unity with other systems and is experienced as a sense of belonging, acceptance, respect, wisdom, and inner peace. In exercising spirituality, healthy humans have the capacity to transcend their immediate environment through a mode of perception that goes beyond logical reasoning to locate target systems that reflect the universal order, unify with them, and sense within the unity the awesome power of the universe.

Stability. The two remaining targets of stability and growth are needed for system survival. The target of stability wards off anxiety about system decay, and growth is needed to counteract anxiety about stagnation and incongruence with a changed environment. Stability addresses the core of a person, character, or personality. It signifies the person's definition of identity that includes body image and self-esteem. Stability is embedded in a set of values, attitudes, and rules of life. The person follows these rules to ward off disturbing influences that might challenge traditional life patterns or attitudes and endanger the system's integrity. It is important to realize that stability is not equivalent to safety or adherence to tradition. Stability includes all of a person's basic values and beliefs, including the flexibility to change if a need arises and the openness to challenge one's own opinions and attitudes. Consequently, a person may change behavior patterns and attitudes without affecting system stability as long as the changes are in concert with the underlying basic pattern of values.

Growth. The target of growth requires a substantial reorganization of basic values and priorities. Growth is necessary in situations in which a person's stability has become incongruent with the environment and results in new behaviors derived from a set of newly adjusted beliefs and attitudes. A true growth process has to overcome great resistance, is disquieting to humans, and is often painful. A threat to a person's basic belief patterns demands a redefinition of identity and purpose. Healthy humans experience growth as a response to a crisis when it becomes evident that traditional system structure and function are no longer adequate. The person struggles to prevent a breakdown of the total human system by reaching for a new level of stability based on a revised set of values and life priorities. Growth can also happen at a slower pace by incorporating new knowledge into the human system that leads to certain flashes of enlightenment and stimulates the person to reexamine traditional values and modify convictions.

If the systemic process is successful, stability and growth as well as control and spirituality are pursued to the extent desired by the individual. Each target represents a separate, independent dimension and all four dimensions concur in bringing about congruence. This balance represents a basic life pattern that serves as a blueprint to all actions, is relatively stable, and distinguishes one person from the other. To understand the system processes fully, the reader needs to put Figure 1.1 in motion. Depending on a person's situation in life, age, or culture, the basic life pattern may vary to some extent, as one target or another gains or loses importance while the strategies within the process dimensions change accordingly. Through a fluctuating movement toward the targets, the system connects with environmental contact systems. Connections are unstable as well, in that many are dropped and others are instated over time and each change carries a potential to provoke anxiety. Consequently, human life signifies a continuing struggle to readjust the four targets and balance them against each other and the environment.

The Process Dimensions

The process dimensions of system maintenance, system change, coherence, and individuation encompass the concrete behaviors necessary to strive toward the abstract targets. On the level of the family system, these dimensions are described in the literature and have been extracted by factor analytic research (Friedemann, 1991a). The same dimensions are applicable to human systems and can be reconciled with existing theories of human functioning. Arrows that form the boundary of the four segments pictured in Figure 1.1 point in two directions, meaning that each group of behaviors leads to two of the targets.

System Maintenance. System maintenance (see Figure 1.1, right-upper quadrant) is directed at stability and control. It includes all actions that maintain the system and protect it from threatening changes. These actions are aimed at meeting physical, emotional, and social needs and are comparable to what Orem (1985) termed *self-care actions*. System maintenance encompasses actions such as sleeping, exercising, eating, working, resting, or enjoying recreational activities. Many are sharply regulated and occur in repetitive patterns or routines. Added to these actions are behaviors aimed at reducing the threat of change, which are based on concepts described in the literature such as "resistance resources" (Antonovsky, 1979), "coping style" (Andrews, Tennant, Hewson, & Vaillant, 1978), or hardiness derived from stress and coping theory. Likewise, defense mechanisms described in psychoanalytic theory are a part of system maintenance, because they are activated in stressful situations (Lazarus & Alfert, 1964).

At the base of system maintenance lies a set of values and beliefs that concerns physical and mental health as well as orientation to time, tradition, and flexibility. Healthy system maintenance represents a controllable order or pattern of life that provides the person with a sense of security and autonomy. Many of the patterns are acquired in early childhood and practiced throughout the adult life span. Consequently, system maintenance is stable but does not preclude changes in the system. If flexibility, openness to examine options, respect for diversity, and doubt about beliefs and attitudes are integrated in system maintenance, the person may change patterns of daily life and attitudes without affecting the basic value structure of system maintenance. In fact, such a person can modify system structure without experiencing the struggle and pain that are often associated with system change.

System Change. System change (see Figure 1.1, right-lower quadrant) is an independent dimension not antithetical to system maintenance. For system change to occur, a person experiences pressure from within or from the environment. Tension or unhappiness with the present situation compels the person to test values and set new priorities in life. Actions of system change lead to the targets of control and growth. System change is brought about by conscious acts controlled by the person that lead to decisions about whether or not to accept and integrate certain information, change, or replace old values and attitudes. Resulting structural and process changes are ultimately incorporated into system maintenance and constitute new patterns to be used on an ongoing basis.

An example of system change is a man who recovers from a coronary infarct. The person has changed those patterns of life that have contributed to the system tension and therefore to the disease. If striving toward perfection was the problem, the person has learned to accept human weakness and has become accepting of himself. Without experiencing radical shifts in values and priorities of life, he would have followed the rehabilitation orders of his physician only to return to his old life as soon as possible, a strategy of system maintenance.

Coherence. The dimension of coherence (see Figure 1.1, left-upper quadrant) signifies the joining of a person's subsystems into a unified whole and all the behaviors necessary to maintain the unity. Values, attitudes, beliefs, and perceptions underlying coherence concern the self and the human purpose in life. Consequently, the most stable components of a person—namely, the body and its organs, as well as psychological constructs, such as personality, self-system, self-esteem, body image, personal identity, self-confidence, and sexual identity—are integral parts of the coherence dimension. Coherence develops in childhood through parental support, acceptance, and encouragement as well as successfully mastered environmental challenges (Erikson, 1950). Coherent persons feel secure and at peace within. They accept their weaknesses but at the same time acknowledge the abilities and talents that they courageously convert into actions.

Figure 1.1 indicates that coherence targets not only stability but also spirituality. Through spirituality the human organism attunes the rhythms and patterns of physical, emotional, and ideological subsystems to a unified entity. In the light of frequent disappointments, setbacks, uncertainties, and conflicts in life, the striving toward a spiritual entity continues throughout a person's lifetime. Actions leading to coherence differ greatly among humans. Examples include reducing tension through exercise, enjoying the beauty of nature, cultural and artistic activities, listening to music, meditation, religious worship, practicing body awareness, finding oneself in sharing thoughts with others, enjoying life through the senses, and so on.

Individuation. Coherence is a requisite for the process of individuation (see Figure 1.1, left-lower quadrant), in that humans need to have inner security to venture out and apply themselves in their environment. Individuation also targets spirituality, this time by attuning the human entity to other systems. As subsystems of environmental systems, humans will adjust their own rhythm and patterns and feel connected to other units of their choice, be it a friendship system, a workplace, an ethnic group, an ideology, a religious community, nature, or the universe. Through such connections, people will develop their talents and ideas, absorb new knowledge, and gain understanding. Consequently, individuation leads to growth, but growth cannot happen in isolation.

Due to the connectedness of all open systems, individuation happens through an interactive process with other systems. If humans assume roles in other systems, they necessarily sacrifice a part of their personal freedom by taking on responsibilities in support of the system. Nevertheless, it is within such connectedness that humans can expand their minds and thoughts. Only by being connected can they be truly free. They take advantage of the system's revelations and have the opportunity to make their own personality felt within the system. This seeming contradiction has been recognized as philosophical truth throughout the ages (Jung, 1953).

Actions of individuation include intellectual and physical activities that expand a person's horizon, teach about the self and others, and lead to a new perspective and sense of purpose in life. Such activities can involve work, social tasks, education, listening to other opinions, reading and thoughtfully integrating literary ideas, critically analyzing the meaning of events, discovering new understanding through travel, exposing oneself to various cultures, and much more.

In summary, humans regulate the earthly conditions of time, space, energy, and materials through actions within the four process dimensions. System maintenance and system change lead to the target of control, coherence and individuation to the target of spirituality, system change and individuation to the target of growth, and system maintenance and coherence to the target of stability. Consequently, each human being needs a repertoire of actions within each dimension to successfully curb anxiety that arises through tension within the human system and at the interface with incongruent systems of the environment. It is important to realize when assessing human system actions that certain actions may pertain to more than one process dimension. For example, within the dimension of system maintenance, reading a book serves as a way to relax and balance daily physical activity with a restful period and intellectual stimulation. The same book may also provide an activity through which persons can ratify their own self and maintain coherence. Likewise, within individuation, the book may lead readers to examine their attitudes and give them an incentive to recognize prejudice and grow by adjusting values. Thus, it is not the action itself but its ascribed meaning that determines the systemic process dimension.

The quadrants of the process dimensions indicated in Figure 1.1 have different sizes. These sizes have been chosen arbitrarily to signify person-to-person differences. Individuals can be distinguished according to their basic life pattern or the emphasis they place on each of the dimensions and consequently on the relative system targets. Furthermore, variations occur in the repertoire of actions within each dimension. Thus, this model is applicable to all cultures in that all people pursue identical targets. Drastically different ethnic and cultural patterns, however, are evidenced within the process dimensions and allow for the distinction and description of ethnic groups.

Health

Propositions
1. Health is the experience of system congruence evidenced in all levels of an individual's system, the subsystems, and the environmental systems of contact.
2. Health is not an absolute. It is never totally absent and never fully present.
3. Physical disease is a condition that refers to the organizational disturbance at the organic system level.
4. Physical disease and poor health are not synonymous and neither are lack of physical disease and good health.
5. Physical disease may mirror an incongruence of life patterns with the order of the universe. It can lead to health if it reveals to the person the path toward congruence.

6. The crucial determinant of a deficiency in health is anxiety that results from system incongruence, whereas well-being is a sign of high-level health.

Perfect health signifies congruence of the systemic temporal and spatial pattern with the universal order. As indicated in Figure 1.1, perfect health is experienced in the center of the inner self through the uninhibited flow of empowering energy as the targets interact. The perpetual rhythms and patterns of energy are calming and soothing and promote a supreme sense of well-being. Such a state is rarely achieved except for limited periods of spiritual tranquility.

Disturbances of energy flow, experienced daily by all persons due to system tension, lack of congruence with other people, and changes within the environment, result in anxiety. Anxiety is basic to all other emotions and is the antithesis to well-being. Anxiety and well-being are unified reactions of the total person in that they encompass both feeling and physical sensation. Systemic health is the product of the two interacting and vacillating as situations change. Thus, health fluctuates but has a certain consistency over time and can be subjectively evaluated by the host person.

Because all parts of a system and all external systems are interrelated, anxiety experienced by the individual at one particular level of the system, if it cannot be curbed successfully, will be integrated in the systemic process. Once the feeling is interpreted, repressed, or converted and put into action, its physical effect on organs may eventually result in symptoms of disease. Outwardly, anxiety is transferred to other humans and social systems through patterns of behavior that reflect system incongruence. Simple linear causality is not applicable (Constantine, 1986). Contact systems react to the change of behavior patterns rather than to the anxiety itself, and their reactions are dependent on their own internal system processes, their targets, and process dimensions. If humans in contact with an anxious person change their own patterns of behavior unfavorably, the anxious recipient of the feedback may perceive that change as a further threat and experience still more anxiety.

Consequently, where uninhibited anxiety takes over, it spreads by a cyclical feedback process not only horizontally to other humans but also vertically, downward to human subsystems, organs, and the microscopic system level and upward to larger contact systems in the environment. This feedback process may endure over long periods of time, represent part of a person's total life pattern, become established in the dimension of system maintenance, and be passed on to the next generation. With prolonged incongruence, it becomes increasingly difficult to pin down the roots of anxiety, the causes or effects, and the original destructive system changes.

Physical disease is defined as a malfunction of one or more human organic systems or microsystems. As such, physical disease is not equivalent to lack of health or the disturbance of congruence between systems and subsystems. On some occasions, disease may occur in the absence of anxiety. For example, physical disease in a body weakened by age or a congenital condition is intrinsic to universal order. Consequently, a weakened person afflicted with disease may have willingly accepted mortality through the process of spirituality, transcending the immediate environment to find congruence with a higher power. Such a diseased person is considered healthy. More frequently, however, disease is a manifestation of incongruent systemic patterns and accompanied by anxiety, or anxiety occurs when the person interprets the disease as a threat to system maintenance, or both.

According to the medical profession, disease is a pathological entity and illness refers to the discomfort manifestations of the disease. The treatment of both requires attention to impaired organs, microsystems, or body parts as well as suppression of the associated symptoms. In contrast, the enhancement of health demands attention to the congruence of systems, rhythms and patterns, and the exchange of energy between humans and their systems of contact.

Family

Propositions
1. The family embedded in the civil system is transmitting culture, the total of human system patterns and values.
2. The family shares with the civil system and the environment at large the responsibility to provide physical necessities and safety, procreate, teach social skills to its members, provide for personal growth and develop-

ment, allow emotional bonding of members, and promote a purpose for life and meaning through spirituality.

3. The family satisfies its members' needs for control over their environment and guides them in finding their place in the network of systems through spirituality.

4. All family processes include collectively accepted and coordinated behaviors or strategies that aim at regulating the earthly conditions of space, time, energy, and matter in pursuing the four systemic targets.

5. Family strategies fall into the four process dimensions of system maintenance, system change, coherence, and individuation. The dimensions share collinearity but exist independently in that none is emphasized at the expense of another in healthy families.

Although families enacted early in history the only existing civil system available to humans, this is no longer true. Today, the family is embedded in a complex civilization consisting of community, economic, and government structures. The responsibility for processes previously owned by families is now shared with systems of the civil structure. The human education and socialization process once unique to the family occur predominantly in schools and social recreational organizations. The assets necessary for economic survival are earned outside the family and managed with the help of community financial institutions. Even basic tasks, such as reproduction or physical care for young or needy family members, may be carried out outside family boundaries with persons other than family members. It follows that the family functions of providing necessities and safety for members, procreating, and the socializing of the young complement those of the larger civil structure.

Nevertheless, the family remains important in that it provides an environment in which many individuals can best meet their need for control and spirituality. Within the family they can assume responsibilities and directly influence the system's decision-making process. Furthermore, individuals can tune into each other's systemic organization through emotional bonding and the free flow of energy, thereby sensing connectedness with other human beings representing images of universal order. A healthy family may represent an oasis within an overwhelming and largely uncontrollable environment in which members feel acknowledged and provided with the necessary support to venture out and apply themselves in the community.

Definition of the Family

According to the framework of systemic organization, the family is a unit with structure and organization that interacts with its environment. Second, the family is a system with interpersonal subsystems of dyads, triads, and larger units defined by emotional bonds and common responsibilities. Third, the family is composed of individuals who each have distinct relationships with family members, the total family, and contact systems in the environment.

Of importance in defining family is the decision about who should belong to the system. The sense of belonging is a prerequisite for individuals to function as a system. Consequently, the definition of family is subjective and differs according to each member's perspective. Members of the family do not need to be biologically related or live in a single household. The family is defined as all persons an individual considers to be family. The family includes all persons who carry family functions and are emotionally connected to the individual. Consequently, the persons who are emotionally connected are those the individual is concerned, worried, or upset about.

This flexible definition is useful for nursing and family counseling. It encourages the exploration of all possibilities to locate a family support system of seemingly lone individuals or even form a family of committed individuals for the purpose of mutual support or goal attainment. Yet the subjective nature of the definition may present a problem in that even members within the same nuclear family may differ in their family definition. For example, a wife may add to the nuclear family her family of origin and her husband's brother, sister, and nephew, but her husband might not feel connected to his wife's parents and refuses to recognize them as members of his family. Whether or not to include them in the nursing process will depend on whose needs are considered the major focus of nursing care.

Family Processes

The aim of the family system is to transmit culture, that is, to endure and adjust in the midst of change and maintain congruence with its environment. Family culture is the sum of all family processes at a given point in time. Over time, stability of culture is maintained through the transmission of stable family patterns and values from one generation to the next. Yet growth is also possible in that new knowledge is acquired and integrated into the system. Thereby, transformed cultural patterns form a new structure and stability that are subsequently transmitted to the next generation (Kantor & Lehr, 1975).

Healthy family processes allow each family member to attain personal congruence and curb anxiety. A representation of the pathways of family processes is shown in Figure 1.2. The family system regulates the earthly conditions of time, space, energy (Kantor & Lehr, 1975), and matter (Constantine, 1986) to accomplish the family tasks pertaining to each of the four process dimensions listed in the middle column. Because these conditions represent an unescapable reality, it is necessary to consider them in planning family strategies and solving problems. Successful solutions will then guide the system toward its desired targets and congruence as indicated on the right side of Figure 1.2. The family processes of striving toward the indicated targets to find congruence are equal to human and other social systems.

The Family Targets

Originally, family therapy theorists described the major goal of the family as a constant striving to establish and reestablish a previously held stability or homeostasis (Bateson, 1961; Haley, 1959; Jackson, 1957). They observed that change of system patterns or second-order change rarely happened. What appeared to be a change in family processes often turned out to be a new way of reinforcing old patterns (Watzlawick, Weakland, & Fisch, 1974). Eventually, however, the family came to be viewed as an evolutionary system in constant interchange with surrounding systems (Auerswald, 1987). The concept of growth or morphogenesis was introduced by Buckley in 1967. Morphogenesis was seen as the evolutionary force that alters families as they adapt to changes in their social environment. The compatibility of stability and growth was suggested by Kantor and Lehr (1975). They concluded that families, like individuals, function according to a basic systemic pattern that acts as a blueprint for all actions. This pattern includes a stable core of traditions and values needed to preserve a sense of identity (Lewis et al., 1976) as well as the openness to make changes (Speer, 1970). Families, adapting to changes within the system

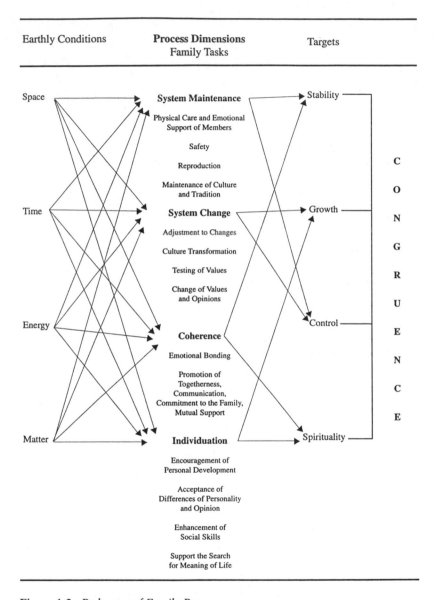

Figure 1.2. Pathways of Family Processes

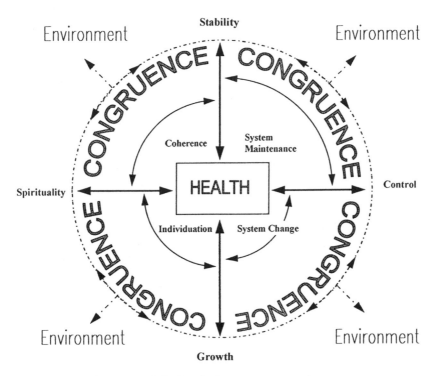

Figure 1.3. Life Process of the Family System

or in the environment, will employ behaviors in concert with their blueprint. Flexibility will allow them to incorporate new knowledge that will gradually lead to change in family structure and process as the system evolves. Consequently, Kantor and Lehr (1975) suggest that healthy families will succeed in keeping the processes' stability and growth in a functional balance.

This suggests that the diagram of system functioning (see Figure 1.3) is as applicable to the family as it is to the person.

Stability. The target of stability in the family addresses traditions and common behavior patterns rooted in basic values and cultural beliefs. Members of healthy families ascribe to family values and respect traditions that provide them, in turn, with a sense of belonging and safety. They are proud of their family identity, which they feel has become part of their inner self. It is through their adherence to these values that they earn their membership in the family and each family adopts explicit and implied rules that the members are to follow. The family maintains its stability and protects the system from extinction in that it teaches its traditional patterns of functioning to the children, who will then pass them on to each generation.

Growth. The target of growth takes form within the process of culture transformation. Through their roles within other systems (e.g., schools, workplace, union, or church), family members gain new ideas, realizations, and knowledge that will influence them and change their personal system. The family may be forced to readjust its own processes to accommodate the changed needs of its members. According to systems theory, significant changes in the members will exert a detectable influence on the structure and processes of the family and lead to growth of the system. Communication is the tool for a healthy growth process in that it enables the family to process new information and adjust to it. Adjustment can happen in two ways. The family can accept new information and integrate it in its own value system or it can decide to live with contradictory values among its members by turning diversity of opinions into a basic family value and appreciating it as a desirable aspect of family maintenance.

Family growth therefore occurs always secondary to change in its members. The family owns the difficult task of finding a balance between stability and growth that leads to congruence among the members and with the environment. Families differ significantly in the emphasis they place on either target. Furthermore, families differ in their interpretation of stability. For example, in one family stability may signify the almost exact replication of life patterns of the past generation. It may therefore select homogeneous friends and send the children to private schools likely to raise the children in a traditional way. Another family may value free thinking and encourage its members to test values. Both families can be healthy and vital as long as they find in their environment systems with which to connect and find congruence.

Members of the family feel anxious about threats to family stability as well as their own. As in personal systems, the buffering of anxiety also happens through the targets of control and spirituality. A close look at the family literature shows that researchers and clinicians of various disciplines describe family functioning processes that can be categorized into these two targets. Family control is expressed by concepts such as power structure (Haley, 1976), boundaries (Minuchin, 1974), coalitions, rules and roles (Haley, 1976; Lewis et al., 1976), family organization and control (Moos, 1986), and adaptability (Olson et al., 1984). In interacting with the environment, families take active control over external influences as well. According to Kantor and Lehr (1975), families open or close their boundaries, screen information, and select what should be incorporated into family knowledge.

Spirituality is also addressed in the family literature with concepts such as differentiation of the self (Bowen, 1976) and cohesion (Moos, 1986; Olson et al., 1984). Furthermore, research in social ecology (Moos, 1974; Roberts & Feetham, 1982) and social learning (Bandura, 1969; Couch, 1970) addresses the interdependence of individuals and families within their environment.

Control. According to the framework of systemic organization, the target of control encompasses the organizational structure of the family that is consciously regulated. Threats from the environment are collectively reduced and energy is carefully channeled to reestablish congruence. Because individuals have little influence on the civil system as a whole, a healthy family may fulfill its need for autonomy better than any other system. It allows the members to take on important roles through which they maintain a minicivil structure of the family that lends perseverance and strength to the system and through which they can gain personal self-confidence. Within these family operations they can plan for the future, make decisions about the acceptance or rejection of new information, or choose environmental systems to connect with. They can set up rules to follow and hold members to the rules. A collective sense of autonomy and commitment thus gained buffers anxiety about uncertainty, vulnerability, and isolation.

Spirituality. Control, to be effective, needs a basis of spirituality. The target of spirituality is an important aspect of family culture. It is rooted in values that concern commitment, love, and affection. Spirituality encompasses all that binds family members emotionally and encourages them to seek personal growth outside the family. Through spirituality, family members reduce their fear of isolation, feel connected, and find comfort and help in difficult times. Spirituality is practiced by individuals. In some families, it is a private matter to be dealt with on a strictly individual level. In others, however, a definition of spirituality or religion is mutually shared and accepted as the members assist each other in interpreting personal experiences and share similar ideas about life. Irrespective of individual differences, each healthy family owns a set of core values expressing togetherness and commitment. They may be rarely mentioned but are strongly felt, and they clarify the members' position in the family and their external world.

The Process Dimensions

Figure 1.3 suggests that, identical to the personal system, the targets of the family system are reached with behaviors falling into the four process dimensions of system maintenance, system change, coherence, and individuation. These dimensions were originally conceptualized based on the findings of Friedemann's (1991a) research in developing a family assessment instrument. They appeared on a factor analysis of 40 items describing possible family strategies.

Strategies within the four process dimensions are determined, as are all behaviors of living systems on Earth, by the basic conditions of space, time, energy, and matter. As Kantor and Lehr (1975) observed, families use specific strategies to regulate each of the four conditions in their struggle to preserve the system from extinction. Thus, behaviors within each dimension can be subdivided according to the conditions of time, space, energy, and matter they are regulating. Table 1.1 shows examples of the categorization of such strategies.

System Maintenance. System maintenance consists of those behavior strategies that are anchored in tradition, refer to family structure and family flexibility, and deal with organizing and operating the family business. The word *strategy* signifies collective actions in that a number of family members participate in performing certain tasks or

TABLE 1.1 Examples of Family Strategies Ordered According to Process Dimensions and Basic Conditions

Process Dimension	Basic Condition	Strategies
System maintenance	Space	Rent apartment, provide home for family meeting, select vacation spot, choose kitchen for family talks, provide a study corner, communicate whereabouts
	Time	Adjust family routines to members' schedules, coordinate vacation times, enforce curfews, buy retirement insurance plan, schedule relaxation time, have regular meal times, reminisce jointly
	Energy	Select family friends, accept or reject information, enjoy recreational activities, make decisions, punish a child, discuss issues, do family chores, play with the children, sleep, reward accomplishments, set and enforce rules, ask for help
	Matter	Buy furniture, pack suitcases, pay bills, wrap presents, cook dinner, wash clothes
System change (applies only if basic values are changed prior to actions)	Space	Provide more private space, give up job to stay home with retarded child, rent out a room to solve financial problems, take in divorced daughter and child, admit parent to a nursing home
	Time	Cut family time due to job responsibilities, change family routines due to odd schedules, shorten vacation time to save money, give up leisure time while caring for chronically ill family member
	Energy	Accept outside help for lack of better options, adjust to a child's being married, accept an unusual career choice of a child, set new priorities in life
	Matter	Sell a vacation cabin due to financial problems, use saved money to send a child to college, decide to respect a child's preferences for unusual clothes

(continued)

TABLE 1.1 (Continued)

Process Dimension	Basic Condition	Strategies
Coherence	Space	Sit around the table and share experiences, go on family trip, keep doors of rooms open, make a visit to grandmother's home, make family room comfortable for all
	Time	Hold regular traditional family celebrations, make time to communicate, spend free time together, agree on times to do work together, adjust mealtimes to various schedules, spend time baby-sitting a sibling
	Energy	Share interests, help each other out, respect family members' opinions, accept others' uniqueness, laugh together, respect family rules, show pride in family
Individuation	Space	Arrange a playroom, excuse adolescents from a family gathering, decorate family room for a birthday party, welcome children's friends in the home, let a child go to camp, visit a museum
	Time	Allow children time to play, provide time for study or community involvement, let members choose times to pursue own interests, cancel picnic to attend a child's ballet recital
	Energy	Support innovative ideas, encourage achievements, listen to unusual ideas, support independent problem solving, allow free choice of friends, enjoy personal differences, get involved in community activities
	Matter	Accept symbolic value objects hold for family members; encourage expression of personality through room decorations, clothes, or hairstyles; provide books for learning; have journals, newspapers, or encyclopedia for family use

assuming mutually dependent roles necessary to reach the intended goals. System maintenance strategies encompass a large part of family life: daily routines of rest, activities, eating, sleeping, rules, communication patterns, sharing of ideas, roles, rituals, decision making, parenting methods, financial management, health maintenance measures and caregiving patterns, planning the future, recreational patterns, religious practices, and many more.

Family activities have to be coordinated if they are to meet the needs of more than one family member. For example, to maintain a stable family, members have to communicate with each other, and to communicate effectively occurs when members are required to make contact with each other. Consequently, they share the same space at the same time. Furthermore, discussions of ideas, making plans, or solving problems concern energy to be channeled and kept under control, and, in addition, certain plans or decisions involve material things such as money, food, or personal belongings to be regulated. This shows that the sum of the coordinated operations aimed at keeping family function in accordance with the family's norms and rules refers to the two targets of stability and control.

System Change. System maintenance operations refer to family culture transmission in that they represent the preservation of traditional patterns (homeostasis). Concurrently, system change leads to the incorporation of new knowledge and the assumption of new family behaviors, structure, and values and therefore encompasses culture transformation (morphogenesis). To facilitate system change, the family allows a free flow of energy and material in and out of the environment, absorbs information into the system, and adjusts its time and spatial arrangements in response to environmental feedback. Thus, the family system reaches the control target by accommodating new needs of members. The outcome of the system change process is a decision about the acceptance or rejection of certain values that can be made only through channeling and absorbing knowledge and information. Because the process involves conscious decision making, it aims at the target of control, whereas the resulting change in family structure targets family growth.

System change refers to significant alterations of system operation with repercussions in the traditional family value system that require the cooperation and agreement of all members. Change of family structure is possible only when system incongruence is severe and difficult to achieve. Often, argumentation and hostility of members who sense a high level of anxiety render the process painful. A high resistance of families to change is experienced by family therapists who, after many sessions of attempting true change, observe that their clients have assumed new behaviors that simply represent another way of executing the same destructive family process. Watzlawick et al. (1974) used the term *second-order change* in explaining system change as a "change from one set of premises to another of the same logical type" (p. 27). Although the first set is established within the system, the second needs to be introduced from outside the family by the environmental system. As a rule, families search fruitlessly for solutions within their own system maintenance operations until tension becomes great and a crisis develops. At a certain breaking point, system change may occur in that members are suddenly able to absorb certain environmental information and apply it to their system. At that point, the solutions that were so hard to achieve seem simple and logical.

Such solutions are listed in Table 1.1. Readers need to recognize that these same strategies could be listed under system maintenance if their enforcement did not involve a change of values, attitudes, or opinions. For example, at certain times in the lives of family members, the need for private space may increase. Families who generally value privacy will automatically back off if a member expresses a need for space. System change, however, may have to occur in a family in which members are tightly bonded. In such a family, a member's attempt to spend time outside the family or refuse talking about his or her problems may be considered an affront and lead to a crisis only to be solved by relaxing the core value of family unison.

All other changes listed in Table 1.1 are to be understood similarly. It follows that system change is less easy to assess than the other process dimensions. Most system change behaviors can be examined only retrospectively. Nevertheless, the readiness of a family to make changes and the prediction of crisis can be estimated by examining the flexibility of the value system anchored in the system maintenance dimension.

The independence of the two dimensions needs to be stressed once more. The dimensions are not negatively correlated or placed on opposite ends of the same continuum. It is a mistake to equate system maintenance with rigidity and lack of change. Instead, included with all other family operating patterns is the flexibility to make changes. In families in which such flexibility is traditionally high, changes can be readily made without affecting core values or family stability.

Coherence. The previous discussion made it clear that the process dimensions of system maintenance and change represent processes of the family system as a whole observed as collective strategies. In contrast to this, the major focus of coherence and individuation is on the activities of the family's subsystems. Coherence relates to the relationships between family members. It includes all processes that lead to spirituality or the process of subsystems attuning their patterns and rhythms to find congruence. Thus, energy is permitted to flow freely between members so that space, time, and matter are regulated in a way to connect the members through a bond of affection.

Coherence targets stability of the family. Its outcome is a sense of unity, belonging, and a mutual commitment to the family system as a whole necessary for the survival of the family system. Through coherence, family members acquire a family identity that becomes integrated in their personal structure. Consequently, the members know what their family signifies and what it stands for. In exchange for safety, belonging, and support from the family, members are expected to commit some of their time, energy, and resources to the system, thereby sacrificing part of their personal autonomy and independence. Coherence is actualized through effective communication. Actions within the dimension include the sharing of experiences and feelings; mutually accepting personal differences; appreciating accomplishments; showing affection; physically expressing sexuality; caring for children, the old, and the weak; and materially assisting the needy. Still others are listed in Table 1.1 according to their categorization along the conditions of space, time, energy, and matter being regulated.

Individuation. A second group of actions addressing spirituality falls within the process dimension of individuation. This time, bonds are established between family members and environmental systems.

A family that stresses individuation encourages the members to acquire new knowledge, establish their roles within systems of the environment, and thereby experience personal growth. Table 1.1 lists actions the family can undertake in support of its members' uniqueness, such as letting them express their personality in selecting their own friends, decorating their room, or assisting them in the pursuit of their interests. Family strategies related to individuation are also categorized along the earthly conditions of space, time, energy, and matter.

Through individuation, new information, values, attitudes, and opinions of family members demand entry into the system. Because all subsystems and systems are connected, a reaction of the family in response to changes within the members has to be expected. Individuation is therefore a first step toward family change.

Family Health

Propositions
1. Family health encompasses four observable criteria: the presence of strategies within all process dimensions, satisfaction of all family members with their family, positive environmental feedback about family members' execution of roles in community systems, and low anxiety level in the family.
2. Family health is a dynamic process that, in response to changing situations, is continually attempting new ways of reestablishing congruence within the system and with the environment.
3. Family style is the product of weighing and emphasizing the process dimensions and choosing certain strategies within them.
4. No family style can be judged effective or ineffective without evaluating the four criteria of family health.

Family health is the experience of congruence in the family. It is achieved through balancing the four targets of stability, growth, control, and spirituality dynamically and in accordance with the changing situation of the family. The system targets are emphasized, combined, and weighed against each other in such a way that none of the family members have to compromise their personal growth and sense of well-being in their interaction with other family members or with environmental contact systems. Consequently, family health is likely if all of the following criteria are met: (a) strategies pertaining to all four process dimensions are present, (b) the family system is congruent with its environmental contact systems, and (c) there is congruence within the system, that is, all family members are reasonably satisfied with their family. Furthermore, a healthy family provides well-being to the members and lowers their anxiety.

Like individuals, families attempt congruence, but perfect health can never be reached entirely. Families do the best they can, considering their circumstances. They have many options of achieving a dynamic equilibrium, and no style of functioning can be judged better than the other without assessing the system along with the above criteria of health. The family's style is defined by the emphasis on the four targets, the family's value structure. As such, it is relatively stable and serves as a blueprint for responses to change (Kantor & Lehr, 1975). During the course of a family's lifetime, some shifts in emphasis and changes in the family strategies will occur within each process dimension as families adjust to specific situations or developmental levels of members. Just like individual life processes, however, family style is generally robust and is altered only by serious shifts of norms and values brought about by the process of system change.

Finally, it needs to be pointed out that this chapter purposefully includes dynamics of healthy family systems only, because practitioners need to establish a firm basis of understanding the healthy family process. Such knowledge is vital if value judgments are to be avoided and families are to be evaluated as subsystems of their environment rather than against a set of arbitrary norms or biased standards of middle-class functioning.

2

Nursing of
Families and Family Members

Since the American Nurses Association (1980) propagated the family as the necessary recipient of nursing service, much progress has been made in conceptualizing the family and its functioning and in deducing nursing interventions that promote health to the family system and its members. Although still in its infancy, family nursing is recognized as a specialty cutting across all nursing areas (Hanson, 1987).

The question of where family nursing should be practiced is still being debated. Barkauskas (1986) describes family nursing as long-term care to be practiced in various sites but excluding acute care settings, and others (Bomar, 1989; Gilliss, Highley, Roberts, & Martinson, 1989) specifically stress the need to strengthen the family focus of care in such sites.

Family nursing depends on the way the practicing clinician views the family. Friedman (1992) maintains that even today the predominant view of the family is that of context for the individual. As such, the family acts as both stressor and resource in providing social support, thereby influencing the individual's health status (Clements & Roberts, 1983; Newman, 1983; Pender, 1987). Viewing the family as the sum of its members is another perspective in nursing, mainly implicit in primary and community health practice (Friedman, 1992), in which efforts of conceptualizing the family system as the recipient of care have been stifled by cost-containment policies (Doherty, 1985). Nevertheless, authors of major textbooks of family nursing today agree that the family system should represent the recipient of care (Friedman, 1992) and that the needs of family members should be addressed as well (Barkauskas, 1986; Bomar, 1989; Gilliss et al., 1989).

Significant progress has been made in defining the process of family nursing. Nursing interventions tend to be categorized along some aspects of family functioning viewed as being important. For example, Wright and Leahy (1984) classified nursing action according to cognitive, affective, and behavioral functioning of the family, using systems and family therapy theories as the basis (Wright & Leahy, 1988). There is consensus among recent authors that nursing interventions should be based on theory, and some excellent efforts have been made to outline assumptions that pertain to various theories useful to nursing, such as systems, developmental, symbolic interaction, ecological, and stress and coping theories (Berkey & Harmon-Hanson, 1991; Bomar, 1989; Gilliss et al., 1989). The concept of health and nursing actions that leads to an umbrella theory encompassing the breadth of family functioning has not been available to family nursing as of yet. Nevertheless, Berkey and Harmon-Hanson's (1991) first step toward an encompassing theory presents a coherent approach of applying the systems model of Betty Neuman (1982) to the nursing process with families.

There is a general understanding that family nursing should be systemic, holistic, and health oriented and include the family's strengths and resources. These premises may be anchored in theory but are often neglected in nursing care plans. Friedman (1992), for example, presents a list of possible family strengths but proceeds with predominantly problem-oriented care planning and interventions. It appears that most of the actual family nursing practice still occurs along the traditional problem-solving nursing process approach using strictly linear thought processes that cannot possibly provide understanding of the richness of family life. A nurse needs to fully grasp the wealth and depth of each family's experience before being able to enhance its health.

It is my opinion that the use of nursing diagnoses based on the work of the North American Nursing Diagnosis Association (NANDA) (Carpenito, 1989) presents a danger to holistic nursing of families in that systemic thinking is not essential to setting goals for interventions. Furthermore, practicing nurses are asked to make professional judgments related to the function versus the dysfunction of families that are necessarily based on a set of norms related to how healthy families should function. Such norms and standards generally assumed to be true for all families seldom take social status, culture, or specific life circumstances into consideration and are highly influenced by the nurse's perception based on his or her own family experiences (Gilliss et al., 1989).

Many observations of marginal inner-city families struggling with incredible problems make me contend that strength and beauty can be found in each family experience. It is found within the family system's resilience against all odds, which deserves one's admiration. There is no good or bad and there is no function or dysfunction. Instead, there is joy and much pain, and by sharing in the family's pain, nurses can soothe it and show the family the way to heal its own wounds.

What follows is a detailed explication of nursing that may clarify some of these issues, help the reader see through the complexity of family life, and suggest ways to use the self in systemic interaction to discover the beauty and meaning of family relationships.

Nursing

Propositions

1. Nursing occurs on the various system levels, from organic systems to the larger social systems in the community.

2. Nursing focused on individuals also includes the family and the environmental systems of contact. Therefore, all nursing is family nursing and is practiced in all clinical settings.

3. All nursing interventions at the level of the family system or the community also heed individuals and their subsystems.

4. Nursing is a process of mutual growth through spirituality.

5. The goal of nursing is the support of the clients' systemic processes leading to health, whereas the clients' goal is health.
6. The art of nursing consists of the nurse's creative ability to shift his or her position from the role of a participant and actor in the system to that of a bystander and shift from one system level to another.

Nursing, according to the framework of systemic organization, is directed at the unified systemic whole, be it the person, the family, or the community. Human pattern and rhythm express the wholeness of universal order and mirror system congruence. Therefore, each system needs to be understood as both an entity and a part of the unity of all systems. A person, for example, does not have a body but is a body in which universal order takes shape. Thus, anxiety or symptoms of disease, family conflict, or loss of well-being serve as expressions of systemic tension and indicate a need for change of direction on the path toward congruence. Symptoms of disease are signs of health, because when physical and emotional pain become intolerable, necessary system change and growth can be initiated.

The only goal of nursing is sharing the pain and support of the process of life unique to each system in its struggle to find health. Therefore, although the goal of health belongs to the client system, nursing's goal is the life process itself that encompasses both nurse and client as active participants.

Nursing is a science because its interventions depend on the understanding of system operation and processes. Nursing is also an art in that nurses temporarily extend themselves to unite with the client system by letting energy flow between them so that their patterns and rhythms adjust to that of the client. In this manner, the client system becomes receptive to individuation by incorporating the information, matter, or energy needed to make changes in the process toward health. Consequently, the art of nursing is the creative expression of the self in reaching the client, but it also encompasses a mutual process of individuation in that both nurse and client expand their self through system growth and spirituality.

Nursing interventions are described in various ways in the family literature. Friedman (1992) proposes that family nurses should change behaviors and modify the environment, whereas Wright and Leahy

(1984) advocate the support of functional processes. Generally, interventions are intended to correct dysfunctions of the family member, the family system, or their interactions. Specifically, activities such as counseling, advocating, role modeling, teaching, and informing are seen as suitable in working with family members.

Nursing actions, according to the framework of systemic organization, differ from these traditional views in rather significant ways. First, they address the systemic whole rather than disconnected pieces or areas of individual and family functioning. Nurses visualize the systemic network in constant movement and address evolving patterns that express the total life process rather than the status of an individual or family system. Consequently, the science of nursing is not limited to knowledge of physiology and normative human functioning but encompasses the understanding of immensely complex systemic processes of interaction between humans, families, and their environment.

Second, family members are not seen as recipients of support or stress from the family system. Instead, individuals are actors within the family system and are involved in mutual processes of giving and receiving. The nurse is therefore not viewed as an expert who is in the position to tell families how they are to support their own system or their members. Instead, the experts are the client systems themselves. The power of change lies within individuals and family systems waiting to be nurtured and kindled. This process of empowerment has been extensively described in other helping disciplines (Dunst, Trivette, & Deal, 1988; Rappaport, 1987). Nurses, although they execute the roles of consultants, teachers, and client advocates, use a personal art of connecting to client systems. Their expertise lies in understanding complexities rather than teaching facts, listening and learning rather than advising, and asking questions rather than answering. A reasonable degree of congruence between nurses and clients is a requirement. By feeling their way into the clients' systemic order, nurses transcend their own rigidity and free themselves from the limits of biased opinions and prejudices. Barriers to the formation of a congruent nursing system are removed by the nurses' openness to be touched by the clients' energy. It is imperative that nurses consider this process of spirituality challenging, especially when they are confronted with families or family members whose appearance or behaviors part from the norm, have difficulties with trust, or consider themselves outcasts in the society. The flow of energy is facilitated through communication, the expression of sincere interest, encouraging words, a caring look, a warm touch, or a friendly gesture. Because spirituality signifies the adjustment of the nurses' own system to that of the clients, the nursing process demands work with the self to overcome anxiety, insecurity, strong values, and prejudices.

Because nursing is to be a mutual process, the process of simply offering interventions or information to a passive client system can be detrimental. Not only does the nurse's scientific expertise smother the client's autonomy, but the helpfulness cannot be returned by the client and, as a result, the nurse gains stature as a parenting figure *vis-à-vis* the client, who becomes increasingly dependent.

There are, however, situations in which clients are necessarily dependent as in the case of an unconscious client who requires total physical care. His or her autonomy is at a minimum. Here, the key to preserving the client's respect and dignity is the nurse's understanding of being a responsible component within the systemic network that includes nurse, client, and family as well as their common environment. This understanding leads to an attitude of respect and veneration and a process of nursing that remains mutual in that it allows a nonverbal exchange of energy. The perceptive nurse will transcend severe functional limitations in search of the client's intact wholeness. Together with the family, the nurse will discover subtle secrets that the client may reveal about finding health through pain and struggle with death. The family is best helped to ease suffering and pain by actively taking part in the process of spirituality and the art of nursing. As long as there is life, no client should be reduced to a body or object. Instead, each nursing contact has the potential of an intense experience through which the nurse is the recipient of systemic health as much as or more so than the client.

Nursing of families will be discussed in two segments. In the first, the focus is on the individual within the family context. The second part concerns nursing of the family system. Here, the roles and contributions of the individuals to the health of the family stand in the foreground. Furthermore, nursing of the family system focuses on the environment's influence, specifically on the process of culture transformation and the family members' involvement with their environment.

Nursing of Individuals Within the Family

The process of nursing family members encompasses all aspects important to nursing individuals but adds to it a strong focus on the systemic interchange of the client with the family and the larger environment. Reasons for family-focused care can be many, for example, disease, emotional pain, adjustment to loss and limitations, interpersonal difficulties, difficult life transitions, or simply the desire to enhance the quality of personal life (health promotion). Because the client goal in nursing signifies systemic health, clients need to acknowledge their need to enhance health and express the willingness to work with the nurse toward self-discovery and adjustment of systemic processes.

Leaders in family nursing agree that goals should be set jointly with clients and that the clients should arrive at their own decision to make changes (Friedman, 1992). Furthermore, Mischke-Berkey, Warner, and Hanson (1989) describe nursing for the purpose of primary prevention as actions to modify or regulate the system's potential for health-promoting activities. These actions agree with the premises of this framework. There is a slight difference in the view of the nursing process in that within this framework all nursing actions are considered health promotion. This includes, for example, hands-on psychomotor tasks provided to support body function. These actions free up some of the client's energy needed to facilitate general healing. Healing is equivalent to regeneration of life processes that lead to systemic health. Therefore, all actions in support of healing also promote health. Nursing of individuals within the family context, or the promotion of systemic life processes leading to individual health, occurs along the following steps:

1. Assess health patterns
2. Describe the systemic diagram
3. Determine need for change
4. Highlight existing strengths
5. Encourage the use of systemic resources
6. Assist in the discovery of new strategies
7. Lead the change process
8. Test results and evaluate health
9. Honor all efforts

Similar steps have been previously published, describing the Congruence Model for mental health nursing of family systems (Friedemann, 1989b, 1991b). The Congruence Model is a structured approach that uses special instruments for assessment and treatment. The model can be adapted to families of varying needs. For example, an eight-session treatment approach with clearly defined session content has been tested with substance-abusing families (Friedemann, 1994). The Congruence Model, however, is only one approach to nursing, whereas others based on the same framework are possible as well.

Nursing, according to the framework of systemic organization, can be provided in all health care settings and with all types of clients. The previously mentioned steps of treatment are commonly applicable. The acronym ADD HEALTH expresses the client's goal to be achieved through the nursing process. The sequence of the steps may be changed as the need arises. Steps 1 and 2, and Steps 5 to 7, usually occur concurrently. There is often a need to reassess health and factors that might prevent it. In difficult cases, the nurse may have to go back to Step 3 to assume a new focus. Also, Step 9 needs to be practiced throughout.

The assessment can take on many different formats, from structured forms to informal conversations with clients. Timing of the assessment can differ significantly according to agency policies or client situation. The following, however, is generally valid for all nursing with this framework: (a) The majority of the assessment represents the client's perception. The nurse's role is to question inconsistencies and draw on family members and friends to gain a broader understanding of strengths and problems. (b) As listed in Step 2, the systemic diagram is explained to client and family at some time during the assessment process. Unless the persons are well educated, the discussion is limited to the four process dimensions that can be explained in very simple terms. The diagram provides a common language, channels the understanding about human functioning and needs, and is used as the rationale to support nursing interventions. (c) The content of the assessment is organized along the process dimensions. The various areas included in each dimension are listed in Table 2.1. According to each client's situation, certain areas take on importance, whereas others may be mentioned briefly or skipped entirely.

TABLE 2.1 Themes for Assessments With Individuals

	Perspective of the Client
System Maintenance	
Body function	Respiration
	Digestion
	Elimination
	Sexual/reproductive function
	Cardiovascular function
	Endocrine function
	Musculoskeletal function
	Sensory function
	Neurological function
	Condition of teeth and skin
Health care measures	Hygiene
	Nutrition
	Exercise
	Sleep measures
	Pharmaceuticals
	Pain relief measures
	Household remedies
	Comfort measures
	Protection from illness
	Accident prevention
Life patterns	Activities of daily living
	Work/employment patterns
	Relaxational patterns
	Personal financial management
	Contribution to household routines
	Contribution to child rearing
	Caregiving responsibility to impaired members
	Social activities
	Participation in holiday celebrations and rituals
Rhythms	Activity/rest
	Social time/private time
	Sleep/wake
	Time orientation (present, past, future)
	Time structuring, planning/lack of structure stage of development
Mental stimulation	Reading/writing
	Involvement with art or music
	Problem solving/reasoning
	Discussions/argumentation
	Interpretation of events and happenings
	Intellectual games

TABLE 2.1 (Continued)

Perspective of the Client	
System Maintenance (Cont'd)	
Recreation	Social events
	Sports/outdoors activities
	Crafts and hobbies
	Vacation travels
	Television/movies/shows
Religious practices	Church/mosque/temple visits
	Prayer/meditation
	Religious holiday rituals
	Social/organizational involvement
Coherence	
Inner peace	Solitude
	Prayer/meditation
	Integrity/morals/principles
	Overcoming anger/resentment
	Explaining pain/suffering
	Practicing tolerance
	Reconciliation with losses/aging
Relationship with the environment	Enjoyment of art/music
	Enjoyment of nature
	Expression through appearance
	Attachment to objects/symbols
	Structuring and decorating living space
Social relationships	Mutual friendships
	Trust
	Mutual respect
	Acceptance of social roles
	Independence/dependence
Values and attitudes	Personal history/identity
	Emphasis on material goods and money
	Emphasis on social life
	Emphasis on spiritual life
Individuation	
Achievements	Work accomplishment
	Family responsibilities
	Community involvement
	Political involvement
	Achievements in sports/arts/music
	Self-development
	Service to others

(continued)

TABLE 2.1 (Continued)

Perspective of the Client	
Individuation (Cont'd)	
Human relationships	Growth through social roles
	Friendships
	Partnership/marriage
	Parent-child relationships
	Caregiving relationships
	Work relationships
	Social status/power
	Exchange of ideas
Environmental interchange	Collection and evaluation of information
	Education/professional training
	Development of skills
	Travel/learning about cultures
	Exploring nature
	Seeking God or a greater power
Philosophy and ideologies	Search for meaning/explanations
	Testing of values
	Gaining insight through books
	Involvement in ideological movements
	Opposition to ideologies
	Belonging to a religious organization
	Participation in social/political organizations
	Choosing detachment
System Change	
Past value changes	Enlightenment through the following:
	Previous tragedies
	Developmental process
	Important events
	Meaningful information
	Value changes due to illness
	Learning from exposure and experiences
Resources for change	Flexibility of attitude
	Feeling of being supported
	Means for living
	Education
	Sense of purpose
	History of previous adjustments
Barriers to change	Fixed patterns of system maintenance
	Low self-confidence/coherence
	Anxiety or related emotions
	Incongruence with people or environment

Step 3 represents the outcome of the nurse's synthesis of the assessment data that is shared and verified with the client. The nurse uses the theoretical knowledge about system functioning to tentatively formulate certain connections between physical symptoms, personal strength, behaviors and emotions, significant changes, and difficulties intervening with the client's pursuit of health and that of the family members. This synthesis constitutes a description of behaviors used to maintain or change the system, support coherence, and allow individuation. As such, it is presented to the client and family. The nurse contributes the rationale for arriving at certain conclusions about the need for change but allows the client to approve or reject these conclusions. Consequently, the client's systemic processes in pursuit of congruence are thought through jointly to determine which behaviors should be strengthened or deemphasized.

Step 4 serves to more closely examine attitudes and behaviors that are successfully used within each process dimension. This discussion will also provide evidence to estimate the importance the client ascribes to the four systemic targets of stability, growth, control, and spirituality. The nurse who understands the client's individual way of striving toward congruence will be able to assist in setting concrete goals and effecting changes of behavior and attitude. For example, stability is of major importance for most people. Clients will take heroic measures to reestablish their previous system maintenance and coherence patterns to become again what they once were. Such efforts can be supported to a certain extent; however, the situation may be such that conditions cannot be reversed and the client is forced to change the system. Here, the client is helped most by a nurse who fully acknowledges the pain and difficulty associated with systemic change. This nurse helps family members to understand and commit themselves to support the client's life process by providing what is needed for systemic growth, be it space to be alone, an ear to listen, or physical assistance. Honest encouragement mentioned in Step 9 gains special importance in such cases and needs to be directed to all individuals involved.

At the time when a client sees a clear path toward health, family members recognize their individual roles in the process, and all have the desire to make changes, Steps 5 to 7 can be enacted. The nurse becomes a guide and consultant in the change process and encourages the client to follow through and keep up hope. Changes are built on existing strengths and the client is encouraged to use those problem-solving behaviors that were successful in the past. At times, adjustments need to be made in that the same resources are used more extensively or in new situations. The introduction of different behaviors is indicated if familiar problem-solving approaches do not lead to the desired solution. In such cases, the nurse helps to explore other options and advises the client in the testing of new strategies.

Before effecting change, the nurse needs to be clear about the necessity of a system change. The simple addition of new behaviors that are in accordance with the existing structure of system maintenance will be easier to accept by the client and less painful. These may involve measures of self-care, communication patterns, methods of parenting, leisure activities, and many others.

System change, however, is required if the situation demands a major shift in values, attitudes, or systemic targets. Noncompliance, resistance, anger, hopelessness, and severe anxiety may indicate the need for system change. Examples in the third part of this book will explain this process of change more fully.

In summary, the synthesis of data is initiated by the nurse and verified with the client and the family. The process of planning care has been said to be mutual and client directed, ascribing to the client the autonomy to determine the path desired. This may seem impossible in the case of clients with severe functional limitations (e.g., aphasic, cognitively impaired, or comatose persons), but in fact, the nursing process follows the same principles. When severely impaired clients' verbal contribution to the assessment is limited or nonexistent, family members and other data sources will be substituted to gain a comprehensive picture of the client and context, and the client's life pattern is observed in terms of reactions and responses. Clients cared for with dignity are assumed to retain a fair share of autonomy, no matter how ill they are. Through the provision of physical care, the nurse assists in the maintenance of the physical system, hoping to free up enough regenerative energy to allow physical healing. On the physical level, client autonomy signifies the will to live or the body's response to nursing care that allows healing. The remaining autonomy has shifted to spiritual targets but is by no means lost. It is assumed that the client's ability to connect remains unimpaired and takes precedence over other goals in life (Sacks, 1987). Effective nurses open up their own system to the client's to be used as a spiritual connection as long as the client hangs on to life. The key to all nursing care is therefore the perception of the client's subtle way of communicating that demands expertise not only on the cognitive level of scientific understanding but also on a covert level of perception in terms of sensing the energy flow among systems.

The evaluation of care refers to Step 8 in the previous list. According to the framework of systemic organization, the evaluation necessarily encompasses an estimation of systemic health at regular points in time during the course of treatment. The clearest indication of overall improvement or effectiveness of care is the reduction of the client's anxiety and an increase in the reported well-being. In addition, it is imperative to evaluate specific interventions, such as physical care and comfort measures, new problem-solving behaviors, communication techniques, interpersonal behavior strategies, or caregiving behaviors. Because these changes are assumed to enhance the client's and the family's systemic processes, the purpose of the evaluation consists of verifying whether expected results actually occurred. This may not be easy because effects are not linear but are hidden within complex processes of the system as a whole. Therefore, it is recommended to discuss again each process dimension separately by using the systemic diagram and let the client determine whether changes within the dimensions are occurring as expected and are perceived as beneficial to the client's health.

Likewise, the level of the client's congruence with the family system is evaluated by assessing the effectiveness of helping and supportive measures in enhancing the client's well-being. In addition, however, each family member's satisfaction or anxiety about the situation needs to be considered. Because all systemic processes are mutual, evaluation of the family context also includes the client's own role in supporting the family and its members. Furthermore, the evaluation should include the entire family. Clinical experience with this theoretical framework has shown that changes may take unexpected turns. For example, surprising effects have been felt even by members who have had no contact with the nurse.

Finally, the nurse needs to use the evaluation as a means to provide positive feedback to the clients. Thus, evaluation is tightly connected with Step 9. Nurses can function as superior motivating agents of clients as they point out subtle system changes that were missed and interpret small changes as significant beginnings of a chain of positive reactions. This interpreting function of the nurse is not to be underestimated. Often, the perception that improvement is occurring is by far more important than measuring visible changes. A positive outlook often renews long-lost hope, kindles love and affection, and provides client and family with a sense of trust and belonging necessary to conquer the odds.

Nursing of the Family System

Nursing at the level of the family system has recently become the definition of family nursing (Friedman, 1992; Gilliss et al., 1989). Although there seems to be general agreement that family nurses should reason systemically, little evidence suggests that systemic thinking is actually used in clinical practice (Bozett & Gibbons, 1983). Instead, the literature is plagued with inconsistencies and confusion, suggesting that linear causality is much more pervasive than admitted. For example, most educational approaches with families assume direct effects of skills taught by nurses, such as parenting behaviors, communication techniques, problem-solving approaches, or health measures on family members or family systems, thereby discounting the unique way families absorb, transform, or reject such information. Finally, the description of the role of the nurse as an agent able to change behavior (Friedman, 1992) indicates that nurses understand the system better than the family itself, which seems preposterous.

Wright and Leahy (1984) have recognized the complexity of true systemic approaches and suggest leaving system-focused family nursing to experts educated in therapeutic approaches. Although I agree with system complexity, the opinion that systemic nursing is therapy does not coincide with the definition of nursing as the facilitation of systemic life processes. The main reason lies in the fact that psychotherapy or family therapy focuses heavily on pathology and aberration from normal functioning, the very biases I attempt to eliminate by using a framework that accentuates health and builds on the clients' own judgment about what constitutes normality or congruence for them. What follows is a description of systemic nursing that can be executed by mature nurses experienced in working with families who are eager to grow and learn and understand themselves, others, and the systems in which they function.

System-focused family nursing considers the family unit as a whole. Nursing of the total family system aims at family strategies within the process dimensions of system maintenance, coherence, system change, and individuation. Family therapy theory claims that healthy family operations will encourage a more healthful adjustment of the individuals and consequently lead to individual health (Minuchin, 1974). This premise is also supported by the concept of systemic interaction in that family members take on roles through which they serve the system and simultaneously strengthen their own personal coherence.

The family system focus is taken in situations in which the reported incongruence affects the operations of the family and its members as is the case with traumatic experiences, financial problems, serious illness, or death. In addition, the support of the family interchange with external systems may be of the essence in situations in which the members' incongruence with environmental systems carries repercussions in the family operation. Cases that warrant such interventions involve, for example, the adjustment of a handicapped child, poverty, drug rehabilitation, or ethnic tension experienced by a client. Interventions may involve systems such as a hospital, school, workplace, church, prison, or a social agency.

The family system is subdivided into coalitions or interactive systems within which two or more family members are united for a common purpose. On occasion, such systems need to be assessed and supported apart from the family as a whole. Examples of interactional subsystems include the partnership system for sexual relations and sharing responsibilities or enjoyment; the parenting system for raising children; sibling systems for mutual support; or the mother-eldest child system for helping with family responsibilities.

Likewise, the individual's specific needs and pains deserve attention. Because family members act as subsystems who partake in family operations, they feel the effects of system incongruence. Furthermore, the family as a whole also needs to be understood as an active subsystem within its larger environment.

The art of systemic family nursing consists not only of the ability to understand the complexity of system functioning but also of the knowledge when and how the nurse should shift the focus from a subsystem to higher system levels and from taking the position of a participant in a system to assuming that of an objective bystander or evaluator. Nurses may fully apply their own self within families to sense the energy flow, the rhythms, and patterns, but to protect their own coherence, they need to recognize when to step out of pain-inflicting dynamics to gain an objective view as an outsider to the system. To be successful with such position shifts, nurses require superior knowledge of their own systemic processes and need to be in control of their impulses.

The initial focus of systemic nursing depends on the presenting problem. For example, an interpersonal system focus is taken if reported problems are particularly threatening to the health of such units. Examples include marital conflict, discipline problems, abuse in a caregiving situation, sibling rivalry, and others. In most situations, several courses of action are possible. Nurses must rely on the direction of the family toward its own priorities and on its own creativity to arrive at strategies palatable to all involved.

Nurses practicing with families will attempt to temporarily gain entry into the family system or one of its interactional systems. Acting as subsystems, they take part directly in shaping new processes and contribute to changing the characteristics of the whole. Interaction with families enhances the nurses' growth process in that it facilitates their own individuation through new experiences, insights, and information. The steps in the nursing process of family systems are the same as the ones listed for individuals (see p. 38).

The assessment includes the perspectives of all family members and possibly of persons representing contact systems in the environment. Again, before initiating interventions, the family members need to understand the way their family functions, their strengths, and their shortcomings. The four dimensions of the systemic diagram, this time focused on the family system, are explained to members to direct the family in categorizing systemic processes accordingly for the purpose of the assessment.

Suggested contents of the family assessment, organized according to the four process dimensions, are listed in Table 2.2. Also in Table 2.2, assessment data specific to interaction subsystems are inserted under each process dimension. In addition, relevant material from

TABLE 2.2 Themes for Assessments With Families

Perspective of the Client	

System Maintenance: Family System

Family structure	Persons in the household(s)
	Other family members
	Children
	Significant persons of support
	Persons who drain resources
Residence(s)	Type, size, age, condition
	Geographic location
	Type of neighborhood
	Furnishings
	Decorations/luxuries
	Availability of space
Role distribution	Decision making
	Household responsibilities
	Financial management
	Rule enforcement
	Child-rearing responsibilities
	Physical care
	Discipline (How strict? Consistency? Age-appropriate changes?)
	Social training
	Intellectual stimulation
	Emotional support
	Caregiving to ill and disabled
Life patterns	Daily activity routine
	Household routine
	Outside work activities
	Religious activities
	Recreational activities
	Shared activities/individual pursuits
	Communication patterns
	Traditional holiday celebration/family rituals
	Time and energy commitment/mutual help
	Flexibility to change roles
Rhythms	Activity/rest
	Sleep/wake
	Time orientation (present, past, future)
	Time structuring, planning/lack of structure
	Stages of development

(continued)

TABLE 2.2 (Continued)

Perspective of the Client

System Maintenance:
Family System (Cont'd)

Conflicts	Contradictory interpretation of roles
	Different opinions about family commitment
	Conflicting individual life patterns
	Conflicting schedules and daily rhythms
	Conflicting values and interests (generation gap)
	Firm structure preventing adaptation
	Lax structure preventing efficient operation

System Maintenance:
Interactional Subsystems

System structure	Persons involved
	Common purpose
	Criteria for acceptance
Roles	Power distribution (leaders/followers)
	Complementarity (balancing responsibilities)
	Negotiation of mutual expectations
Conflicts	Power struggles/controlling others
	Conflicting expectations

Coherence: Family System

Belonging	Maintaining a family identity
	Mutual caring
	Being together
	Respecting uniqueness of members
	Sharing/communicating
	Providing safety and security
Relationship with the environment	Sharing outside interests
	Sharing experiences (listening, discussing)
	Sharing resources
Values and attitudes	Representing a common vision
	Respecting differences of opinion
	Maintaining tradition
	Compromising individual wants
	Honoring rituals and symbols of unity
Conflicts	Resentment about expectations
	Value conflicts
	Lack of mutual acceptance
	Attempts to control others

TABLE 2.2 (Continued)

Perspective of the Client	
Coherence: Interpersonal Subsystem	
Belonging	Agreement on common purpose
	Motivation to contribute
	Disagreement about purpose
	Forced suppression of personal needs
	Resentment/interpersonal abuse
Individuation: Family System	
Introduction of new knowledge acquired by family members	Sharing of knowledge based on the following:
	Work accomplishments
	Community involvement
	Political involvement
	Achievements in sports/arts/music
	Self-development
	Service to others
	Sharing insights about human relationship
Environmental interchange among family members	Education or professional training
	Skill development
	Experiences with cultures through travel
	Exploring nature
	Seeking God or a greater power
Philosophy and ideologies of family members	Search for meaning/explanations
	Testing of values
	Discussing insights through books
	Sharing views about ideologies
	Discussing religious views
	Discussing views about social/political issues
System Change: Family System	
Past value changes	Family changes due to the following:
	Previous family tragedies
	Important events
	Serious illnesses
	Value changes in family members
	Adjustment to members' development
	Development of new family skills
Resources for change	Flexibility of attitudes
	Strong coherence
	Material resources
	Past successful experience with change
	Effective problem-solving process
	Capacity to learn new family strategies
Barriers to change	Fixed values/system maintenance patterns
	Inflexible roles and attitudes of members
	Threat to coherence

Table 2.1 needs to be added when focusing on the individuals and their influence on the system. The list of systemic behaviors and strategies is too vast to be clinically useful in its entirety. The assessment is made efficacious by trimming and limiting information to essentials reported as problems and, above all, the systemic strengths likely to assist in solving problems. The alert nurse may also search for clues suggesting covert dynamics not reported by the unaware family that may need to be brought to the surface to effect change.

Systemic assessments are rarely completed after one or two meetings. An initial assessment may describe the situation at a specific point in time. Because patterns evolve over time and the nursing process itself contributes to its evolution, assessments have to be supplemented and modified after each meeting with the clients.

Ideally, all available family members are allowed input in the assessment. As a result, multiple perceptions are obtained of the same system, and the nurse's challenge presented in Step 3 of the nursing process consists of constructing a total family perspective in collaboration with the members. The bricks for this construction include shared views, values and understandings, strategies and repetitive patterns, topics of agreement or conflict, and emphasis on behaviors within the process dimensions. The synthesis of existing family processes needs to be compared to a vision of the ideal if an agreement is to be made about necessary changes and desired goals. The ideal family picture must be discussed, collectively understood, agreed on, and remembered at all times during the course of intervention. I have used various techniques to ingrain the ideal family vision in the members' memory, such as written descriptions, drawings, role-plays, family sculpting, or imaging of the family with symbols or metaphors (Friedemann, 1992).

Step 4 signifies the beginning of systemic interventions. As many members as possible should take part in the process, depending on the size of the family and availability of the members. Nonparticipation does not preclude nursing of the family system. As a last resort, family system nursing is possible with only one family member by helping the individual modify responses to the family and by observing the reactions of fellow members between sessions. The aim in Step 4 is to detect processes compatible with existing system maintenance mechanisms that have been found useful in the past.

In Step 5, these strategies are accentuated as family strengths, assets, or resources to be mobilized to reach the desired goals and enhance family congruence. Family members are encouraged to use these useful behaviors more often or in new situations.

New interactive or system approaches may be needed to approach their family vision. In Step 6, the nurse assists the family in examining options by brainstorming and questioning possible effects of suggested new behaviors. To approach the vision of their ideal family, the members mutually explore their paths of change and begin to set short-term goals with the assistance of the nurse.

Step 7 is concerned with implementing the planned changes. New strategies may require a particular change in an individual or a new way of communicating within an interactive subsystem. Because each person who is required to change needs to feel supported and motivated, the nurse will make a shift to the individual system level or interactive systems temporarily as the need arises. Likewise, work at the individual level with the support fairly equalized among members is vital to ensure impartiality and prevent competition and conflict. The nurse must avoid contributing to the victimization of family members and discourage all blaming or attributing fault for problems to certain members. Families need to be reminded repeatedly that family process is a collective phenomenon in which each person carries a role needed to maintain the process. If they desire change, not just one but all roles need to be shifted and adjusted to each other. Much encouragement and honest praise for effort are supplied by enacting Step 9 of the nursing process throughout.

Evaluation is marked as Step 8. As members practice new behaviors, they begin to react differently to each other and to family members not involved in the nursing process. Changes are observed and felt on all levels. The evaluation involves the assessment of the members' perception of change for better or worse, specifically, their level of anxiety, felt relief, or happiness. Furthermore, the level of attainment of specific behavioral goals is estimated and decisions are made whether behaviors instituted should be maintained, discontinued, or modified. The process of reflecting on changes will lead to further motivation if the family responds positively to its chosen path.

In summary, nursing of families along the framework of systemic organization concentrates on assets and resources rather than problems. Nurses discover health in each system and assist in building new self-confidence and a better image of the self and family. They treat each family as normal, considering its particular circumstances and assuming that all families and persons will adjust to difficult situations to the best of their ability, depending on their resources. Instead of attempting to shape a family into a mold of normality, the nurse will let the family members decide what system will work for them and assist them in their struggle toward congruence and health. By joining family systems and participating with them in their systemic processes, the nurse experiences personal individuation and growth, expands consciousness and tolerance, and opens the mind to new alternatives applicable to both private and professional lives.

Finally, it is important to keep in mind that by following the nursing process as described, failure of a nurse is not possible. Because the decision to be helped and to change is the family's and the pursuit of the goals is the family's, failure to do so is the family's responsibility as well. Nurses, by offering their assistance in participating in the family's struggle toward health, become learners instead of teachers. Failure does occur, however, by not following the suggested process. Nurses may force their entry into family systems and prescribe changes and thereby encounter resistance and mistrust. They may teach and advise without listening, thereby discounting the clients' worth and autonomy. They may look at their clients as dysfunctional systems, thereby encountering anger and rejection, or they may consider their clients helpless victims and render them weak and dependent.

Furthermore, using skills and sensitivity to human needs and following the above guidelines do not ensure that needed change takes place. Nurses will not always succeed in engaging individuals or families in the nursing process. This should not be considered a failure, however, because clients have many reasons for not seeking or accepting help. They may not have reached the point of distress at which change is inevitable or have developed the necessary trust required for mutual involvement in the nursing process. Nurses who do not give up offering their time to listen and keep showing genuine concern are often surprised to be sought out by reluctant clients, who, at some unexpected time, are ready to face their problems.

PART

2

Influential Factors in the
Family Process and Research

3

Family Type Considerations

In critiquing a review and analysis of recent divorce literature (Amato, 1993), Kurdek (1993) suggests that the field of family science has had a long-standing obsession with family structure and researchers have erred in treating the family type (e.g., the single-parent family, nuclear family, stepfamily) as an independent variable in their largely atheoretical search for causal mechanisms. Recently, several other authors (Baron & Kenney, 1986; Grynch & Fincham, 1990) have also recognized the futility of searching for unambiguous causal relationships. Kurdek (1993) joins these authors in proposing that family structure, among other family factors, may in fact represent a dynamic process rather than a variable and urges to explore process-oriented models of interpretation. This realization, however, is an outcome of a long journey of the social sciences through family history.

Although there is almost unanimous agreement among researchers, politicians, clinicians, and therapists that today's families have serious problems, some claim that today's families are the problem, based on high rates of illegitimate births (Santi, 1987), high rates of divorce (Glick, 1988), increasing numbers of stepfamilies (Glick, 1989), widespread antisocial behaviors (Patterson & Capaldi, 1991), and psychological problems in children (Hetherington, Cox, & Cox, 1981). According to Aries (1962), any process, phenomenon, or system may be defined as a problem if it functions contrary to the norms generally judged to be right and good. Consequently, the family system became a problem during the Age of Enlightenment in the 18th century, when writers such as Locke, Rousseau, and Paine introduced the idea of a family reform through which children were to be socialized by their parents to achieve a personal lifestyle commensurate with their intellectual potential (Zimmerman, 1947).

Families in the 19th century experienced fundamental changes. Influenced by ideas of human development and principles of education by 18th-century thinkers, the educational process slowly shifted out of the family into a growing system of educational institutions (Ravitch, 1974). Having lost much of its function as a training organization, the family of the industrial bourgeoisie proclaimed personality development of children as the family's primary mission and thereby developed the family ideal further. High moral standards, a special focus on the well-being of children and their development, strict rules about behaviors and attitudes that lead to economic success and social aptitude, and appreciation of the humanities and religious practices constituted these families' impetus (Bergier, 1971; Shorter, 1975).

Women took the opportunity to enact the ideal Victorian family style in the American middle class. In fact, one of the most important aspects of this style was the role of family women guardians of solid morals, not only by promoting them among the children but also by being involved with the Protestant clergy in the missionary endeavor within the community. The problem was ascribed to those families whose values and attitudes did not reflect the noble cause, namely, the families of lower status (Douglas, 1977).

Social developments assisted in the perpetuation of the Victorian family ideal. Economic difficulties created increasing numbers of "bad fathers" who abandoned family responsibilities (Furstenberg, 1990). Furthermore, women's employment outside the family became a problem because it stood in contrast to the glorification of motherhood as a woman's career and was viewed as detrimental to children's development (Aries, 1962). The fact that 97% of all married women, including immigrants, at the turn of the century did not work outside the home despite increased employment opportunities in industrial centers made accessible through public transportation showed the pervasiveness of the ideal of domesticity (Tilly & Scott, 1978). Later, the idea of salvation of the noncompliant working-class families was maintained within the religious and humanitarian tradition despite enormous social changes brought on by two world wars (Douglas, 1977). This rather simplistic synopsis of family history is by no means complete but illustrates how the idea of a problem becomes embedded in the society's value system. Nonconforming families have long suffered unfair accusations and victimization as their difficulties, viewed through a Utopian lens, have lent themselves to easy interpretation as decay and decadence (Hareven, 1987).

Today, lifestyles in our society are increasingly heterogeneous (Rubin, 1983). Groups of oppositional ideologies are involved in a battle of ideas and emotions that have serious repercussions on family values. Women's rights activists, pro-life and pro-choice groups, religious fundamentalists, and groups embracing Eastern philosophies and religions as well as individualism, self-actualization, or cultural pride join a multitude of professionals, researchers, and academics in claiming to have the right answer to the problems. All these ideological, cultural, and social variances are reflected in a multitude of family forms or processes that constitute adaptations to vastly different environments to which people are subjected or that they tend to choose for themselves (Roth, 1989b).

Given the multitude of environments, alternative family structures may soon become the rule rather than the exception. Nevertheless, families deviant from the idealized two-parent ideal still run the risk of being compared with traditional norms, judged accordingly, and declared a problem. This is likely to create unnecessary hardship and confusion and result in a loss of family competence and motivation in alternative families who can be as healthy as nuclear two-parent families (Gershwin & Nilsen, 1989).

If we refer back to the opening of this chapter, Kurdek's suggestion that family structure should be viewed as process seems plausible. Consequently, this chapter will use the framework of systemic organization to help the reader grasp the complexity of systemic processes, among which family structure constitutes only one factor.

From the perspective of the framework of systemic organization, families aim to reach the four systemic targets through a varying mix of behavioral processes. Although the structural family types may indicate the composition of the family and the availability of members to carry out processes, the resulting processes and patterns are of superior importance. If a family strives to maintain its stability, it can be successful with any type of structure that promotes a firm membership, clearly defined rules and roles for the members, and an efficient decision-making process. A sense of togetherness and commitment to the family are prerogatives, and both qualities are independent of the family's basic structure. Likewise, if the members desire a strong family commitment toward individuation, any type of family can have flexible rules and accept a diversity of attitudes, irrespective of its structure.

Furthermore, the definition of the family advanced by this framework is inconsistent with the concept of structural family types. Terms such as *nuclear family, single-parent family,* or *extended family* refer to the people living in the same household rather than to the members who feel emotionally bonded by a sense of belonging to a family system, irrespective of their geographical location. If the latter definition is used, it becomes obvious that there may be few truly nuclear families. Instead, many nuclear families actually constitute extended systems with members dispersed in various households. Because these members are likely to contribute to the family process, sometimes in a significant manner, it seems reasonable to use the family's extended constellation to assess systemic family health. It follows that nurses need to focus on contributions of all family members, rather than on the structural composition of households, by assessing family health or the family's success in reaching its desired targets through the behaviors embedded within the process dimensions.

The Nuclear Family System

Professionals have clearly voiced their concern about the "vanishing" traditional nuclear families. Census figures from 1990 show 24.4 million households in the category of two parents with children under 18 amounting to 25.1% of all households. Compared to this, in 1970, the nuclear family constituted 40.3% of all households in the United States. This diminishing number seems to have various reasons. Most important, households in 1990 had an average of 2.62 people compared to 3.14 in 1970. Consequently, families with fewer children remain in the category of households with children under 18 for a shorter period of time. Furthermore, other household categories have increased in numbers, such as people living alone and single-parent families.

Nevertheless, among families with children, the two-parent system seems the most common even today, with 74.6% of families falling into this category. Two-parent households, however, are not necessarily traditional families but instead include a considerable number of married couples who are not in their first marriage and mothers or fathers who are not the biological parents of the children in their household. Divorce rates had peaked around 1980 with 40 divorces per 1,000 married women, with an estimate of 49% of all first-time marriages to end in divorce (Glick, 1983). Since then, the rates have leveled off or have slightly declined to 37 per 1,000 women, according to the 1990 census. Taking into account that up to 80% of divorced parents may remarry, sometimes more than once (Baker, Druckman, & Flagle, 1980), it seems reasonable to assume that the traditional family, even if it should become outnumbered by stepfamilies by the year 2000 (Herndon, 1982), remains the ideal to be recreated after one or more failures.

The figures suggest that today's nuclear family should be described in terms of variability instead of commonality and in terms of process rather than structure. When two people join to build a family, they need to work out a systemic process that is satisfactory to them and to the children who may follow. The major difficulty in succeeding with this task is a general confusion about conflicting values. The following example illuminates this point.

Paul and Heather have been married for 2 years. Their baby is 6 months old. When they were married, they had high ideals. Their family was to meet their emotional needs and render them united and strong to face life's challenges. Heather was to be a mother dedicated to foster her child's development to the fullest extent. She had read books on parenting, taken her own mother's advice, and thought she was fully prepared for what was to come. Paul had started a promising career as a lawyer and was confident that he could support his family.

Today, Heather wonders why the happiness she had envisioned did not really occur. She remembers that before meeting Paul she was determined to remain single to be independent, develop her individuality, and have a career as a lawyer who fights for the equality of women. Somehow, these expectations nag her now because they make her aware of stark discrepancies with everyday reality. Instead of self-development, she practices self-sacrifice; instead of being supported, she finds herself cheering up her tired husband; and instead of being revitalized through sexual excitement, she is tired from dragging herself to the baby's room at night to rock him to sleep. Equal sharing of labor was another illusion. Paul sleeps too well to even wake up when the baby cries. His career has utmost importance and his good intentions of spending quality time with his child are often forgotten in the light of professional obligations. Heather has been trying to compromise her values: She reduced her career aspirations by temporarily working part-time and assuming low-key employment to give more time to the baby's developmental needs, and she lives with less income to further her family's ideals. On the other hand, it seems as if she alone has had to make all the sacrifices, thereby losing her cherished equality. Suddenly, economic aspects come into focus as well, because family resources are more limited and Heather's freedom to seek recreational opportunities, travel, and entertainment is restricted.

Paul, too, finds that their marriage no longer provides the emotional support he envisioned. Communication breaks down when both are tired. Heather's expectations of him are too high. Paul is supposed to read Heather's wishes and relieve her of duties, neglect his career for the family and still provide more money, and be empathetic to Heather's complaints and accusations and subsequently inundate her with romance and sexual desire.

The example shows the beginning of a vicious cycle fed by resentment and mutual anger about shortcomings in meeting the expectations of happiness through marriage. The core problem of family systems that aspire to traditional models is that the ideology of marital romance is out of sync with reality. The impetus to emphasize personal happiness within the marital institution has gained full expression only in the 20th century (Staples, 1989). Marriage was originally intended to be an arrangement to jointly provide for physical, social, and sexual needs. As the example shows, even family systems of today are preoccupied with finances, health problems, social functions, and daily hassles that have little to do with romance and fulfillment. Consequently, families become increasingly fragile when they set the expectation of happiness too high. Such marriages are likely to fail due to the imperfections of the people involved (Staples, 1989).

According to the framework of systemic organization, Heather and Paul will need to realize that their happiness depends not on external factors but instead on their own personal coherence nurtured by the process of spirituality. Happiness does not depend on certain characteristics, qualifications, or appropriate behaviors in living an idealized role. Instead, happiness arises through unconditional acceptance and involves one's own adjustment to the other person by seeking within that person the pattern of wholeness that reflects universal order.

The ideal of the traditional family prescribes behaviors that often conflict with other needs and personal priorities. Failure to live up to the ideal arouses guilt over one's own shortcomings. Instead of admitting their conflicts and weaknesses, most humans will attempt to protect their ego by seeking fault in their significant others. This destroys the very basis of family coherence necessary to work out a satisfactory systemic process. In the past, the function of working together to survive has served as a binding force. Today, however, the high divorce rate testifies to the fragility of marital unions. For a large number of people, the first year in marriage seems to be the happiest (Blood & Wolfe, 1960), and stressors that arise in the marital relationship or the family system seem to affect people's happiness more than others (Glenn, 1975).

The best professional advice for Heather and Paul may be to drop their unreasonable ideals and search within themselves for what is truly important to them. They should relax and smile about their own shortcomings and learn from the other person's insights. In terms of the framework of systemic organization, they should shift their emphasis from control of each other to spirituality, and from stability and adherence to rigid defenses to growth or tolerance of differing values. Heather and Paul are hardly an exception. Disillusion with marriage is rampant and pessimism about the stability of families is expressed by professionals such as Staples (1989), who expects that the predominant family type of the future will be a series of monogamous relationships of progressively shorter duration.

Today's growing number of stepfamilies seems to indicate that people are looking for satisfaction in recreating a nuclear system after divorce. Statistics indicate that 16% of all families with children have at least one stepchild (Moorman & Hernandez, 1989). Stepfamilies are even more vulnerable to failure than first marriages, with 60% ending in a second divorce (Kantrowitz & Wingert, 1990). One may speculate that the failing families, in creating their new system, still cling to the traditional family ideal. They place even higher expectations on the marital relationship, hoping for support and healing of their emotional wounds.

Dainton (1993) suggests that stepfamilies need to reconcile themselves with a popular myth of instant love. The myth seems to be an extension of the ideal mothering role, resulting in society's expectation that stepmothers immediately and easily accommodate to this role. Consequently, the children are believed to automatically and genuinely return the stepmother's love (Visher & Visher, 1988). In reality, the adjustment process in stepfamilies is difficult and complex. Child-related problems make it difficult to achieve family coherence. Although young children are generally quite adaptive (Hetherington et al., 1981), adolescents who carry much resentment and deal concurrently with separation issues may have a serious negative impact on family operations (Visher & Visher, 1978).

Pill's (1990) study of 29 successful stepfamilies with adolescents sheds some light on the challenging adjustment process. Generally, family cohesion measured with FACES III (Olson, Portner, & Lavee, 1985) was low for these families and adaptability was extremely high. The families reported a loose structure, allowing the growing children considerable space and personal freedom. Individuation was emphasized with respect to each person's uniqueness. In concert with ideal family expectations and the myth of instant love, mothers more than other family members expressed disappointment about lack of emotional closeness. They reported that it was hard work and a constant struggle to build a sense of family identity that eventually developed through the sharing of experiences and life events.

It follows that stepfamilies seek closeness and strength within a new marital relationship but need to put equal emphasis on individuation of all members. Stepfamilies have the formidable task of creating a system maintenance process that determines family boundaries, power relationships, loyalties, and daily patterns that respect the individuals' uniqueness and needs (Visher & Visher, 1982). Nurses ought to refrain from judging stepmothers if they fall short of the traditional mothering ideal but should reward the stepmothers' flexibility to move away from the ideal to pilot test new and unconventional processes likely to promote growth.

In summary, the overwhelming motivation to form two-parent families seems to be love and commitment. For parents in their first marriage as well as those in their second or third marriage, the key to family survival is to maintain this commitment by responding to changes with creativity that allows growth. It is not family structure that predicts failure, but the inability of individuals to find their own congruence within the family process. Success is less a matter of adjusting the family maintenance process to one's individual needs than of shifting from a paradigm of self-actualization to one of systemic belonging and to enact one's individual process of spirituality in adjusting one's own systemic process to that of the family and its members.

Nontraditional Family Systems

What has been said earlier is generally true for all family structures. Nontraditional structures such as single-parent families, multigenerational systems, kinship networks, and unions of nonrelated adults and others are neither better nor worse than nuclear families (Gershwin & Nilsen, 1989). Again, the professional's task is to explore the family's process, commitment, and flexibility to estimate their health or congruence.

Studies of single-parent families report contradictory evidence in terms of effects on the children (Staples, 1989). Much of this research has reflected biases and misassumptions, declaring single-parent families as pathogenic or an ailment of society (Mednick, 1987). Although newer literature takes a more liberal stance (Demo, 1993), there is general agreement that single-parent families suffer more stress and more economic hardship than nuclear families. From this, the assumption is deduced that the family structure leads to hardship due to its misfit with existing social arrangements (Allen, 1993). There may be some truth to this; however, more needs to be known about the problem before reaching conclusions (Amato, 1993).

The framework of systemic organization advances an alternative explanation: If families are institutions of culture transformation, it is likely that they adapt their process to internal and environmental conditions and that structure follows secondary to the system process that is optimal for survival and growth. For example, if single parenthood follows a divorce, the divorce may have been the adaptive process in reducing internal conflict and finding coherence within a newly structured family system. If single parenthood remains the long-term condition of choice for a parent who targets personal stability and growth, it is less a matter of adjusting to this family structure than of adjusting the family processes and the interactions with environmental systems in such a way that they lead to health of all individual family members and the system as a whole.

Sociological history of the family clearly shows that adaptation of the family systems to the social and economic environment takes place. Although the purpose of building families has changed over time and differs according to cultural understanding, individuals' aims to actualize these purposes have remained constant. Although the middle-class family or the adult partnership is to fulfill emotional needs above all others, in the lower-socioeconomic bracket, family forms such as the kinship systems or multigenerational families have developed as superior alternatives in ensuring survival. Among the poor, single-parent families have definite economic advantages as well, and these will be discussed in Chapter 5. Still other family forms, such as communes or cults, are products of disillusionment with societal norms.

Family forms arise from an innate need for togetherness and mutual support in braving the challenges of life. With more heterogeneity in our environment, more diversity of family forms should be expected. The few forms listed earlier do not comprise the existing variety of creative arrangements to meet individuals' needs. The family definition within this framework demands an expansion of the concept of family structure so that if membership is to include all people who influence the systemic process, various households, friends, and extended relatives may form a countless variety of structures. These expanded functional structures gain legitimacy because they constitute the entire available team of individuals who manage the family process. The following example illustrates such a situation.

Tanya was divorced 3 years ago and has custody of her 5-year-old daughter Chelsea. Her son stays with his father in a different state. Her financial means are meager. She produces handmade crafts sold in stores that appeal to people interested in alternative lifestyles. In addition, she receives a small alimony. She lives in a large, old, inner-city house shared by four young men and one woman. Their living arrangement is primarily economically motivated. The young men are artists who accept temporary jobs to support themselves. Rent and expenses are shared. The two women have agreed to keep house in exchange for a reduction in their monthly rent. Although each member has the freedom to live his or her own life, the household suffers from a lack of structure. Because income is sporadic, bills do not get paid on time. The telephone is disconnected periodically and there is tension among members who do not live up to their financial obligations. Although the young men rarely eat at home, the two women like to cook healthy foods they buy on discount at the market in the hour before closing. Tanya knows where to get used clothes and toys for Chelsea, takes her to the library, works with her in the garden behind the house, and lets her take care of a stray cat. In addition to the two of them, Tanya considers her family to consist of her son, whom she misses, the young woman in the house, a boyfriend of 6 months who lives three blocks away, her mother in another city, and two close women friends. Other than providing emotional support and an open ear to listen to her problems, these family members have practical functions. Her housemate baby-sits without charge. Her boyfriend has a car and takes her to visit her mother or brings her to a doctor. One of the women friends works in a store that sells Tanya's articles and the other takes Tanya to poetry readings she enjoys. Tanya cooks for her friends, crafts useful things for them, brings them vegetables from the market, or watches their kids. Tanya wishes for more resources, a more stable life, and her son's presence, but she is reasonably happy.

The example shows two different pictures, depending on which perspective is taken when defining the family. Although the household harbors many problems, Tanya's functional family shows definite strengths. Her family's structure lacks stability, but at the same time Tanya seems to have adaptability and resiliency that should not be underestimated. The example makes one suspect that functional structures might yield higher correlations with individual and family health variables than the traditional structural constructs research studies have used. It is important to bear in mind, however, that for such correlations, family teams would have to function effectively. In reality, interactions among certain family members often render it difficult to achieve family congruence and individual health. Therefore, although functional structures may have an advantage over the traditional categorization of family types taken as variables, they cannot be objectively evaluated without also looking closely at the consistency of family processes.

Research has contributed little to understanding systemic complexity. Two studies of divorced families may come closest (Healy, Malley, & Stewart, 1990; Hetherington, Cox, & Cox, 1982). Both report that spending time with noncustodial fathers had a positive effect on the adjustment of children only if these fathers were recognized as contributing family members. With high interparental conflict, however, children's time spent with the father had negative repercussions. Furthermore, several researchers documented positive child development outcomes if other adults were assisting the single custodial mother (Cochran, Larner, Riley, Gunnarsson, & Henderson, 1990; Dornbush et al., 1985; Santrock & Warshak, 1979), but the findings of Friedemann and Andrews's (1990) study suggested that the effect on the child was relative to the quality of the relationship the mother had with the helping adult.

In summary, although family structure has some bearing on the systemic process, or the process may be a driving force to modify the structure, structure alone should not be judged as good or bad, or positive or negative. Instead, nurses should first consider supporting the family structure as it is and assist the members in creating system maintenance processes that are in concert with the structure. In some cases, however, the functional family structure may be inadequate to reach the desired systemic targets. Only then should nurses, together with the family, examine the possibility of changing the functions of some members, adding new members, or employing external assistance.

4

Life Span Considerations

As individuals in the family develop over time, their perceptions and needs change and require an adjustment in the family process, specifically in the way members relate to each other. Developmental theory has been used extensively to explain such changes over time. This chapter will first examine the relevance of developmental theory in light of the structural complexity of today's families. Second, it will present the developmental phenomenon from the perspective of the framework of systemic organization.

Chapter 3 has pointed out the pervasiveness of the traditional family ideal and its resiliency over time. Developmental theory has had a major function in enhancing and perpetuating this ideal. It may not be by chance that the sociologist Glick (1947) introduced the concept of the family life cycle at a time when women's efforts were no longer needed to support the war machine. There was a need to teach women how to be professional mothers and homemakers and teach fathers how to support the family to optimize the children's personality and vocational development. The family life cycle, based on traditional family norms, has served as a concrete teaching tool with which one could deduce the tasks families had to master within certain predictable phases of family life, the length of which was calculated with the help of demographic statistics. Thus, couples aspiring to the traditional family ideal could be given specific instructions on how to over-come developmentally induced stresses and improve their spousal relationship and parenting skills.

Developmental theory applied to individuals and the family system has shaped sociological and psychological thinking over several decades and is still heavily used. It depicts a model of distinct phases with significant transitions to be mastered between each phase and the next. The most popular family developmental theories in nursing are the Duvall (1977) eight-stage model and the Carter and McGoldrick (1980, 1988) paradigm of six stages developed for family therapists. Both delineate a series of normative events during a family's life cycle and the adjustments to be made to move from one stage to the next. Although these theories may have served their purpose during a time when most families followed the traditional model, many problems with these theories have been discussed recently.

McGoldrick and Carter (1982) have recognized the need for theory adjustment for complex families because "normality" of families is difficult to determine. They have developed a list of additional developmental tasks for divorced and remarried families, the most frequent nontraditional variations. Teachman, Polonko, and Scanzoni (1987), however, claim that the life cycle model is limited in its clinical applicability, not only due to the great variations in families and living arrangements today, but also because the nature, timing, and sequencing of life events in ethnic and poor families do not follow the described norm.

New theories related to normative versus nonnormative transitions are presently being developed on the basis of the work of Neugarten (1979), who found that individuals develop expectations of life cycle events. As long as changes fall within the expected norm, families are reasonably able to adjust, whereas nonnormative or unexpected events may lead to crises. Although this theory provides helpful guidelines to practicing nurses, it also raises a series of questions. First, just as in the description of life stages, inter- and intrastage normative transitions cannot be valid for all families. For example, "a young mother working" could be a normative transition for a lower-middle-class family, a nonnormative transition for a traditional family with an unemployed father (Kelly & Voydanoff, 1985), or no transition at all for a mother who had worked all along. Other related transitions would be markedly different for the three women as well. Child care in the first family may be provided by a grandmother or a neighbor, and the third woman may have explored child care facilities before deciding to become pregnant. Leaving the baby with a sitter would be considered normative for both and result in minimal guilt. The traditional mother, however, would experience great difficulty leaving her child with a stranger. The example points out the futility of declaring one course of events as normative. Nevertheless, ideals have been mistaken for norms and are declared as desirable by the media, entertainment industry, politicians, or commercial advertisements. Families are led to believe that they can realize such normal things as "the American dream," wealth and happiness, healthy and professionally successful children, or a leisurely retirement age. But today's reality looks drastically different for the majority of families who fall short of such norms. Much despair could be eliminated if families could see their course of life as a continuing struggle with challenging situations, such as the loss of a job, a learning disability of a child, illness, or giving care to aging parents, instead of a pursuit of happiness.

This points to another shortcoming of family life cycle models. Until recently, developmental theory was based on the assumption that in healthy families, positive relationships were needed for smooth transitions to new phases and remained positive despite developmental changes. Research on intrafamily relationships, however, has long demonstrated that such unchanging relatedness is a fallacy. Marital satisfaction, for example, seems to continuously decrease after the first child is born (Feldman, 1971; Ryder, 1973) and reaches its lowest point when the children are in adolescence (Burr, 1970; Stattin & Klackenberg, 1992). Most parents report some disharmonious relations with their children at one or more age levels (Stattin & Klackenberg, 1992).

These findings suggest that family development is a fluid process that is infinitely more complex in nature than the stereotypical nuclear family life cycle models present it to be (Breunlin, 1988).

Breunlin (1988) describes the process of adjustment to a child's development. The parents, siblings, grandparents, and other relatives adjust to the higher competence of a child with a series of microtransitions. Because development occurs continuously and time does not stand still, many changes in the relationships with the child take place, but at certain points in the child's development, an intensification of the change process, a "nodal transition" (p. 134), is required. Breunlin argues that nodal transitions occur as "discontinuous leaps" (1988, p. 138) and are brought on by an oscillation of family behaviors in that the family experiments with higher-level behaviors (e.g., giving an adolescent freedom of choice rather than setting strict rules to obey; letting a child decide his or her bedtime rather than enforcing a strict napping routine) to reverse symptoms of stress and dysfunction but keeps slipping back to its habitual behaviors. The transition is completed once the oscillation is stabilized at the higher level. What Breunlin neglects to mention are the secondary changes in the relationships between parents, siblings, and the extended family who attempt to also negotiate new rules, roles, discipline, and child-rearing methods to regain equilibrium in the family process.

In terms of the framework of systemic organization, a nodal transition signifies system change or second-order change. The oscillation vividly illustrates the intense struggle between stability and change in families whose system maintenance repertoire does not include the behaviors necessary to accommodate the change. However, several authors have given tribute to large differences among families in the ease of transitions. Although some families report difficulties, many seem to move through time without encountering major hurdles (Burr, 1972; Rankin, 1989). The theory of systemic organization explains this difference as pertaining to the nature of system maintenance processes and underlying values.

The values and behavior patterns of system maintenance of a family comprise not only the behaviors pertaining to the currently activated developmental phase. System maintenance also includes values and expectations that give rise to their relative behaviors throughout the entire course of the family's life.

The foundation for these behaviors is laid by the adults joining to form a family. They bring together two sets of expectations and values to be mutually reconciled. This is true for married couples as well as partnerships, homosexual unions, or adult-family groups. What McGoldrick and Carter (1982) describe for spouses is valid for all others: Adults have acquired values from their parents and have defined issues and shaped attitudes about a multitude of behaviors, from daily activities to caring for others to rearing children. A multitude of values as well as life and communication patterns are learned from the family of origin, the media, books, neighbors, or friends.

Consequently, young adults planning to raise children have certain attitudes about the meaning of children, timing of pregnancy or adoption, number of children, the rights and responsibilities of adults and children at various ages, gender roles, sexuality, and so forth. These attitudes are closely intertwined with religious beliefs, cultural patterns, and ideologies such as women's rights, materialism, or individualism. Built into this complex system of attitudes and beliefs is the notion of flexibility to make changes. In fact, processes of change, testing of values, and tolerance of diversity are learned from early childhood on just like their more stable counterparts. It follows that when developmental changes occur in children, parents will take action in accordance with their own expectations about system maintenance, their own values, beliefs, and ideologies. In a family whose system maintenance pattern includes the necessary behavior patterns needed in the various stages of development, much adjustment will occur subconsciously, intuitively, and successfully without a need for system change.

Difficulties arise if system maintenance expectations are inadequate in meeting family needs. Such individuals may have been raised in families of origin that lacked health and gave them little opportunity to learn patterns of family coherence. Other adults involved in child rearing clash if their expectations or attitudes differ drastically. In still other families, living conditions have significantly changed and system maintenance values have not been adjusted to allow for such changes.

The latter example suggests that developmental changes in the family constitute only one of many types of possible changes that confront families concurrently. They have to be viewed as one component of the family's current life situation that interacts with all others and exerts a combined influence on the total process of seeking health. Whether or not developmental changes or any other factors demand family system change depends on the resilience of system maintenance patterns. It follows that the issue of normative versus nonnormative changes is irrelevant because each family carries its own "norm" imprinted in its system maintenance dimension. Each demand for change is evaluated against this "norm" and perceived as easy or overwhelming accordingly.

TABLE 4.1 Assessment of Developmental Factors of Children and Elders

---

System Maintenance

Level of assistance needed in
- . basic physical care
- hygiene
- play/learning
- social interaction

Family adjustment to
- sleep/wake rhythm
- eating patterns
- elimination patterns
- entertainment/recreation schedule
- health care needs

Caregiving roles (Who? How?)
- basic physical care
- entertainment/recreation
- stimulation/learning/tutoring
- discipline
- baby-sitting/adult-sitting
- transportation
- illness care
- religious guidance

Adjustment of
- family social activities
- recreational activities
- work schedules

The framework of systemic organization suggests to the practicing nurse to assess and assist families as was described in Chapter 2. Here, the interplay between individual needs, based on personal development and the family's accommodation of these needs, is the focus. Although the assessment guide for individuals in Chapter 2 sufficiently addresses the life patterns of independently functioning adults, children, elders, or chronically ill adults who request care and support from the family need an additional set of items added to the assessment. The nurse needs to determine the extent of physical care and emotional support needed by the family and, more important, the family's reaction to these developmental needs. Table 4.1 presents a short summary of the topics relative to family developmental issues.

TABLE 4.1 (Continued)

Coherence

Needs to develop or maintain
- gross motor skills
- fine motor skills
- social skills
- affection/emotional control
- learning/intellect
- self-confidence
- identity/direction

Individuation

Support of
- motivation to learn
- special interests
- expression of personality
- preferences and choices
- decision making
- problem solving

System Change

Encourage
- adjustment of approaches to changing situations
- independent thinking

Critically discuss
- decisions
- values and attitudes
- behavioral consequences

The following examples illustrate the interplay of developmental issues and other family circumstances in the formulation of nursing goals.

Families With Young Children

Deanna is 19 years old. She left her abusive family at age 15. After living with a maternal aunt for a year, she dropped out of school, moved in with a man, became pregnant, and had a baby boy. Shortly after the birth the relationship broke up. Deanna received help from a shelter for the homeless in finding a small apartment and getting food stamps and Aid for Dependent Children. Encouraged by her social worker, Deanna took classes to earn a high school equivalency diploma. This, however, came to a standstill when she met Duane, who vowed to support her and be her child's father. Duane now lives with her and provides her with modest financial help from his earnings as a part-time security guard. He takes classes at the community college to become a mechanic. Deanna is pregnant with his child. They hope to get legally married after completing his education. Meanwhile, they need the child support to pull them through.

Justin, Deanna's son, is 14 months old, has grown normally, and is well nourished. He has started to walk and is very inquisitive. Deanna takes him along wherever she goes, and he has adjusted by taking naps anywhere, in friends' houses, in grocery stores, in the park, or in a car seat. Deanna lets him explore his environment almost to the point of carelessness, but if he bothers her when she is busy, she wants him to mind and respect her private space. Duane is good at distracting Justin in situations like that. He throws him a ball or picks him up to play rough. He tells Deanna that Justin does not understand respect yet.

Duane is looking forward to the birth of his child. He loves children because he grew up in a large family and took care of his younger siblings because his mother worked. Deanna is more skeptical about a second child. She has suffered intense morning sickness and is afraid that this may be a bad omen for the things to come. She feels discouraged about her goal of becoming a legal secretary. Two children will be so much work. Sometimes, she sees herself as sliding into the same predicament as her mother, who felt overwhelmed by responsibilities and never handled her life very well. But then, she attributes that to the fact that there was never a caring man in the house and, all the more, Deanna's hope is Duane. If he makes it economically, maybe he can help her and they will both be happy. The thought of losing him frightens her.

Discussion

This family rests on rather shaky ground but exhibits some remarkable strengths. That the partners' relationship is pivotal to family stability has been generally recognized. Much has been written about intimacy, but the concept has been poorly defined and its relationship to the overall family process is far from being clarified (Schaefer & Olson, 1981). Wynne (1988) observed that modern couples are commonly preoccupied with the maintenance of intimacy to the point of neglecting everyday necessities and the development of mutual problem-solving skills. Intimacy rests on personal autonomy and the skill to communicate and continuously adjust to one another within the relationship (Wynne, 1988). It is glorified in the traditional family ideal and it seems that Deanna, in her dreams, has ascribed to this ideal. She expects Duane to play the role of Prince Charming and liberate her from her predicament that has been a generational pattern in her family of origin. Although Duane has many assets, Deanna's clinging dependency is dangerous, because it defies autonomy and mutual growth. Being in a state of emotional deprivation, Deanna has many needs but insufficient ability to give of herself.

Deanna has not fully completed her adolescent development. Her disruptive past has prevented her from gaining enough personal coherence to sustain her health. She made a solid attempt to gain self-esteem by taking the high school equivalency classes. She still has visions of being a legal secretary but is plagued by much self-doubt and low coherence. Instead of relying on herself, she counts on Duane's help. She invests inordinate amounts of energy in the attempt to reach her target of spirituality through the relationship with Duane. Individuation and personal growth become difficult. All the more, she seems to interpret her child's attempts to gain her attention as an interference with her individuation process or maliciousness. Trying to balance this shortcoming, she resorts to the control target and reacts to the threat in a punitive manner. Duane acts as a catalyst in such situations by recognizing Justin's needs. He may serve as a role model but there is a danger that Deanne may interpret this as competing for Justin's love, which she requires to maintain her coherence.

Although Duane's personal coherence and commitment to the family seem to compensate for some of Deanna's insecurities, long-term family coherence can blossom only if Deanna is able to grow stronger as a person. In addition to a supportive environment, the growth process requires personal system change in that Deanna's thinking of herself as a helpless victim needs to shift to trust in her abilities.

A nurse expert working with this family consequently devises ways for Duane to employ his remarkable abilities in the support of Deanna's individuation and reward her for moves toward independent decisions or contributions to joint problem solving. Simultaneously, the nurse helps Deanna understand her personal life processes as well as her child's developmental needs by using the system diagram. Justin, at age 14 months, needs much help with system maintenance. Deanna and Duane are responsible for most of his physical management, teaching him to relate to people and his environment. They need to carefully monitor the development of his coherence through individuation and accommodate his need to manipulate and explore objects, practice his motor skills, and find excitement in the developing expertise in language and communication. Duane and Deanna represent the major systems with whom Justin can exchange information and affection to actualize his individuation process. To be able to do this, Deanna needs to have sufficient personal congruence and would benefit from the nurse's assistance in setting personal goals for her own growth and individuation. Increased coherence through autonomy will allow Deanna to demand less from Duane. At the same time, she will learn to focus on Duane's needs, give of herself within their relationship, and prepare for the new baby's arrival.

In summary, the example shows the interdependency of individual and family needs and suggests a nursing approach of assisting the partners to work jointly in helping each other to grow so that the family as a system has a reasonable chance to survive the changes imposed by the addition of another child. Research generally shows a decrease in happiness within the parental dyad throughout the childhood years of the children (Burr, 1970; Spanier & Lewis, 1980). This may indicate a need to refocus expectations of young couples from the traditional, romantic ideal to a partnership that centers around the challenge of instituting a generally effective, flexible, and supportive system maintenance operation. This means that satisfaction should not be based on meeting one's ever-increasing individual wants and desires. Instead, this period in family life particularly represents a time of mutual support and consolidation. Adults committed to raising children need to learn to understand the differences in each other's life processes, accommodate through spirituality, and reward themselves for their success in solving complex problems.

Families With Adolescents

Brian is 16 years old and lives with his single mother, Pat, in a small apartment. Pat is a diabetic and legally blind. His father is an alcoholic who left the family when Brian was 5 and his whereabouts are unknown. Throughout his childhood, Brian has hated his father for deserting him. Brian has always felt very close to his mother. He supported her emotionally, because she underwent several surgical attempts of retinal reattachment that eventually failed. Since age 11, he has taken on many family responsibilities. He cleans the apartment, runs errands, and does some cooking. Pat's parents live close by. They take her shopping and her father helps her with the mail, banking, and paying bills.

Brian has been a good student. He and his mother used to sit together to do homework for school. He particularly liked science and read the chapters in his science book to Pat, who discussed the topic with him and asked him questions that made him think a little more deeply about the subject. Presently, however, things are not going well. Brian refuses to be supervised with homework. Pat was called by the school principal, who told her Brian was failing. Brian had lied to her about his school grades. He is belligerent whenever Pat reminds him of his duties and he refuses her help with schoolwork. Pat fears that she cannot keep things under control because of her handicap and feels devastated about having lost her son's love and trust.

One night, Pat discovers that Brian has gone without telling her where. She is afraid that he may be into drugs or sexual relationships and waits up for him until he enters at four in the morning. When he gets home, she tells him how worried she is and how disappointed she is that he has misused her trust. Then she sends him off to bed. Later in the day, Pat receives the monthly visit of the public health nurse. She shares her problems with her. She tells her that Brian has had difficulties with the kids at school for some time and has been beaten up several times and teased. Pat feels that it is because of her. Since age 14, Brian has never brought classmates home because he seems ashamed of his mother. At that point, Brian enters the room in pajamas and tells Pat that she neglected putting out his clothes for the day. The nurse feels a strong impulse to tell Brian that he is old enough to do that himself, but then she thinks a second and asks, "Is it important to you that your mother does this for you?" Brian answers, "Yes, she knows best." It turns out that this odd occurrence is the key to the nurse's understanding of their relationship. In a flash of enlightenment, she senses a deep sense of caring from both sides. Brian lets his mother do this for him because he still feels a need to be taken care of. In so many other aspects of his life he has taken on responsibilities beyond the ordinary for his age. At the same time he acts contrary to his natural urge to be independent and something tells the nurse that he does this for the sake of Pat. Deep down, Brian is proud of Pat for overcoming her many obstacles. When Pat goes shopping for his clothes, she wants to be in control. Her parents explain what the colors and patterns are and what the clothing looks like on Brian. Brian may choose what he likes. Pat then feels the texture and shape and forms a mental image of each piece of clothing. Every morning, by getting his clothes ready, Pat has control over Brian's appearance. For her, this action has a symbolic value. As she shapes the appearance of her son, he becomes part of her. Pat carries his mental image with her throughout the day.

By talking about this to the nurse, Pat and Brian recognize the symbolic meaning for the first time. It all had happened intuitively before, but now they feel mutual appreciation for each other. This gives Brian a chance to take a look at his own issues and he feels ashamed about his behaviors of the night before. The problems in school are discussed, and after Pat expresses her true concerns about his future, he willingly accepts the idea of arranging tutoring sessions with the teachers to catch up in his classes.

Discussion

Adolescence is a difficult time in many families. Earlier developmental theory (Erikson, 1968) claims that for adolescents to gain independence, they need to detach from their families and replace their parents with other systems. Out of this arose the family stage of the unattached young adult launched from his or her family of origin and ready to start a new family (Carter & McGoldrick, 1980, 1988). Recently, social scientists have taken a less definite stance. Steinberg (1990) denies that young people abandon their families of origin. Instead, the relationships to parents and other family members are redefined to gain a new sense of connectedness (Gilligan, 1987;

Steinberg, 1990). It appears that adolescents in emotionally supportive families overcome difficulties more easily and gain more stable identities than those that lack closeness (Adams & Jones, 1983; Josselson, 1987). Clinical accounts are available about families with overinvolvement (Minuchin, 1974), but research on long-term consequences is lacking (Fullinwider-Bush & Jacobvitz, 1993).

Although the last example seems like a classic picture of a dysfunctional family at first sight, the nurse used her intuitive sense and refrained from a premature judgment. The family system exhibited signs of health that could easily be interpreted as problems if judged against norms. Pat, Brian, and his grandparents formed a system struggling with unusual circumstances. There was a mutual commitment to support each other. Brian, as an adolescent, had the need to conform to his peers. Their acceptance was of prime importance, because previous problems he had with peers probably threatened his coherence. To gain entry into a group of peers with whom he was impressed, he had to deny his strong attachment to his mother and could not honestly admit his family commitment. Furthermore, being studious and conscientious were not desirable qualities in this particular group of adolescents.

According to the framework of systemic organization, individuals seek congruence with those people or systems in the environment who allow them to maintain or build coherence in the line of their values. Young people who lack coherence are easily impressed and pursue certain ideologies and images of power or material wealth, thereby suppressing or rebelling against family values acquired earlier. This conflict came to light in the previous example in that Brian suddenly experienced guilt as he realized that he had disavowed his family and the values it stands for. The incident with his clothes was the key to recognizing the true meaning of his emotional ties.

In summary, nurses need to guard themselves against quick judgments based on all kinds of norms. A diagnosis of overinvolvement or enmeshment does not serve a purpose other than labeling a family as "sick." Following this framework, the nurse examines the role of emotional bonds within the total individual and family process. Health is threatened if any of the four process dimensions are curtailed, as was the case with Deanna in the first example. It remains to be seen if Pat and Brian succeed in adjusting to Brian's strivings toward autonomy and finding coherence personally and within the family. The role of grandparents in this process is of importance as well. It is hoped that they will listen, facilitate communication, and mediate if there should be misunderstandings. The nurse may decide to include them in a family session during which roles within family system maintenance are redefined to accommodate the changed needs of the individual members.

Families With Adult Members

Life cycle and developmental literature put their major emphasis on the child-rearing stages, but in reality most people in industrialized countries may spend half of their lifetime in families with adult members only. Census figures from 1990 show that close to one third of the households in the United States are young married couples who have decided against or postponed having children. The other fraction is composed of couples whose children have reached independence. Both groups have grown in size due to factors such as increasing career options for women, better opportunities to limit and space pregnancies, and the generally increased life span of people that allows many productive and independent years after the launching of children.

Life cycle literature takes the reader through the launching stage during which the children disengage and leave the middle-aged spouses alone again (Carter & McGoldrick, 1980). Although this stage is viewed as providing new chances for growth, especially for the woman (Abbott & Brody, 1985), it can also bring the problems of the empty-nest syndrome or retirement stress due to suddenly being devoid of responsibilities (Atchley, 1980; Golan, 1981). Several recent trends suggest, however, that the happily retired couple who focuses its main energy on renewing the relationship and reaping the fruits of labor is becoming a relic or illusion. Launching of children has become increasingly difficult due to the need for many years of extensive education or job training and increasing problems for young adults to become economically independent. These difficulties have led to unstable and complex transitory family structures and to moving in and out of the parental home as young people explore their options of partially dependent styles of living (Avery, Goldscheider, & Speare,

1992; Goldscheider & Da Vanzo, 1989; Thornton, Young-DeMarco, & Goldscheider, 1993). The problems are accelerated in the economically deprived minority community, in which dependent jobless adults, especially males up to their 30s, frequently live with their families of origin or other relatives (Anderson, 1989).

Furthermore, many middle-aged adults have little opportunity to enjoy themselves in retirement, as they are burdened by enormous responsibilities not only for their children but also for chronically ill and frail parents who need to be supported and cared for in their homes or in nursing homes. All this renders it impossible to establish norms for adult family living. Developmental needs, for example, young people's gaining of independence or middle-aged parents' adjustment to new goals and social activities, are by no means the sole factors determining family development. Instead, each family, on the basis of its basic systemic pattern, will react to its particular situation and will make adjustments, compromises, and sacrifices in the attempt to meet the needs of all members and find systemic health.

The nurse working with the framework of systemic organization is advised to use developmental guidelines on the level of each individual in the family and evaluate the system's ability to accommodate to these various needs. Again, it needs to be stressed that families are not to be equalled with households. Adult families, especially, are often dispersed in several households, as in the case of elderly parents and their various children with families or a young adult living in an informal partnership arrangement and being closely connected to the family of origin who offers financial support, does the laundry, and cooks frequent meals. The following example gives some clarification.

Rosemary is a 51-year-old director of a day care center. She lives alone in a city apartment. Her brief marriage ended in divorce when she was still in her 20s. Since then, she has dedicated her life to the cultural enrichment of people's lives, working with television and radio, organizing literary circles, and developing a pilot educational program for small children. She has a strong belief in people's basic right to uninhibited growth and self-development. She has social ties to many of the community's intellectuals, artists, and independent thinkers.

Rosemary was the younger of two children in a working-class family. Her father was an almost tyrannical head of household who denied his wife any formal attempt to put her extraordinary creativity to work. He used physical discipline methods liberally in the attempt to control the children and keep them in line with standards. Rosemary's brother had broken his ties with the family after the mother died 10 years ago, because he harbors deep resentment toward his father. Rosemary's early marriage was motivated by her urge to break away from her family. She remained aloof for many years since.

Through the illness and subsequent death of her mother, Rosemary renewed her involvement with her family. Having rid herself of personal resentments through the spirituality process, she has gained an understanding for her father, in whom she has discovered valuable human qualities. In fact, she has started to appreciate his stubborn peculiarities because she realizes how much she actually means to him even though he has never been able to express this in words. Being almost 90 years old now, he lives alone in his little cluttered apartment. Rosemary looks after him daily and is the only person allowed entry. She had previously tried to engage a home care service but several well-meaning women were ordered out rudely by her father. Rosemary can sense how much his independence means to him. He hangs on to his favorite activities, reading the paper, watching TV, and taking walks. Rosemary acts as her father's advocate. She calmed down the neighbors when they complained about loud noise from the TV and were cursed out by the "deaf old man" who did not understand their concern. Then she went to buy him earphones. Rosemary weighs his independence against safety with a liberal and open mind. She knows that if she forces her father to move into a nursing home, his spirit will die. Independence and the ability to master difficult situations have been the pride of his life. So he fights any threat to his coherence with incredible determination.

Recently, he has adjusted to increasing disabilities by creating a reality that preserves his integrity, and a mild confusion allows him to relive his better days in the past without losing touch with reality to a great extent. He is particularly attached to a child from Rosemary's center who bears a resemblance to Rosemary as a little girl. Rosemary takes the child for visits occasionally and is almost moved to tears when she watches her father talk to her. It is as if her father reexperiences the affection he has always had for Rosemary, only now he can express it freely without feeling the need to discipline and control. The same confusion carries inherent dangers, however. Twice it has compelled Rosemary's father to step down from the curb onto a busy street, upon which he was hit by a passing car. Rosemary has doctored his bruises and done some hard thinking about his future. She has decided to let him carry on despite the danger and will not feel guilty in case of a serious accident. She feels that she is in no way entitled to rob him of his dignity and lock him in a home like a caged animal.

Discussion

The example shows the remarkable adjustment of two people to a difficult situation. Rosemary, like many people in midlife, has gone through a period of reexamining the meaning of her life and her values. Taking on a changed perspective, she started to appreciate her father and recognized his iron determination and passion for life in the same patterns that used to inflict pain on her in younger years and have estranged her brother. The relationship with her father has become a spiritual process of renewed adjustment of her own patterns to his to honor his needs and preserve his dignity. Through the process of individuation, Rosemary has matured and grown to understand the depth of her own life and the process of aging.

It was the intent of this chapter to increase the readers' awareness of the complexity of developmental factors interacting with the structure of the family and the total life situation. Instead of comparing families in treatment with a norm that in today's times has little in common with reality, the framework of systemic organization gives the nurse guidance in assessing the developmental needs of individuals and the family's systemic accommodation based on its very individual history, pattern of functioning, and environmental situation.

5

Cultural Considerations

Maintenance and
Transformation of Family Culture

As described in Chapter 1, the process of transformation of cultural patterns is a central issue in the framework of systemic organization. Culture is defined as the totality of the human way of life (Hartog & Hartog, 1983) that includes the control of natural forces to meet physical and safety needs of people. Furthermore, culture entails the institutionalization of social, interactional, and spiritual practices in families. The definition stands in no conflict with the sociological understanding of ethnicity as those stable cultural patterns shared by a group of families who have the same historical past, race, religion, and national origin (Kumabe, Nishida, & Hepworth, 1985). Ethnic groups of families perceive themselves as distinctly different from others (Glazier & Moynihan, 1975) in that they have a unique understanding of the essence of humanity (Devore & Schlesinger, 1987), the self, and its difference from other groups (McAdoo, 1993).

Ablon and Ames (1989) maintain that all human societies have established a blueprint that represents their culture—namely, beliefs, attitudes, and behaviors people are expected to ascribe to or follow. The family systems have the task of implementing these cultural expectations. Experts in the family field have recognized that ethnicity is strongly reflected in family functioning and that, in fact, it may be a superficial overlay. That is, ethnicity as a unique variable may be of minor importance compared to the more basic family processes that subsume its effects (Bowen, 1976). Thus, families establish a unique process through which they can accomplish the task of living the culture of the group they represent.

The primary socialization process of a child occurs within the family and entails the adoption of a set of values and life patterns imprinted by the family's ethnicity (Ablon & Ames, 1989). Cultural stability or the maintenance of ethnic patterns occurs also at the level of the family system in that values and beliefs are mutually guarded against conflicting environmental trends and ideals. Ethnicity can be maintained in a relatively pure state if the environment supports the families in maintaining their long-established systemic patterns and if these patterns remain functional and beneficial for the families.

Culture in the family, being synonymous with the total family process, represents a stable core of beliefs, values, and their relative behaviors that also has the capacity to change. If environmental patterns and ideologies conflict with the patterns anchored in system maintenance, families will adapt slowly under pressure as they seek congruence with changed environmental conditions.

Within the American urban society, individuals and families are continuously exposed to widely differing and quickly changing beliefs and attitudes (Ablon & Ames, 1989). To adjust to such changes, families need to incorporate some new knowledge and compromise many of their usual behaviors, a process that inevitably leads to system change and culture transformation. Families who migrate or suddenly find themselves in a drastically different economic situation or social status experience severe incongruence that forces them to change rapidly to avoid a crisis. According to the framework of systemic organization, culture transformation processes can be divided into three components: (a) acquisition of knowledge from the environment and revision of values and beliefs through individuation and system change, (b) integration into system maintenance of new behavior patterns with concurrent elimination of patterns that are no longer relevant, and (c) transmission of the total system maintenance pattern, including newly adopted behaviors, to each new generation.

These theoretical elaborations do not conflict with recent research and the literature. For example, the anthropologist Lewis (1965) similarly describes the development of personality within the family context. He sees the family as a mediator between the culture of the society and the individual person in that each family adopts and transmits a collection of societal values suitable to meet the needs of its members. Therefore, each family develops its own distinct culture, depending on how the system interacts with and applies the information to its daily pattern.

Because ethnicity entails identity based on historical continuity (Giordano & Giordano, 1977), no family is without ethnicity. However, distinct ethnic identification often becomes difficult due to the above-described culture transformation process. Tripp-Reimer and Lauer (1987) point out that diversity within ethnic groups is considerable and warn nurses to avoid stereotyping. The concept of mainstream culture rests on the idea of the "melting pot." This theory assumes that immigrants to the United States are becoming homogeneous by adopting mainstream American values and life patterns, thereby relinquishing their traditional life patterns. This process of intermeshing cultural patterns has been termed *acculturation,* whereas the replacement of ethnic values with mainstream values is called *assimilation* (Kumabe et al., 1985; Spector, 1979).

The American mainstream culture in reality represents an adaptation of Northern European cultures to the living conditions found in the new country. One may be justified in questioning the existence of a homogeneous culture, based on vast differences in religious and social values as well as customs and behavioral rules among various ethnic immigrant groups. Nevertheless, acculturation has taken place as economic goals have been pursued and a common government and legal system have been defined as guidelines for all. McAdoo (1993) claims that the pursuit of common ideals, "the American Dream," has worked for white Europeans and highly educated Asian immigrants (Kikumura & Kitano, 1973), but other ethnic groups are denied access. Instead of assimilating, ethnic minorities are prevented from participating in the mainstream culture and forced to become bicultural, that is, carriers of two cultures (Gillian, 1990). Thus, they have adopted a set of mainstream ideals while living by another reality and suffering from their inability to reach the ideal.

Other authors claim that the melting pot theory is a fallacy altogether in that assimilation occurs for all groups only partially and at differing rates, leading to a great diversity that has been ignored by science for too many years (Staples & Mirande, 1980). That the process is greatly influenced by other factors, such as the economic situation or the educational level of the people, has been shown extensively by research. For example, Cromwell and Cromwell (1978) failed to find significant differences in decision-making patterns between Caucasians, African Americans, and Chicanos based on ethnicity alone. Likewise, differences in the use of the health care system tend to be minimal if the socioeconomic status and geographical access problems of the subjects are controlled for in the studies (Alston & Aguire, 1987). This phenomenon points to an assimilation process, a blurring of ethnic patterns and intercultural differences among previously distinct ethnic groups who share the same environment (Staples & Mirande, 1980), but representatives of the same ethnic background become increasingly diversified, depending on their environment and living conditions.

In summary, the framework of systemic organization supported by literature and research suggests that families tend to maintain a core of ethnically based values that are strongly intertwined with the way they define their identity. These values tend to be modified over time and replaced by more functional ones, if the family experiences incongruence based on its living situation. Depending on the flexibility built into their system maintenance, ethnic groups differ in the extent to which they maintain or change values. A common core of values has been established by early European immigrants, developed over time, and perceived to be American. These mainstream values, strongly related to personal achievement and economic success, are accessed and adhered to by successful families but have remained ideals beyond reach for many others. Although minorities are particularly disadvantaged for many reasons (McAdoo, 1993), increasing numbers of impoverished Caucasians share their economic plight.

This discussion shows the enormous complexity of the dynamics occurring at the interface of ethnic family patterns and personal characteristics of individuals with the environmental factors that determine the conditions of life. The rest of this chapter will cite examples to explain particular problems encountered by recent immigrants from various cultures and the African American population segment.

Culture Transformation in
Immigrant Families

Ahmed Aljahmi, age 45, emigrated with his family from Lebanon 10 years ago with the help of his older brother who had lived in the Detroit metropolitan area for some time. Ahmed's brother managed to find him a job in a Lebanese bakery to get started. While living in a small apartment with his wife Mona and four young children, Ahmed worked every hour he could but had severe difficulties making ends meet. Ahmed had acquired some basic English language skills in his home country and now took evening classes at a community college nearby. Because he did not want to depend on his brother's resources for long, he soon found a higher-paying job in a tooling company. This required, however, moving his family closer to the new workplace to keep transportation costs down. Ahmed had just succeeded in getting a driver's license and bought an old car in fair condition. This move, however, meant that the family had to leave the brother's community, where there was strong support among people from various Arab countries who lived in the vicinity of a mosque that served as a cultural and community center.

In his new workplace, Ahmed became an outsider. Because he refused to try the beer offered to him at work and never joined his coworkers in the bar after work, they started to tease him about his religion and later shunned him and became outright hostile as they discovered that Ahmed worked better and harder and earned himself a small pay raise. Ahmed felt displaced, lonely, and hurt. At home, expenses for the children grew and his wife demanded more money than he was willing to give her. Struggles ensued about how to manage the budget and about the failure to exercise frugality.

Ahmed's coherence was seriously threatened because he had lost autonomy and personal control. He had failed in living his ascribed role of providing for the family. To compensate for this inadequacy and helplessness he sensed about himself, he attempted to claim for himself that part of his cultural role that was still available, namely, to lead the family and make decisions. However, the culturally justified protection of wife and children took on the character of dictatorial control of their behaviors. Any resistance on their part awoke in him severe anxiety about losing the last support in his life and he resorted to severe disciplinary methods, including occasional physical abuse. The worst incident occurred when his wife announced that she wanted to look for a job to have enough money for the children.

His eldest son, now in first grade, presented another problem. Ahmed was forced to watch him adopt American habits, because his son was now exposed to different ways of thinking by the educational system and through his classmates. Ahmed realized that the school was the key to his son's success in life, but at the same time he felt strong competition in rearing his children.

Mona felt deeply troubled. She had little support in the community and the scarf she wore made her feel like a foreign object. In the school she sensed discrimination as teachers seemed to assume that she was incompetent in supporting her son's education. Her language skills were deficient and she was homesick for her extended family in Lebanon. Although life back home was filled with hardship, it somehow seemed less complicated. She knew her role and her place within the family system. She could talk to people about problems, and conflicts seldom got out of hand. Here, she had difficulties even in supermarkets, where she could not locate the ingredients of dishes she was used to preparing. She had to ask Ahmed's brother to get them at a specialty store and bring them over periodically.

Conditions started to improve after a serious talk between Ahmed and his brother during a visit. When Ahmed told him about Mona's wish to work, his brother answered, "Why not!" He told Ahmed of other families with working wives, especially a friend who, because his wife worked, could take classes in accounting and a few years later was able to make a good living. He also pointed out to him that Mona's unhappiness was due to isolation and was likely to improve if he let her get out of the house and be involved. Ahmed hesitantly touched the subject with Mona and expressed his fear about her being tempted by other men. At that point she laughed and assured him faithfulness. She then assumed a job as an aide in a group home with elderly residents.

As a result, Mona feels happier and is enthusiastic about taking evening English classes. She begs Ahmed to let her learn to drive and feels that he will consent as soon as he gets tired of driving her to too many places. Meanwhile, Ahmed has set himself the goal of becoming an auto mechanic and is taking classes. Although the children have little difficulty in adapting to the new world, both Mona and Ahmed need to keep adjusting their cultural values and patterns. The children, who are now watched by neighbors with children of similar ages, encounter frequent problems with their parents if they behave like Americans. The parents at times interpret demands for new clothes as immodest and the voicing of opinions or preferences as disrespectful or conceited. Mutual understanding demands open communication channels and the maintenance of coherence within the family system while flexibility is built into the family's system maintenance mechanisms.

Discussion

The example outlines only a few of the many immense problems families encounter in adjusting to a new environment. At the same time, it shows how system change may come about under pressure and severe incongruence. Because culture defines the self and provides identity, it is no surprise that immigrants are reluctant to change these defining characteristics about themselves and their family. Consequently, Ahmed and his family initially moved into a neighborhood where their culture was amply represented. This allowed them to continue their life patterns at least to some extent. This trend is observable with most immigrant groups and has led to Chinatowns, Mexican barrios, Greektowns, and Puerto Rican districts within large cities. Within such cultural enclaves, people can protect their system maintenance by interacting with those components in the environment that are congruent with their patterns and values. Some groups (e.g., the Amish in Pennsylvania or the Cubans in Miami) (Suarez, 1993) have been remarkably successful.

Although there are large differences in the flexibility to adjust and change values or to allow intermarriage among ethnic groups, some accommodation will take place over time as these groups are forced to interact with institutions that represent a contrasting cultural orientation, such as the schools, the workplace, and health care facilities. Because the children of immigrants are more likely to adopt the customs of their host country, intergenerational conflicts are common in many different immigrant groups. For Muslims, youth behaviors such as dating or drinking are particularly threatening, and marriage outside the faith is forbidden (Nanji, 1993). Young Asians experience a value conflict between professional success and family commitment that implies their unwillingness to compromise personal freedom and traditional loyalty to their parents (Lin & Liu, 1993). In Hispanic families, intergenerational conflicts similar to Ahmed's problem tend to concern the status of women and their participation in the work world, which would result in neglecting their traditional family and parental duties (Suarez, 1993).

Recent literature, however, warns practitioners to stay away from cultural stereotyping, because each family reacts to a changed environment in a unique way. The previous example also shows that the reaction is greatly influenced by factors other than ethnicity, such as economic conditions, social isolation, and accessibility of religious institutions, as well as individual factors, such as education, motivation to become American, developmental needs, range of coping behaviors, health factors, and many more. Because of this complexity, it seems reasonable for nurses to engage in an assessment of the life process for each individual family. The framework of systemic organization is culturally consistent in that the targets are equal for all families, but the emphasis placed on the targets and the patterns used to reach the targets are culture based. Nurses are advised to assess ethnically rooted patterns within the four process dimensions and consequently estimate the effectiveness of the patterns in reaching desired targets and satisfying the needs of individual family members.

As previously mentioned, family health is a dynamic process based on the perception of congruence. Thus, many families such as Ahmed's, who are exposed to discrimination and cultural stereotyping, have additional difficulties to overcome.

The Problems of Minorities

A minority group not only is represented in smaller numbers than the majority group but also signifies a socially, politically, and economically subordinated status (McAdoo, 1993). This implies that minority groups are given less power and fewer opportunities. In the past, ethnicity, minority, and race were treated similarly. Only recently, mounting evidence of the remarkable diversity within each racial group has led to the realization that racial designations commonly used are artificial labels and preclude the broader ethnocultural distinctions (Valle, 1989). Recently, research has focused on ethnic differences within the racial groups. For example, Gelfand and Fandetti (1980) have compared caregiving patterns of various segments of Euro-Anglo families, whereas Valle (1989) has discussed the diversity of historical family patterns among blacks from English and French colonies in the Caribbean. Valle (1989) has further demonstrated that to determine a true picture of the culture of a particular group, it is necessary to include not only the historical ethnic distinction of family life, but also the families' socioeconomic status and their perception of the level of discrimination they experience daily. The interaction of all three gives rise to the culture of the family and shapes its patterns of behavior. The following example of an African American family in poverty most clearly illustrates this point.

Rochelle is 42 years old and rents an inner-city, three-bedroom apartment. She lives with her two daughters and a grandchild. Her daughter Teney is unemployed and Sallie, the younger daughter, is pregnant with her second child and supported by Aid for Dependent Children. Her eldest son, Tyrone, is presently in a drug rehabilitation center run for the indigent by the Salvation Army. Rochelle has a remarkable history. Rochelle was 16 when she had Tyrone. She stayed with the baby in her mother's house until she married an automotive worker 2 years later, when she became pregnant with his child. The man was an alcoholic and Rochelle started drinking with him to avoid conflict. Rochelle admitted that the family situation was chaotic, especially when Sallie was born and her husband was fired due to his drinking. She applied for public support, but the funds went mainly for alcohol and there was never enough money for necessities. Rochelle's mother helped out with the rent to prevent eviction, but often the family went without electricity and heat in the winter.

Rochelle reports that one day, 2 years later, she woke up and decided to change. She went to church and talked to the minister. That evening she stopped drinking "cold turkey." She demanded that her husband leave the house and filed for divorce. With the help of her social worker she enrolled in courses to become a secretary and learned to drive. With incredible determination she endured hardships but never let her goal out of sight. She found strength in talking to her mother, who also supported her with child care, and in church. Two years later, she launched an office job in the suburbs and bought an old car.

At this time, Rochelle is worried about her children. Tyrone, who has a mild learning disability but never received help in school, dropped out of school at age 16 and roamed the streets. He has never worked longer than a few days, and for the past 2 years he has lost control over his life, being dependent on crack cocaine and caught in a relationship with a much-older alcoholic woman. He was involved in criminal activities and had robbed the family of funds and objects he could sell. Rochelle is relieved that he is in treatment at the moment but doubts his ability to pull his life together. Her daughters are aimless and depressed. They lack self-confidence, hoping for a man to pull them out of misery, but have become disillusioned over time. Teney is working part-time as a bagger in a grocery store but her assets are insufficient for her to become independent. Sallie has been making plans to move out for some time, but each time she saves up her support money for a rent down payment, the family has an emergency, such as a car repair or a doctor's bill, and she ends up staying at home. Rochelle seems exhausted from working, watching her grandchild, and organizing the household and is upset about getting little appreciation from her daughters, who let her do all the cleaning, shopping, washing, and cooking.

Discussion

This family lives in a harsh and largely unsupportive environment devoid of resources needed for living. The example, however, shows several family qualities that contribute to the resilience of families and are needed for survival. As recently as in the 1960s, African American families have been considered pathological, because their predominant matriarchal structure presents a stark contrast to the traditional family ideal (Moynihan, 1986). More recently, this view has changed but is still disputed. Authors disagree on whether or not mother-led families, who are ever-increasing in number, present a problem or an adaptation (Stack, 1986; Sullivan, 1989). Many authors (e.g., Billingsley, 1968; Boyd-Franklin, 1989; Willie, 1988) describe today's African American families in terms of their historical and ethnic patterns that are passed on from generation to generation. Family patterns are believed to have been formed in Africa, during slavery, and after the Civil War. Basically, women have learned to fend for themselves, because their husbands were often sold or placed elsewhere. An extraordinary loyalty to the community had existed already in African tribal villages and was maintained over time. To survive in the United States, families have learned to form kinship networks for the purpose of sharing resources, nurturing orphaned children and young mothers, and providing emotional support. The church as a social institution plays a strong role in fulfilling material, social, and emotional needs (Boyd-Franklin, 1989).

Other investigators (e.g., Norton & Glick, 1986; Stack, 1986; Staples, 1986) explain family development in terms of adaptation in that families exposed to new situations process information and adapt their lifestyles in an effort to survive. For example, Peters and deFord (1986) note that although men's family roles were curtailed by historical happenings, today they are being legislated out of their families by the welfare system that denies assistance to unemployed fathers. Carol Stack (1986) makes the point that the harsh economic environment is largely responsible for the African American family structure in the inner cities. Generational welfare dependence and a lack of an economic role by unemployed men have given rise to financial power being held by females. Thus, the literature describes African American inner-city families as having two major features: single mothers and disengaged fathers. The one-parent, female-headed family functions within the context of a large, extended system of kin and friends, if they are available. Meanwhile, economic constraints and high unemployment, hopelessness, drug abuse, discrimination, and a strong desire for the material ideals that are out of reach have affected the role of men.

The fact that middle-class African American families are predominantly two-parent nuclear systems that strongly emphasize the fathers' provider role (Bowman, 1993) seems to support the "Africanity" model set forth by Staples (1974) and described by Nobles (1978).

Like the framework of systemic organization, this model explains ethnic patterns played out in the family to represent African traits maintained in the system. However, these uniquely African patterns have been blurred and adapted to the present-day reality (Staples & Mirande, 1980) through system change. The earlier example alludes to kinship assistance. The role of grandmother was important when Rochelle had young children, and the same responsibility is now being taken on by her in support of her grandchildren. Women have carried the load of family responsibility for at least two generations. The strengths that suddenly arose in Rochelle seemed to be derived from her strong values based on historical roots. Because she now sets a positive example for her daughters, she hopes and prays that one day they will recognize within themselves their budding strengths and capabilities.

Rochelle's family supports Tyrone as well. In fact, many African American families tolerate lifestyle deviances that would throw most middle-class systems into a crisis. This tolerance is based on their ability to live by multiple sets of values, a cultural schizophrenia. Gillian (1990) notes that African Americans and other minorities interfacing with the mainstream have become bicultural in that they have internalized mainstream values while they live by other values that represent their environment. Consequently, Rochelle dreams of living comfortably without serious problems. This goal would be within reach if it were not for her other obligations. Her ethnic set of values, supported by religious principles, obliges her to support her economically dependent adult children. Rochelle understands Tyrone's problems and those of her daughters and supports them, but at the same time she recognizes her limits and feels extreme frustration because her reality in no way approaches the ideals of a comfortable life, no matter how hard she tries. Her predicament is one of the many destructive forces in her environment that stretch her outstanding resiliency to the limits.

The example shows with clarity the interaction of economic factors, ethnic patterns, and the feeling of hopelessness and discrimination or the anger of being denied access to a life worth living. The situation of ethnic immigrants is comparable because their plight is also relative to the resources of their own people and their environment. Consequently, among Hispanics there are considerable differences in the ability to reach mainstream ideals. Although long-established, highly educated, and mutually supportive Cubans have built a culturally congruent community that supports their needs (Suarez, 1993), Puerto Ricans have been living in poverty as they experience severe racial discrimination and unemployment (Delgado, 1987).

In summary, understanding culture is of major importance because it does not simply influence family patterns, but it represents the family's life pattern, the essence of being, and the identity. Through system change, families adapt some of their values in many ways and at different rates while they cling to others. The process of adaptation is relative to the environment in which the family lives and seeks congruence. Consequently, a cultural assessment is not a list of historical traits and peculiarities but a description of how the family conducts its daily business, maintains coherence, and grows and changes when faced with problems. The family's health and the success of reaching congruence with society and its institutions are greatly influenced by the family's ascribed status and experience of discrimination. Nurses who understand the dynamics of culture will appreciate the strengths of diversity and act as advocates for families who are subjected to stereotyping and denied access to needed resources.

6

Research With the
Framework of Systemic Organization:
Basic Considerations and Issues

ROSANNA DeMARCO
MARIE-LUISE FRIEDEMANN

The purpose of this chapter is to raise fundamental questions concerning the function and process of family research and the use of knowledge relative to families. The first part will address the tenets of positivist-empiricist science and its assumptions of predictive regularity and empirical validation. This will be followed by a discussion of the influence of these assumptions on current philosophical and theoretical debates. Next, an introduction to research triangulation as a possible methodological perspective to be used with this framework is followed by a discussion of current research paradigm debates between quantitative and qualitative methods and ethical considerations related to diversity in research. Finally, the conclusion of this chapter refers to the creation of midrange family theories commensurate with the framework of systemic organization and the challenges to operationalize and test them.

Philosophical and Theoretical Issues

The failure to comprehend can be discomforting. The effort to make sense and organize phenomena of interest increases the likelihood that concepts and theoretical assertions can be made understandable. Thus, knowledge development is an important goal for family research.

From an empirical standpoint, the three major functions of scientific family theory are *description, explanation,* and *prediction.* Scientific description and understanding are created through the construction of systematic abstractions (theories) that offer a cognitive map of family phenomena. These phenomena need to reoccur reliably and remain stable over time to maintain accuracy in description. Families, however, are in a continuous state of unfolding (a process), and the likelihood of predicting anything within the systemic complexities described so far in this book seems to be small. Theories that enable reliable predictions at one point in time may lose their capacity for prediction and their relevance for control in the next.

The implications this has for how research methods based on family theory should be carried out are revolutionary and open to significant creativity. Within the discipline of nursing, the philosophical basis of the "regularity" of knowledge immediately leads scholars to spirited debates. One basic issue appearing implicitly and explicitly in the writings of nurse scholars over the past decade concerns the question about the relative importance of knowledge and research methods. A brief anthology of concerns and encouragements relative to this issue is presented here as a fertile ground to rethink family research.

Silva and Rothbart (1984) raise concern about the "contradictory, divergent and confusing points of view" (p. 1) that lead to probing questions about the nature of nursing science. Comparing logical empiricism and historicism as two separate viewpoints, they support historicism as "the forefront of science today" (p. 2), based on a definition of science as a culture-bound process rather than as a product. Consequently, theories should no longer be true or false and mutually undermine each other. Instead, they should serve as "collaborators toward the goal of solving scientific problems" (p. 3). Similarly, Suppe and Jacox (1985), as well as Sarter (1990), recommend multiple approaches to theory development and testing. They emphasize that both quantitative and qualitative methods are appropriate depending on the nature of the problems, and diversity of methods and their interrelationship must be tolerated in the development of knowledge. Philosophical integration is also advocated by Dzurec and Abraham (1993), who list six pursuits applicable across paradigms: (a) mastery of self and the world, (b) understanding through recomposition, (c) reduction of complexity, (d) innovation, (e) meaningfulness, and (f) truthfulness (p. 116). Yet today's research falls considerably short of this goal of integration.

Using the work of Belenky, Clinchy, Goldberger, and Turule (1986), Kidd and Morrison (1988) predict that nursing knowledge development is currently in a "procedural knowledge" developmental stage distinguished by a dichotomous use of quantitative and qualitative methods. According to these authors, knowledge is being constructed but fails to be hierarchically achieved.

What is needed next is a "flexible synthesis and integration of grand and middle range theories" (Kidd & Morrison, 1988, p. 223). Theories from multiple patterns of family-knowing may serve well to connect self-knowledge, intuition, empirical studies, prior theoretical formulations, and patient perceptions and provide links between the worlds of practice and theory. Although a theoretical foundation for family nursing that can accommodate all the above has not yet been found, the framework of systemic organization may constitute an important stepping stone. According to Reigel and her associates (1992), an integrating foundation promotes growth by bringing ideas into focus and forming and developing them.

Furthermore, such a foundation needs to include experiential dimensions in research (Newman, 1992). The values and norms of traditional research that are firmly embedded in the presently used paradigms need to be questioned to explicate phenomena beyond the observable, and avenues for new creativity need to be opened. However, because of requirements of methodological rigor, demands for certain designs and data analyses create a dissonance between formal research and the experience of nursing practice. Silva and Sorrel (1992) explain that nurses who practice integrate their experience, but research and theory testing require that they discount their lived experiences as practitioners. It follows that some rigorous methodologies may be incongruent with actual practice and therefore unsuitable for the testing of nursing theory.

In summary, many nurse authors and researchers offer perspectives that address differing or contradictory views of the nature of validity or "truth." Truth in nursing relates to complex human experiences from which the discipline generates knowledge. If family research knowledge gives meaning to the methods, then multiple ways of knowing may ultimately propel nursing family epistemology by means of creative structures and processes. It is up to nurse scholars to pave the way to knowing families. Creating opportunities to receive several views of the phenomena within research is called *triangulation.*

Research Triangulation

Campbell and Fiske (1959), Jicks (1979), Sohier (1988), and Denzin (1989) define triangulation as the combined use of two or more investigators, theories, methods, data sources, or analyses of methods in a study of phenomena. Multiple triangulations involve the use of more than one type of triangulation. The major goal of triangulation is to obliterate bias and compensate for deficiencies that are inevitable in a single investigator, theory, method, data set, and analysis. In addition, validity as a measure of the truth value of knowledge is acknowledged as the motivating factor in building science and knowledge for the discipline of nursing through the use of this approach.

Triangulation of investigators, theories, methods, and data sources is highly relevant for the testing of the framework of systemic organization at the midrange level. Investigator triangulation exists when multiple analysts, observers, or interviewers analyze the same data set (Duffy, 1987; Kimchi, Polivka, & Stevenson, 1991; Mitchell, 1986). The advantage of using this approach is presumably the reduction of bias because multiple analysts will rule out some validity threats derived from each investigator's own viewpoints. According to the framework of systemic organization, researchers, as they interpret their findings, find meaning and truth through an individuation process. What makes sense to investigators depends on their own life process and, specifically, on their mode of perception. Therefore, one expects substantial differences in the interpretation of data between investigators of divergent backgrounds, disciplines, and expertise. The advantage of interviewer triangulation is a broader understanding of phenomena through the integration of various worldviews and reference points (Kimchi et al., 1991).

Theory triangulation involves the use of different theories as competing perspectives of analysis for the same data set. In addition, it involves testing through research the theories that may have opposing hypotheses or a different way of looking at phenomena (Duffy, 1987; Kimchi et al., 1991), for example, hypotheses derived from the theory of systemic organization versus those based on stress and coping models. The advantage is clarification of which theory better describes, explains, or predicts the area of research.

Method triangulation is the use of two methods, usually quantitative and qualitative, to explore the same phenomenon or research question for the purpose of complementarity, not replication (Duffy, 1987; Kimchi et al., 1991; Morse, 1991). Two types of method triangulation are described in the literature: between-methods and within-method triangulation (Duffy, 1987; Kimchi et al., 1991). Within-method triangulation is used when the phenomena under study are complex and the researcher attempts to use two or more types of quantitative or qualitative methods together. In quantitative within-method usage, more than one scale can be used; in qualitative usage, several ways of interviewing or observing processes could be combined. The data are expected to be similar.

In contrast, in between-methods triangulation a certain degree of divergence is expected due to the differing perspectives promoted by the methods. Convergent validity obtained by grouping data generated by more than one method, therefore, may best accommodate the complexity of phenomena studied by nurses and strengthen arguments (Duffy, 1987). However, Duffy (1987) warns that between-methods triangulation may obscure the differences between the methods, and Leininger (1985) claims that triangulation fails to use the full benefit of qualitative research. Nevertheless, the complexity of the holistic nature of things may be illuminated and enriched by using this approach in a creative and methodologically sound way.

Close attention to methodology is imperative. Floyd (1993), discussing qualitative and quantitative between-methods triangulation used in her study of sleep patterns, notes potential methodological problems based on sampling procedures, sequencing of the two methods, and interpretation of the results as convergent or disparate. As investigators become increasingly aware of such issues and learn to prevent problems, their research findings will allow for better interpretation of effects of multiple intervening variables and the process as a whole.

Data triangulation attempts to test theory in more than one way, for example, using multiple data sources derived over time from different geographic locations or from varying samples (Denzin, 1989; Duffy, 1987; Kimchi et al., 1991; Mitchell, 1986). Kimchi et al. (1991) point out that data triangulation over time differs from longitudinal research in that its purpose is validation of the process of interest if it shows persistence and stability, whereas longitudinal research examines change.

Analysis triangulation compares results of data sets using different statistical tests or qualitative analysis methods. At present, there are many unresolved issues around data integration, because the findings cannot be mathematically interpreted and depend greatly on logically derived and theoretically based thought processes.

In summary, triangulation methods seem to be particularly beneficial for theory development (Knafl, Pettengill, Bevis, & Kirchhoff, 1988), theory testing and the enhancement of credibility of a process (Corner, 1991; Hinds, 1989; Murphy, 1989), and overcoming psychometric problems (Aroian & Patsdaughter, 1989). Breitmayer, Ayres, and Knafl (1993) suggest that the ultimate benefit in using triangulation is a push to become vigorously self-aware of researchers' motives in purposely linking methods to find answers. Despite the sampling of benefits, there are serious constraints. The lack of common units of analysis between methods, time, money, and a large amount of data and data analysis restrictions are pragmatic challenges (Corner, 1991; Hugentobler, Israel, & Schurman, 1992; Mitchell, 1986).

Paradigm Debate and Ethical Considerations With Triangulation

Research traditions are evolutionary. Because research tradition and theory are contingent on each other, tensions between assumptions of theory and methodological norms may lead to modifications of either the theory or the methodology or both (Gorenberg, 1983). If congruence of theory and method constitutes a prerequisite for valid findings, triangulation presents an inherent dilemma in that it seems difficult to reconcile diverse methodological assumptions to match the theoretical framework.

Differences between the various research traditions are considerable. Duffy (1987) and Leininger (1992) have capitalized on different derivations of the qualitative and quantitative paradigms, listing side-by-side foci, scope, goals, and anonyms of perspectives ranging from insider/outsider to controlled/ naturalistic. Both authors oppose the combining of methods, stating that researchers use doubtful and vague rationale or practice defensive research. Phillips (1988) claims that triangulation violates coherence within the design, because the data sets are incompatible.

Other authors promote more flexibility. Within the qualitative paradigm, Wilson and Hutchinson (1991) demonstrate complementarity between two methods: Heideggerian hermeneutics and grounded theory. They note the differences in conceptual density and the rich detail each method brings to the research question and point out that both methods have integrity and provide distinct but complementary outcomes. Hermeneutics yield depth of understanding, but grounded theory guides and stimulates further research and clinical interventions.

In the discussion about combining the quantitative and qualitative paradigms, Haase and Myers (1988) acknowledge significant differences but suggest that consistency can be achieved by reinterpreting subjectivity to apply to a common value system. They suggest that equal valuing will reconcile the two traditions and allow nurses to view both as complementary. They conclude that integration is more productive than mixing paradigms. Similarly, Wolfer (1993) asserts that holding to one paradigm only discounts the reality of the other and proposes a new complementary paradigm with three strands. The first is instrumental, which includes methods specific to research questions and ontologically matched hypotheses with a particular type of inquiry. The second strand is called the illumination, in which those who followed different methods could compare what is experientially known. The third strand is referred to as communal. Consensual agreement through shared experience builds a body of knowledge.

The above bears witness to the present discussion that tends to tip the scale increasingly toward the integration of paradigms for certain types of research studies. In addition, a related and equally relevant topic of discussion is knowledge validation. Research validity is a measure of truth of a claim within the research design process (Burns & Grove, 1993). Fundamentally, one wants to know if theoretically generated questions or propositions accurately reflect reality.

According to Burns and Grove (1993), Cook and Campbell (1979), Polit and Hungler (1989), and Woods and Catanzaro (1988), there are four types of study validity: statistical conclusion validity, internal validity, construct validity, and external validity. Statistical conclusion validity addresses the question of whether conclusions about the relationships between variables from specific analyses accurately reflect the real world. Internal validity is the extent to which the effects detected in the study are a true reflection of reality, rather than effects from other variables. Construct validity refers to the fit between conceptual definitions and operational definitions of variables. Finally, external validity addresses the extent of generalizability of the sample (Burns & Grove, 1993).

According to Burns and Grove (1993), controversy still surrounds the relative validity of various research approaches. Whether various theoretical methods are used singularly or combined to enrich theory building and knowledge, what continues to be unresolved is how to achieve truth. When threats to validity are addressed within unitary or holistic worldviews of phenomena, the choice of investigator(s), research questions, propositions, hypotheses, sample, design, method and analysis, and conflicts are inter- or intraparadigmatic. Haase and Myers (1988) noted that efforts to combine the paradigms often lack the valuing of both approaches. For example, quantitative studies may include open-ended questions as a way to insert qualitative data. The analysis of such data, however, may address only surface themes rather than meanings. Likewise, qualitative studies may develop a theory (grounded theory) and then not follow through with further theory building or refining. These defects lead to lack of logical consistency and validity within programs of research and become garbled even more when "integration" means a combination of shortcomings.

Speaking for the integration of the two paradigms, both Duffy (1987) and Coward (1990) claim that validity can be increased by the appropriate use of triangulation. According to Coward (1990), construct validity is enhanced when the results are stable across both methods. Likewise, statistical conclusion validity is more likely when results are similar for various data sets and methods of analysis. Internal validity is also enhanced when results across methods are resistant to threats of causal inference and, finally, the stability of results derived from multiple samples, settings, and time frames suggests a greater likelihood of external validity.

In summary, the evolution of research tradition has not occurred merely within each paradigm but seems to have expanded to cross paradigm boundaries. Dichotomous ontologies, epistemologies, and methodologies have discouraged interparadigmatic valuing, but new developments suggest claims for enhanced validity by the appropriate integration of both perspectives. Despite the methodological inadequacies experienced by many nurse researchers at the philosophical, paradigmatic, and methodological levels of debate, dichotomous (right/wrong) ontologies have been replaced by the promotion of tolerance. Tolerance of diversity as a way to keep open the debate surrounding methodological triangulation also needs to be applied to ethical domains. It is here that one looks at diversity from the point of view of responsibility.

Research choices and decisions are made on the basis of the ethical principles of beneficence and justice set forth by the National Commission of the Protection of Human Subjects of Biomedical and Behavioral Research. According to Woods and Catanzaro (1988), researchers have an obligation to maximize possible benefits and minimize potential harms. Usually, the conception of risk includes physical, psychological, and social factors. The conception of benefits is often directed to knowledge acquired and gains experienced by the study participants.

Scientists have long tried to understand the functions of the human mind through magic, psychology, sociology, anthropology, religion, and medicine (Lazear, 1991). Various theories of knowing and learning point to differing intelligence skills, not all of which are developed equally in individuals. If this is the case, using formats of exploring phenomena that engage only one or a few of those skills will only benefit those participants with strengths in these areas and will therefore be unethical.

It follows that an ethical consideration in family research is the benefits afforded to participants with multiple ways of knowing and describing their experiences. Perhaps research has "progressed from knowledge for its own sake to science for its own sake to methodology for its own sake" without consideration of the life processes of the knowers (Kaplan & Kaplan, 1981, p. 199), leading to an ethical dilemma. The dilemma can be resolved by respect for diversity of intelligences if multiple methods are provided for participants to learn about and describe the phenomena of interest from their own perspective.

Chinn (1985) offers a serious warning to all who approach the context of nursing phenomena with the anticipation of coming "to know" more:

> The myth of the perfect method results in compulsive orderliness, repetitiveness, and a fixation on minute details. It encourages us toward mental laziness in envisioning alternative methods, alternative approaches, and alternative assumptions. We re-search and re-search to the point that we know less and less about more and more. (p. 47)

Rhetoric calls us to our hopes and ideals but experience shows what our ideals demand. Meaningfulness of research and beneficence to research participants must encourage bipartisan outlooks. Conducting research from the perspective of human science and the context of everyday practices of nurses will bring meaning to knowledge that builds the discipline.

In accordance with the framework of systemic organization, family nursing research must consider the researchers themselves as part of the same context. Values, education, beliefs, and experiences affect research, practice, scholarship, and the tenor of controversy in each of these areas. The methodological assumptions that nurse researchers hold are often, paradoxically, the anchors that bind and may preclude movement to other directions and experiences. Mythologies can be created in the anchoring of supportive contexts that are familiar and known. Ultimately, however, enthusiasm about the phenomena studied, participant needs, and the different giftedness of researchers will beckon exploration of diversity, not from a perspective of tolerating questions, but from living the questions of discovery. The framework of systemic organization promises to provoke thought and lead researchers toward novel paths of exploration while providing the necessary coherence that promotes validity in their research designs.

Operationalizing Midrange Family Theories Within the Framework of Systemic Organization

Every theory needs the support of research to become legitimate and, likewise, theory has to serve as a basis for research to validate its findings (Fawcett, 1975; Whall, 1993). Nursing frameworks, sometimes labeled as *conceptual models* (Riehl & Roy, 1980) or *grand theories* (Stevens, 1979), generally have a high level of abstraction and cannot be tested directly. It is therefore essential to deduce testable midrange theories that include concrete and observable variables to be operationalized and measured. Numerous midrange theories derived from the framework of systemic organization can describe the life processes of individuals and families. Some examples include the following:

- The resolution of a crisis entails a strong focus on coherence behaviors and subsequent individuation.
- Addiction compensates for lack of human connectedness (spirituality).
- Caregivers who grow in the relationship with the patient (individuation) do not perceive caregiving as a "burden."

These theories describe systematic processes, the variables of which are not simply related in a linear relationship but are in movement, constantly changing, and adjusting to each other. None of the processes have been tested directly by employing a conventional research process, because quantitative methods cannot address the circular causality of systemic processes. At the level of the systemic diagram that explains behaviors and their motivations, the framework of systemic organization represents midrange theory. It is based on fundamental assumptions of open systems, that is, envisioning change at any system level as influencing the entire system and beyond the limits of a particular system. As an individual strives toward congruence, patterns and rhythms of response (behaviors) occur in the complexity of multiple influences in families and social groups. Concurrently, these larger systems exert influence on the individual acting within them in an equally complex manner.

Open systems assumptions lead to further deductions. For example, within the pursuit of targets, the families' patterns of functioning are learned by individuals over time and may prevail in various systems simultaneously. Specifically, a caregiver who values controlling behaviors as a means of decreasing anxiety in relation to the care of a terminally ill partner at home may also value control in the workplace as a style of management or in relationships. Furthermore, relationships are influenced by perception or cognitive appraisals of how one detects tension/incongruence and one's identity and belief in the meaning of one's existence (coherence) in relation to one's environment (individuation). Therefore, relationships are complex patterns of energy, space, and rhythm within and between systems of contact that are difficult to describe, explain, or predict.

Patterns of space and energy require nurse researchers to examine distancing and coming close or attraction and rejection in family or group relationships. For example, distancing may be evidenced by patterns of behaviors that keep members away from home or allow them to avoid vulnerable emotional connections, whereas coming close can be exhibited by common activities or making efforts to submit to another person's control. Similarly, rhythmical patterns require nurse researchers to examine sequencing of movement through space, frequency, and intervals. If no system change occurs, the rhythm of patterns, a component of the basic life process, is transferred from one relationship to others, because one's perception of self (coherence) persists in multiple relationships.

Patterns of space as a simultaneous system experience can be explored at a particular cross-section of time, but rhythm can be explored only longitudinally. The development and use of midrange theories with the framework of systemic organization beckon nurse scholars and researchers to begin to create cross-sectional and longitudinal studies that use several views of phenomena for comparison as a means for experiential validation of the process. For example, the scores of family functioning obtained with a composite scale instrument (which demonstrates both validity and reliability in various population groups) do not provide full comprehension of the phenomenon, because they fail to express each family member's lived experience. Family researchers will be enlightened to the meaning of experiences behind the scores, however, if the scores are compared with transcribed responses to open-ended questions regarding each individual's perception of the family. Thus, linear quantitative measures can be given shape and texture by adding qualitative data for a more complete understanding of family phenomena.

In summary, the deduction of research questions and the testing of assumptions based on systemic processes demand creativity and a multiplicity of methods. Because systems are in constant movement, continuously adjusting to multiple influences and changing to strive toward renewed congruence, studies of individual and family life processes need to be designed to overcome simultaneously at least to some extent, assumptions of linear causality basic to all quantitative methods and minimize observer bias and maximize objectivity despite direct and often intimate interaction with systems in the process of collecting qualitative data. Discussions of such issues and others that are specific to the family processes in focus are in the research chapters that conclude Parts 3 through 5 of this book.

PART
3

Families in Crisis: Crises Arising Within the Family Life Process

Introduction

The first two parts of this book have focused mainly on health in families and the ability to adjust to changes by reestablishing congruence between family, family members, and the environment. Knowledge of healthy processes is vital for all nurses. Following the process outlined in Chapter 2, nurses engaged in family health promotion and primary prevention explore with their clients healthful living patterns that are congruent with their unique way of balancing stability, growth, control, and spirituality. Nurses help clients use the resources they already own to enhance some of their life patterns or shift priorities if a system change is needed. The promotion of health usually includes anticipating changes thought to be normative for the specific family by thinking through possible approaches of adjusting family strategies to the expected developments.

In contrast, examples in the second part of this book show nursing approaches with families who struggle with more serious problems. Nurses can be instrumental in avoiding crises by reversing a life process headed toward destruction, before it is too late. Many family members show remarkable strength in that they are active participants in the social process and have learned to adjust their values in dealing with novel situations. Nurses can be successful if they follow the nursing process described previously. They support and encourage clients to use more intensively those individual and family strategies that fit their life process. Having gained the family's trust, nurses can then proceed to provide guidance in the enhancement of patterns that the family assesses as being in need of change. Such families need understanding, sensitivity to their cultural interpretation of the world, and encouragement to follow through with their own ideas for change. The outcome of such nursing care is the family members' trust in their own abilities and successful problem solving.

Unfortunately, however, many families find their way into the health care or mental health systems only at the point of a serious crisis. The nurse then is confronted with the complex task of assessing the family's resources for crisis resolution and the extent of their need for guidance. The meaning of crisis needs to be well understood to accomplish this.

The theoretical understanding of crisis derived from the literature rests mainly on stress and coping concepts. A crisis is said to start when regular problem solving loses its effectiveness (Caplan, 1964). Pittman (1987) describes a crisis as a situation in which a family system requires change but fails to have at its disposition the necessary behavior strategies to make the change. Having observed a large number of families in daily life, Kantor and Lehr (1975) realized that most families who sensed tension responded by using more and more intensively those behavioral strategies to which they were accustomed. They continued enforcing ineffective patterns without changing them, which led to the point of crisis.

Once in crisis, families are unable to conduct their usual business because of emotional upheaval and the resulting chaos. The members sense severe tension and anxiety, become highly irritable, and communicate ineffectively (Curran, 1985).

Crises can happen in all types of families. Healthy families may temporarily crumble under immense pressure or a severe shock that overtaxes the system's resources and demands radical change of values. Healthy families will be able, however, to resolve the crisis eventually. Caplan (1964) cites a time frame of 6 weeks to pull out of the immediate paralysis. Within that time, the healthy family is supposed to have reached a new equilibrium of its systemic targets. Crisis resolution has three essential components. First, family members need to understand what has happened to them and ascribe meaning to the painful experience. Next, they pull together, share the meaning, and communicate on a more intimate level. Finally, they examine and adjust their values and beliefs. Having these tasks completed, they can then embark on joint problem solving and experimentation with new behaviors (Jacobson, 1974).

This process suggests a positive quality of crisis. By way of a crisis, families thrown into chaos may gain the awareness that the status quo is more painful than change. This awareness opens them to system change, or the basic restructuring of their family patterns (Rapoport, 1963). As the meaning of the Chinese symbols for crisis suggest, the concept signifies both danger and opportunity. Thus, clinicians have observed repeatedly that a culminating family crisis is comparable to the crisis in an infectious process. It signifies the decision point that determines life or death of the organism. In families who pull together, communicate, and reach internal congruence, a crisis leads to growth and new health through which alternative ways of problem solving become suddenly evident. In systems that lack this ability, a blind effort to protect the injured self and the pursuit of individual desires create victims through misuse of control and eventually lead to the destruction of the existing family structure.

Pittman (1988) describes four types of crises: bolts from the blue, developmental, structural, and caretaker crises. These categories suggest that crises can be induced either from the environment or from within the family system. Pittman (1988) remarks that at times it may be difficult to determine the roots of a crisis. He uses the example of a partner's infidelity, which may come as a "bolt from the blue" but is also the gradual outcome of a family structure that inhibits growth and a family process through which the family members are unable to meet developmental needs.

Not only is it difficult to pinpoint the onset of a crisis, but it is equally troublesome to predict its outcome. It has long been recognized that families react differently to disasters or abrupt changes (Lindemann, 1944). Although even serious disasters will not break the resiliency of some families, others crumble under normal developmental changes of their child. The determining factor is the degree of family health at the time a crisis develops or the effectiveness of the family's general life process through time.

Most crises develop insidiously over time (Joselevich, 1988). If a family experiences a disaster and also deals with the residues of previously experienced and unresolved crises, its systemic process may break. The double ABCX Model (McCubbin & Patterson, 1983) suggests that such unresolved crises result in family system maintenance behavior patterns that perpetuate incongruence over time. The ABCX model introduces a concept called *pile-up* that represents all demands for change a family encounters at a given point in time, including the remaining tensions and incongruence based on previous unresolved crises. Within the theory of systemic organization, the pile-up factor is detected as chronic anxiety among family members that is harmful to family coherence. The anxiety is played out in the members' interpersonal patterns. Irrespective of its origin, such incongruence takes on its own life. It is maintained through complex systemic interactions between external and internal conditions and between the family system and its members, sometimes over generations.

Focusing on the full complexity of the systemic family process, Part 3 will describe crises arising from within the family. Specifically, Chapter 7 discusses examples of developmental crises. Chapter 8 focuses on family structural changes leading or responding to crises, and the topic of Chapter 9 is the problem of addictions and family violence. This is followed by a fourth chapter on the practical implications for research.

Family crisis with disease or illness will be covered in Part 4, and crises due to influences from the environment are the topic of Part 5. Using examples of real-life situations, all three remaining parts will bear evidence that no single causative agent is to be held responsible for most crises. Instead, the family life process, in particular intimate relationships, communication patterns, and interactions among family members and between family and environment, represent the battleground of each crisis irrespective of its roots. Here, too, the usual steps of the nursing process will be advocated; however, the nurse's success in joining the system, assessing the presence of destructive patterns, and interpreting their influence on the health of the individual and interactional subsystems is critical. In families who lack the resources to consolidate and resolve their crisis, nursing means supporting the members in breaking cycles of self-reinforcing destructive behavior patterns.

7

Crises With
Developmental Transitions

The reader can prepare for this chapter by referring to Chapter 4, "Life Span Considerations." Of particular relevance in situations of developmental crises is the discussion of system maintenance and its flexibility to change family strategies as the needs of the members change over time. Family changes of structure and process in response to the members' development and maturation are extensive. They involve changes in family composition as members are added or leave, as well as changes in age composition that affect roles, decision making, communication, or affectional patterns (Roth, 1989a). Clinicians and researchers agree about the need for change in the family organization as developmental needs of the members unfold, but the research literature is devoid of identifying the nature of such processes (Mederer & Hill, 1983). Some authors, such as Rapoport (1963), who describe the "normal crisis" of parenthood, suggest that each developmental transition presents a crisis. This is countered by others who present evidence that transitions to parenthood (Hobbs, 1968), adolescence (Steinberg, 1990), or retirement (Atchley, 1982) occur in the majority of cases as relatively painless processes. Miller and Myers-Walls (1983) conclude that the need for change cannot be considered a crisis unless the family is substantially bothered by its demands.

It follows that for a crisis to develop from within, the family's life process must be marred with some preexisting incongruence. Such incongruence may arise from discrepancies in perceptions between adults in the family or between parent and child (Olson et al., 1984). Disillusions based on unrealistic expectations about the partnership, parenting, or family life (Kidwell, Fischer, Dunham, & Baranowski, 1983) also result in incongruence, the core of which seems to be a clash of values or ideologies played out in relationships. Incongruence or family conflict is felt as uncertainty, anxiety, and a sense of loss (Olson et al., 1984) and touches all members, but each in a different way (Joselevich, 1988). Issues of conflict, such as independence or domination, affiliation with family members and outside systems, and safety needs or role expectations (Chandler, 1982), are seldom anticipated or discussed before partners unite and have children. When the children pose increasing demands on the family, such issues come into focus on the individual and interpersonal levels as family members fiercely defend themselves against threats to their coherence. This is clarified in the following four brief situations, which outline examples of the family process relative to major developmental stages heading toward and culminating in a crisis.

Example 1: A New Baby

Carl and Kristen married 11 years ago. Both teach and conduct research at a major university—Carl in physics, Kristen in sociology. Their families of origin and all of their relatives live in other states. Carl has minimal contact with his parents and siblings. He has not visited since the death of his uncle 6 years ago. Kristen's parents call monthly, and a visit takes place about every other year. Carl has earned himself a name nationally, has written a book, and is invited frequently to scientific meetings. A year ago, Kristen, at the age of 36, frustrated about a rejection of a research proposal by a funding agency and afraid of getting too old, decided to have a child. She did not plan on giving up her career and explored child care possibilities that would permit her to work just as before. But events took an unexpected turn. Kristen suffered from preeclampsia, had a Caesarean section, and delivered a premature infant girl of less than five pounds. Kristen reacted with a major bout of postpartum depression. Her mother flew in to assist, but Kristen's crying spells, outbreaks of anger, and accusations were more than she could handle. She helped Carl to arrange for psychiatric care. Because Kristen repeatedly threatened to kill the baby, her mother waited until the infant was released from the hospital and subsequently took the baby to her home state to care for her until the situation improved. With the help of medications and psychotherapy, Kristen calmed down but kept being haunted by anger and resentment. She was fiercely jealous of Carl's career and considered herself a bitter failure. It seemed that she had lost control over her professional and private life and was consumed by guilt about the baby. Her relationship with Carl was ambivalent, because she was torn between total dependence and desire to control him. Carl was in an equally desperate situation. He was plagued by guilt and helplessness, because he had felt his affection for Kristen vanish. About 2 years ago, he fell in love with another woman, whom he contacted frequently under the pretext of work. At the time Kristen announced her wish to become pregnant, he felt new hope for the marriage and tried to end the relationship but did not succeed.

The nurse's assessment revealed that Kristen's life had been directed toward the target of control: an organized routine, career goals, and hard work. Her misguided spirituality entailed the seeking of professional rewards devoid of a broader personal or religious meaning. She defined her coherence within the academic environment but had no sense of connectedness with other systems. Kristen's individuation was deficient. Although she acquired professional knowledge and skills, she was missing out on life and had difficulties connecting with people. She felt isolated and unable to share or even recognize her human needs. She had married Carl to have a partner with whom she could share her interests. He was similarly oriented and seemed to understand her, but neither had ever discussed anything other than work issues and politics. Their sexual relationship was not satisfactory, and both resented the lack of passion and awkward sexual performance. Kristen's relationship with her mother was similarly cool and formal.

Assessment of the Family

The family consists of two people living parallel lives, sharing nothing more than their inability to relate and a competitive struggle for power. Family coherence is at an all-time low. The existing emotional bonds are maintained by Kristen's dependency needs and Carl's guilt. Although Carl found some closeness with another woman who is devoted to him, Kristen desired a child for a similar reason to compensate for the void in her marriage. Feeling the baby stir in her body triggered intense anxiety and ambivalence, however. On the one hand, the baby seemed like a parasite, sucking energy out of her system and demanding commitment from her, possibly causing the ruin of her career; on the other hand, she needed a person of her own flesh and blood who would truly understand her.

Family system maintenance is oriented toward getting tasks done efficiently. The division of tasks is no problem; much is done with outside help: cleaning, laundry, yard work, and dining out. After the baby's delivery, Kristen was unable to perform any tasks and Carl took over all responsibilities.

Kristen's and Carl's individuation are not tied to the family process, and their external involvement has become increasingly impaired due to the rigid family process. Family values are fixed to the point where any strive toward a new outlook has the potential to create severe repercussions. Carl, recognizing the extreme vulnerability of the system, carefully keeps his dark secret to himself.

Figure 7.1 pictures the family diagram already compromised before the baby's birth (a), and in crisis after the birth (b). The new baby demands a family reorientation, adjustment of roles, reassignment of responsibilities, and, most important, a shift from values related to intellect and power to values of connectedness and giving. The new baby needs to become the common focus and requires family coherence or emotional togetherness. Kristen fell apart under the demands to change her values that seemed indispensable to preserving her personal coherence. The grandmother took the baby out of a sense of obligation. She is likely to experience resentment and anger about the interference in her own life unless the baby presents an opportunity for her to meet some of her emotional needs.

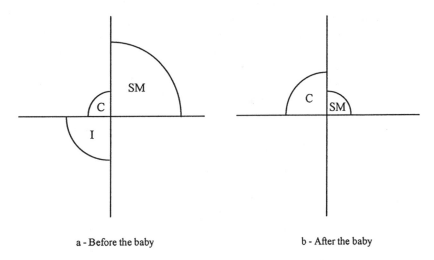

a - Before the baby   b - After the baby

Figure 7.1. Systemic Process of Carl and Kristen's Family

Example 2: Adolescence to Adulthood

Sandy, now divorced, was married for 20 years. As a wife and a mother, she fits the traditional family ideal. She worked as a schoolteacher to finance her ex-husband Eric's education. Without her, Eric would never have undertaken graduate and doctoral studies in political science. Sandy set goals for him, pushed him, removed the obstacles, and found the right professional connections for him. He pursued the career she had planned for him and succeeded to become a department head at a junior college. The financial situation made it necessary for the family to live in Eric's parents' house. Eric's mother seemed to compete with Sandy for the attention of Eric, who felt obliged to spend time with her every evening. Sandy felt enslaved by her mother-in-law, because she had to do work for her without getting recognition and was unhappy about Eric's lack of support for her.

After Eric completed his education, they had two children and lived in an apartment of their own. Sandy gave up her career and dedicated herself fully to ensure the children's healthy development. She played with them, stimulated their thinking and creativity, took them to museums and parks, did crafts with them, had them learn a musical instrument, invited the right kind of friends as playmates, sewed their clothes, cooked healthy meals, and stood behind them whenever they encountered difficulties with other children. Eric did little with the children. In fact, he felt useless most of the time in view of Sandy's efficiency. Sandy was remarkable in other ways as well. Sandy was active in community organizations, schools, and the church. She counseled new immigrants and helped them adjust, dealt with social service agencies, and codirected a neighborhood organization. Everybody knew Sandy and asked her for help.

Despite her dedication to her family, there were problems. Her eldest son, Peter, was an extremely sensitive child. He was small in stature, looked awkward, and wore glasses at an early age. Therefore, he became a target for hostilities and teasing by classmates. Sandy went to school with him daily. She volunteered in the classroom, but each day she could not be with him, Peter suffered abdominal pains. Because the teacher did not seem to understand his problem, Sandy sent Peter to a private school, where he seemed to blend in quite well. To help him adjust, Sandy had long talks with him every evening about his concerns. The school was a financial strain on the family, however, and Sandy had to help make ends meet by being a substitute teacher.

Joel, the younger of the two sons, was easygoing and never caused problems. Because he was well organized, intelligent, and orderly, he often helped Sandy with tasks in the house. Meanwhile, Eric's career was unfolding, but he still needed everybody's support. Eric brought his work home and while he was working, Sandy made sure the children were quiet. Disturbances caused angry outbreaks that frightened the children. Eric respected neither Sandy's nor the children's needs. He seldom participated in family activities. Sandy, always supportive and cheerful, suppressed her disillusion about the marital relationship. Although she responded to Eric's sexual approaches, she was repulsed by the physical contact and suffered periodic migraine headaches or bouts of nausea and vomiting. Sexual intercourse became torture and occurred less and less frequently. Sandy's discovery of Eric's affair came as a bolt from the blue. Sandy felt devastated and unable to forgive him. She divorced Eric and declared her independence but remained emotionally torn between hatred and dependence.

As the boys became older, family subsystems shifted. Eric's mother became Sandy's new target for caring. The two reconciled and reinforced each other in blaming Eric for irresponsibility. Joel also supported his mother. After the divorce, he refused any contact with his father but maintained a warm relationship with his grandmother, whom he brought little presents. Peter's life since age 18 had been in turmoil. An age-appropriate, dependence-independence conflict was greatly magnified by the happenings. Targeting Sandy, Peter broke with her strongest values: religion, sexual morals, self-control, and frugality. He refused any involvement with the church, avoided the celebration of religious holidays, sided with his father, and explored his sexuality. He spent more money than his low-paying office job could provide, drank, gambled, and moved away from the family. Sandy, deeply hurt and angry, was plagued by ambivalence. She felt compelled to withdraw her support but kept giving him money out of fear of losing him. Peter married at age 20. When his wife filed for divorce 1 year later, Peter committed suicide.

The nurse assesses a family in covert crisis. Sandy does not express grief and keeps her composure in her daily routine. In fact, she acts as if this burden had been cast on her to test her strength. She suppresses guilt feelings and openly blames Eric for Peter's death, because she has done everything humanly possible to assist Peter. There is bitterness mixed in with a repressed satisfaction that her secret wish for retaliation for Peter's splitting off and rejecting her was granted. People admire her for her strength. Nevertheless, she suffers from severe back pains, headaches, nightmares, nighttime anxiety attacks, and exhaustion and has difficulties concentrating.

Eric experiences feelings of isolation and loneliness he cannot admit to himself. He has severe problems with coworkers and, as a result, was demoted. Joel, age 17, remains aloof and closed-up, putting his entire energy into succeeding in school and supporting his mother. After a bitter disappointment with a girl, he keeps to himself and spends his free time alone in his room watching TV. Sometimes, Sandy hears him having a conversation with his teddy bear. In this family, caring is a mechanism of control and has served to maintain the system. This family is starved for true relatedness or spirituality. Caring serves as pseudospirituality that is in fact a way to control others. The system is maintained by caring, and Sandy is the expert. Deep down she is terrified that, if the truth was admitted, there would be no family. At the surface, family coherence seems strong. It is the image of Sandy as the ideal and powerful mother, however, that each family member has resisted in his own way. Eric found another target to which to connect, and Peter resisted by ascribing to opposite extremes, the spiritual targets of alcohol, sex, and money—all of which failed to bring the relief he desired. Even Joel resists Sandy's control. He has learned to mirror Sandy's caring pattern and competes for the same type of control by redefining her image as weak and in need of his competent care. Although both assume that the image of weakness held by the other is illusory, they mutually accept it to preserve the other's integrity, fulfill their dependency need, and stop the fear of losing each other. Joel is engaged in learning scientific facts in school that may lead to power and success. He has not learned to make healthy contacts with girls, and his friendships are superficial. Nevertheless, he sees no need for change because his true commitment is to his mother.

Assessment of the Family

The family dynamics are condensed in the diagram pictured in Figure 7.2. The diagram represents the family during the time Eric lived there and remains the same, even though the structure of the family has changed drastically with Eric's exit and Peter's death. Because neither Joel nor Sandy is able to question his or her mutual values, bitter anger remains without a chance of reconciliation of the two camps. After the crisis, Sandy sees family health in the changed structure of the two-person family, the harmonious relationship with Joel, and the extensive involvement of both in the world around them. Eric's continued emotional presence, however, interferes with family coherence. Sandy feels that Eric has inflicted wounds she is trying to heal. Forgiving and understanding Eric are not possible, especially because anger and resentment are a binding force for Sandy and Joel. Sandy feels herself drawn to Eric, even though she despises his very being. Sandy knows that this represents one area in her life in which she has little control and recognizes that her feelings of anxiety and chronic pain are associated with this incongruence. She exercises control in managing her symptoms through dismissing their importance, increasing her tolerance of pain, and influencing doc-

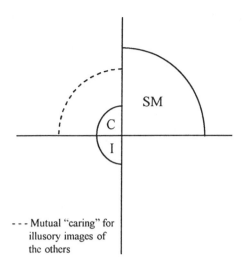

Figure 7.2. Systemic Process of Sandy's Family

tors in medical decisions. Concurrently, she diverts her attention to the pain through long conversations with friends, by reading books, and feeling other people's pain.

Example 3: Assuming Societal Roles

Elizabeth, age 45, lives in a crowded apartment in a poor city neighborhood. Since her divorce from her alcoholic husband, she has completed nursing school and raised three children—two daughters and a son—to adulthood. She was looking forward to reaping the rewards of her labor, but today she is exhausted and depressed. Her expectations have not materialized. The older daughter, Cynthia, divorced from her alcoholic husband, has moved back in with Elizabeth, bringing three children with her. Cynthia receives welfare payments. Elizabeth's son has been arrested for breaking and entering and is serving 2 years in jail; her youngest daughter, Minnie, age 14, is pregnant. Elizabeth also cares for her widowed mother who lives on the same block. Her mother is blind due to diabetes and needs help with shopping, cooking, and cleaning as well as transportation to doctor's appointments and church activities. To earn her living, Elizabeth cleans offices at night. During the day, she needs to sleep but is disturbed by the noise of the children and the TV. Elizabeth is upset about this and the lack of support from the daughters.

Elizabeth does not have the energy to fight with Minnie about going to school. In addition, she is not entirely convinced that she should force Minnie to go to school. She understands that Minnie does not want to be seen pregnant by her friends. The school social worker, however, threatens to take Minnie to a juvenile home if Elizabeth cannot control her. Cynthia is supposedly looking for work and is gone most days. Minnie uses this as an excuse for having to stay home to baby-sit. Neither Cynthia nor Minnie helps with household tasks. In fact, they don't even pick up the children's toys and often leave dirty diapers on the living room floor. Elizabeth has been raised in an orderly house and cannot understand their carelessness. There is much arguing in the house, and Elizabeth has threatened to throw them both out. Another crisis has ensued with Elizabeth's diagnosis of uterine cancer with advanced metastasis. Elizabeth finds some comfort among the women at church who advise her to pray and trust God.

Assessment of the Family

Figure 7.3 shows that the family is deficient in system maintenance. There is strong coherence, however, based on cultural values of belonging and the obligation to care for each other. This coherence is threatened by opposing ideals at the individual level, such as a value of status, self-reliance, and independence. These values promote dissatisfaction and the urge to break out of the family system in which members feel held captive. The daughters refuse to see Elizabeth as a role model in her state of being overworked, exhausted, and irritable. They attempt other ways of controlling their environment to gain recognition but fail. The diagram shows a deficiency in individuation that seems related to the family process as well as the lack of opportunities in the environment. Miserably frustrated, the daughters meet their dependency needs in unfulfilling sexual relationships, and the son has entered into a subculture that promises him peer recognition and status through wealth. With each failure, the members are pulled back into the family system, and this pattern of failure to reach environmental congruence seems to maintain the family system as both a spiritual refuge and a prison for its members.

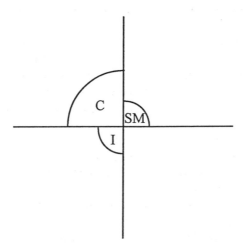

Figure 7.3. Systemic Process of Elizabeth's Family

This new crisis has two possible outcomes: complete resignation and despair of the young members, or a new family structure in which the young members assume the necessary leadership to maintain the system and replace Elizabeth. For this to happen, the daughters need to respect Elizabeth's contribution to the family, accept her as a role model, change their values, and ascribe to family commitment. At the moment, the family as well as each individual has lost control. Outside organizations, the penal system, the school social worker, the welfare system, and the medical system are involved and assume control for the family in the attempt to render the family congruent with their expectations.

Example 4: Retirement

Frank and Dorothy, in their 70s, live in a rural home. Frank worked as a postmaster until age 65, and Dorothy was a homemaker and raised five children, who are all married and scattered. Frank, an excellent craftsman, had been looking forward to his retirement to have time to do home repairs and build furniture. Dorothy had failed to adjust after her children left home. Too young to join a senior citizens organization, she felt there was nothing to do in the small community. She loved to cook and bake but had few takers. She felt bitter about the children not visiting as often as they should. Furthermore, the closest neighbors lived two miles away and it seemed that they were all too busy for social visits. After some time Dorothy felt old, useless, and without energy or joy. When her children visited or called, Dorothy lamented about her loneliness and reprimanded them. Her behavior resulted in even fewer visits and phone calls. Dorothy sat and watched TV most of the day. Frank's retirement did not bring much relief. At first, they went shopping together and visited some places. Then, during the long winter, Frank was cranky and scolded Dorothy for little things, such as being late with dinner or sleeping too long. He was particularly upset when she asked him for favors. The last thing he wanted to be was her "maid." Frank never talked about his own resentments. He felt useless and lonely, and his old friends at work did not seem to care about him any more. By the end of winter, he became seriously depressed. After Dorothy observed him in his carpentry shop taking out a shotgun he had not used in years and cleaning it carefully, she called the doctor. Frank was put on an antidepressant; however, he still moped listlessly around the house. Dorothy, on the other hand, responded by being helpful. Miraculously, her depression disappeared when she felt the need to help Frank. After a long talk with his doctor, Frank volunteered for a service agency, delivering meals to seniors at home. Although Frank's condition improved due to a new purpose in his life, Dorothy regressed to a state of deep depression. She was unable to do housework, take care of her physical needs, and at times she was even incontinent and unable to communicate.

Assessment of the Family

When Dorothy was hospitalized, the nurse assessed the family and arrived at the diagram pictured in Figure 7.4. She noticed Frank's and Dorothy's mutual dependency and their inability to find a common meaning or purpose. That purpose may have been the children some time ago, for Dorothy to raise them and for Frank to provide the necessary resources and enforce family rules. Emotionally, Dorothy was unable to let the children go and she failed to experience growth in her changed relationship with Frank. Because their common purpose was lost when the children

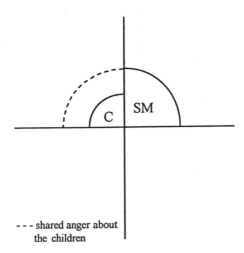

Figure 7.4. Systemic Process of Dorothy and Frank's Family

left, Dorothy's anger about the children's lack of gratefulness has served as a substitute for lack of anything better to hold her relationship with Frank together. Dorothy emphasized stability, coherence of the family, and system maintenance. She derived individuation only through the process of caring for others. Frank's regression to the level of a child returned Dorothy temporarily back to the mother role and consequently lifted her depression as system maintenance was restored. She was all the more devastated when Frank found a new purpose and usefulness. Without a source for individuation and a function in their relationship, Dorothy reverted back to the role of a child.

Assessment of Health

All four situations have certain characteristics in common. All families have ceased to grow. Each individual attempts to control his or her own situation, but the resulting life process is incompatible with the needs of the family system and the developmental needs of the other members. Experiencing serious incongruence and lack of coherence, family members are unable to assume new roles in the family and adjust to changed relationships. In such family crises there are no winners. Instead, all members turn out to be victims wounded by the process they are unable to control. They yearn for spirituality, but their inability to give of themselves within relationships makes them helplessly weak and dependent.

Developmental needs differ in each situation. In the first example, the needs of the new baby overwhelmed Kristen and Carl. The two were in a personal struggle for power and recognition in the professional world but were unable to meet their own developmental needs for mutual affection and intimacy. Sandy and Eric in the second situation similarly were unable to have a sharing, intimate relationship. Eric accepted Sandy's help to establish himself in academia, and Sandy gained respect and admiration by self-sacrifice and control that rendered others helpless. The adolescent boys were caught in the struggle and their development was stifled. Peter's desperate search for an identity, independence from his mother, and connectedness ended in death, and Joel fell into Sandy's pattern of efficiency with equal blindness. The third example showed a middle-aged woman in need of redirecting her goals and who was devastated by her children's inability to establish independent lives in their harsh environment. Finally, Frank and Dorothy, involved in the process of aging and unable to find a mutual purpose beyond work productivity and parenthood, were caught in a pattern of rigidly adhering to roles that were no longer functional.

All families illustrate the interplay of multiple developmental needs, but the situation is such that all members' growth and individuation are thwarted. Some members are particularly vulnerable, depending on the extent of their incongruence with the family and their environment. The family process, unless turned around promptly, has embarked on a path to self-destruction. A nurse offering guidance may make a critical difference in the outcome.

Determination of Need for Change

In Elizabeth's family (Example 3), the existing healthy coherence may elicit the members to move closer and find each other after being jolted by Elizabeth's impending death. The nurse has an opportunity to support the development of the two daughters as they perceive a sudden sense of being needed for the support of the family system. The threat of losing the family may be strong enough to compete with their ideals of individual freedom and wealth. The nurse will need to help them create an environment in which to gain courage and self-confidence in handling their own lives and supporting the family.

In the fourth example, Frank had made a healthy attempt to move toward a useful goal. One would hope that, through treatment for her depression, Dorothy will see the need for change. She may be ready to work with a nurse in redefining the family operation and possibly team up with Frank in pursuing her own growth. Coherence is even more of an essence for Carl and Kristen in the first example. They cannot build the needed foundation for a larger family unless they find each other. If that is not possible, a divorce will demand a new family structure within which the roles of both Carl and Kristen, the baby, and possibly the grandmother's family will have to be clearly defined. A new structure is no guarantee for success, however. Pivotal for family health within the old or a new family structure is Carl's and Kristen's ability to individuate and grow in an intimate relationship.

Nursing Care

In all of these examples, the framework of systemic organization can be used as a tool to help clients visualize their individual and family process. There is hope that Dorothy will find new coherence, hope, and goals through therapy and treatment and that she will sit together with Frank and discuss with him the use of the diagram and how the daily family routine could be enhanced to satisfy their needs and provide new experiences for growth. Likewise, Elizabeth and her daughters may be assisted in the development of a useful family operation in anticipation of Minnie's baby, Cynthia's plans for independent living, and Elizabeth's increasing needs for care. The family needs to gain control of its own operation, and the individuals need to set and pursue personal goals. Taking care of Elizabeth may give the family a purpose and break the cycle of the daughters' acting out due to frustration with their lives. Successful nursing interventions may embark the family on a path toward growth.

In Kristen's situation, traditional therapy would advise an individual focus for Kristen to gain insight and understanding of her limitations within her life process. Nevertheless, because Carl, the grandmother, and Kristen are in need of a family solution, an open systems approach that also addresses each individual's needs may be most appropriate. Kristen's strengths can be built by deciding jointly with Carl and the nurse what her role as mother should look like. As a system maintenance routine is discussed, the marital relationship will come into focus in terms of mutual commitment and ways to find each other emotionally and help each other in building a future. Carl's affair should not be revealed, at least for the time being, due to the devastating effect of such a disclosure. Instead, the nurse should encourage Carl to set family goals, such as sharing his daily events with Kristen, assisting with household tasks, or enjoying a hobby together in the hope that he will gain satisfaction and a brighter outlook for the future. Once the baby is introduced into the family, both parents need much encouragement to gain the necessary confidence in caring and responding to the baby. System maintenance will need to be redefined to include the new tasks, and the nurse will help them gain coherence through awareness and mutual enjoyment of the baby's responses.

The strong, interdependent relationship in Sandy and Joel's family presents the greatest resistance in moving toward system change. Eric is likely to remain outside the family, and Sandy will persevere in the patterns that gain so many rewards. Because no individuation took place as a result of the crisis, Sandy has found a new balance by redefining her family in terms of Joel and herself, thereby excluding Eric and the "ghost" of Peter. This resolution is painful to accept for the nurse who visualizes striving toward family health through a process of healing Sandy's wounds by letting go of anger, hatred, and self-pity. The nurse has hoped that Sandy could gain understanding of Eric's needs and Peter's struggle. Nevertheless, she can do nothing more than gently point out the ideal alternative of reconciliation. If Sandy and Joel reject it, the nurse may want to ensure continued support. The example shows one of many families and individuals who do not change through crisis but pursue their path with blind perseverance. The situation in such families is fragile, as it depends on rigid execution of prescribed roles. Any aberration (e.g., Joel finding a sexual partner or a change in Sandy's health status preventing her social involvement) could disrupt the family life process and trigger a new crisis. A nurse who has the opportunity to maintain long-term contact with resistant families would be wise to reevaluate the situation periodically, thereby looking out for increased tension and conflicts that may open an opportunity to join the system to facilitate needed change.

In summary, developmental crises arise through the family's inability to change its strategies to accommodate developmental needs and changes in the individuals. No different from healthy families in need of guidance, families who experience crises in their adjustment to developmental needs are guided through the nursing process. The initial pivotal task, however, is the assessment of the family's openness to system change so that the necessary development of each member can take place. The resolution of all crises requires working together in finding a redefinition of certain values that guide a new process and support the members' growth. Nurses can do nothing more than remind family members of emotional bonds that once existed and of their need for each other. They interpret signs of affection and encourage sharing and open communication. In families who are ready to change, nurses can reduce resistance and gain trust through the nursing process described in Part 1. Nurses, however, need to reconcile themselves with their own limitations in working with individuals and families who cannot drop their defenses and continue to blindly pursue an obviously destructive path. Nevertheless, a crisis should be recognized as a moment of openness and a time when some families will turn around and accept guidance, provided that such guidance corresponds with their understanding of the world, is free of judgment, and is nourished by empathy. The process, applicable to all crises, will be described further in the next part.

8

Crises With
Change in Family Structure

Three propositions that are of relevance here can be advanced by using the framework of systemic organization and the preceding discussions of family structure (Chapter 3) and crisis (Part 3, Introduction): (a) Family structure is a process (Minuchin, 1974) in that individuals, to the best of their ability, build those types of families that promise to safeguard them and allow them to best meet their developmental needs. (b) Being an attribute of process, structural changes are considered normative transitions and occur in each family as it moves through time; as members are born or otherwise added to the household, leave the family, or die; and as the family seeks congruence with its environment. In a rapidly changing environment, however, healthy families may be those whose trajectory of development encompasses structural changes beyond normative transitions (Staples, 1989). The existing diversity of environments requests a variety of family forms to interact with a multitude of environmental systems that are driven by sometimes incompatible ideologies. (c) If structural changes are attributes of family process, it follows that crises related to structural changes are also developmental crises for the individuals involved and are not distinguishable from the cases described in the preceding part. Because structure is fluent, nurses need to deemphasize it as a distinguishing variable and instead focus on the overall family life process. Of specific importance in evaluating family health and the need for nursing care are the target of growth and the process of system change.

Structural transitions can be categorized in various ways. Although some are desirable or pleasant, others, even normative transitions, are unpleasant and may present difficult challenges with a potential for crises. One such example is widowhood accompanied by severe feelings of loss and grief. Furthermore, transitions can be deliberate family strategies or occur as an act of fate. The latter category encompasses events such as deaths and unexpected births or additions to the household of family members in need of care or financial support. Deliberate changes in family structure include those driven by dissatisfied individuals searching for alternative family options to better meet their developmental needs. The category includes divorces, broken ties with the family of origin, formation of stepfamilies, homosexual unions, or communes as well as the association of isolates with alternative groups or subcultures to serve as family substitutes.

A third way to categorize structural changes is by their outcome, that is, system change and improved health or crisis. The desired outcome of a structural change is system change and growth. System change has the potential for growth and congruence as a new family structure evolves that better meets the members' need for spirituality and control. Examples of this group of families include an elderly mother moving into her daughter's house to be better cared for, a homosexual union with the commitment to share resources and affection, and remarriage with a stepfather's support in raising and disciplining children. A second group of families experiences crises with their structural change and is unable to resolve them. It has been observed, however, that more families have a highly unstable structure marked by the repeated formation and dissolution of partnerships, none of which meets the needs of the partners (Etzioni, 1974). These families may experience system change, but the changes fail to promote progress. A third group of families, still different, experiences often radical structural changes without concurrent growth or system change. The example of Sandy in the preceding chapter belongs to this category. The families survive a chain of crises and changes in structure, throughout which they maintain a remarkable resistance to changing their operation. The second and third groups of families are further explained here.

The Resolution of Structural Crises

As in all crises, structural crises inhibit individuation and system change. Therefore, they are also developmental crises in that the painful struggle to find congruence blocks the members' development and creates intense anxiety. The family dynamics of the developmental crises and the crisis resolution with system change cited in the three examples in the preceding chapter are applicable here as well. The first example of Kristen and Carl showed a couple who decided to add a baby to their family. The structural change compounded the already existing developmental difficulties in the family and culminated in a crisis. The resolution of their crisis is seen in a system change that supports the new structure and includes a mutual commitment to the family and parenting that promotes growth and individuation in the parents. If this fails, a new structure, a family split up by divorce, needs to be developed and tested with the aim of meeting the needs of the people involved.

In the third example, Elizabeth opted for a structural change in terms of accepting her older daughter and children back into the household. Although the option was based on feelings of family commitment and obligation to help, the new structure had serious repercussions because ideals clashed and members moved apart. Elizabeth's cancer diagnosis brought the crisis to a culmination and possibly triggered its resolution. Here, the new structure had the potential of being useful for the family's future. The resolution of the crisis is seen in coordinated system maintenance and mutual assistance in household chores and a common purpose—the care for Elizabeth.

Dorothy and Frank, in the last example, experienced a normative structural change when their children left the house. The resulting structure left a void; Dorothy was unable to adjust her role to find a new purpose, and Frank was caught between the obligation to attend to Dorothy and defining a new individuation process in the adjustment to his retirement. The resolution of their crisis lies in new individuation for both, combined with mutual sharing of their experiences.

Common to the resolution of all crises is the need to pull together, find new solutions, and promote learning and new growth for the members involved. The reader is referred to the preceding chapter for the discussion of nursing care with crises.

Structural Crisis
Based on Inability to Change

This type of developmental crisis refers to the group of families distinguished by their rigid adherence to family maintenance. For example, Sandy's family, described in Chapter 7, was unable to meet developmental needs and experienced an abrupt structural change when Eric sought a way out through divorce. The family's key players, Sandy and Joel, remained resistant to a change of operations that would have accommodated Peter's developmental needs and granted Eric continued family involvement beyond providing financial support. The result was a second crisis, Peter's suicide. The incredibly strong resistance to change could be observed as the family continued to operate in the same format even after Peter's death, rigidly adhering to the old values and beliefs.

Families like Sandy's are by no means rare. In fact, such families exist on all socioeconomic levels. A qualitative study conducted by Friedemann and Musgrove (1994) revealed that 8 out of 12 substance-abusing families in the inner cities pursued a family life pattern that made them highly vulnerable to crises. These people suffered a chain of serious traumatic events, including murder, accidents, serious illnesses, violence, abuse, arrests, and eviction. The reaction to each crisis, as well as the impetus for each consecutive crisis, was a rigid maintenance of the addictive pattern (for an in-depth discussion of addictions, see Chapter 9). In these families, structural changes were incidental as members died, went to prison, took to the streets, or returned home. Although roles were redistributed when members were gained or lost, the families experienced little change within their system of beliefs and the overall pattern of functioning. As mentioned in the preceding chapter, working with multiproblem families presents special challenges to nurses who see what a change toward a more healthful life process should be while the family blindly pursues the old path. The framework of systemic organization can help. By exploring the family life process, nurses learn to understand the resistance that is part of the basic family pattern and thereby reduce expectations for change and frustration. Nurses who truly understand the family system will, if the work situation allows, plant the seeds of new ideas and wait for the family's readiness to move. Unfortunately, strong personal needs cloud the family members' perception, and the moment of clear vision may not arrive until it is too late.

Again, structure or change of structure does not induce crises; instead, it is the family's failure to meet the individuals' developmental needs within the existing or changed family process. Structural change is a by-product of process and as such includes multiple changes during the family's life course. Although some of the changes represent the normative developmental progression of the family, others occur as a result of traumatic experiences, such as accidents or illnesses, and are often accompanied by a crisis. Finally, structural changes may be purposefully undertaken to relieve developmental crises occurring in the family, but, at times, the changes fail the system and lead to further crises.

The following example describes a family passing through a series of crises without finding a way to reverse the destructive trend. The example folds in what was discussed about crises following developmental transitions (see Chapter 7) and illustrates the attempt to resolve crises by changing the family structure. Nursing care involves the participation as an observer to gain a keen understanding of the family's needs and pitfalls and, alternatively, as an actor involved in effecting system change together with the family members. This case is presented in detail and serves as an example to show how family nursing interventions are derived. The same nursing process is also valid in cases pertaining to later chapters.

Barbara, age 29, is presently in a neuropsychiatric institute with the diagnosis of bipolar affective disorder. She has been told that she has a biochemical disorder that has a good chance of being controlled if she takes her medicine regularly. Barbara complains to her nurse about not being listened to and she states after a little probing that she does not see any reason for swallowing these pills, because her life is hardly worth living. She is a failure, she says, and her children would be better off without her. "Do you want to tell me about your life?" asks the nurse, who sits down next to her. So, Barbara tells her story.

"I hate my mom," she says. "All the time I had to do stuff for her and she never appreciated it. She used me, but she did not love me. She got divorced twice, and I had to be there and help her out, watch my two brothers, clean, cook—nothing was ever good enough. In school, I worked hard, and that wasn't good enough either. When mom divorced the first time, I thought it was OK. I didn't like my dad either because he didn't care about us, and he bummed around with other women. My stepdad was much nicer. For awhile, there was order in the house and there was food on the table at dinner time. He made my mom do it. He was strict with us, but he liked me, because I was the most responsible, and he could trust me. He let me play with my friends, even if my mom wanted me to work for her. Then things went wrong between the two of them. I guess my mom wanted more freedom, and I know she resented it that I liked my stepdad more than her. Every once in a while she sneaked out of the house, and several times she came home drunk. My stepdad beat her up for that, and I thought she deserved it. But then, when he beat her real hard, she packed our bags and took us away to live with grandma. We lived there for 2 years. It was crowded, and my mom and grandma always yelled at each other. I hated the new school, because the kids were mean. My mom took a job and finally had enough money saved to move to an apartment. Then I was supposed to do all the work again, and my mom was constantly after me. I hated it. Then I got to know a boy in high school. We were in love and a few months later, when I turned 16, I was pregnant and in trouble. My mom said she had no money to raise another kid. She wanted me to have an abortion and I said no. I cried a lot and went to see the social worker at school. She enrolled me in another school, where they have a baby care program, and filled out the forms for welfare.

"When the baby was born, I lived in a small apartment. Money was tight, but it was OK, because I got food at school and I could take the baby to the school's nursery. The baby's dad stayed with us quite a bit, even though he lived with his parents officially. I was actually pretty happy and proud that I could handle the baby, school, and everything. Then, a month later, I found the baby dead next to me in bed. It was the worst thing that ever happened to me. They said it was crib death, and it was not my fault. Mom said it must run in the family, because she had lost her first child the same way. I was very depressed. I had to move back in with mom. The baby's dad was so shook up, he stopped coming to see me after awhile, and I couldn't take it any more. I ran away and hitchhiked to this state. Then, I wandered around and lived in the street, looking for somebody nice I could trust. It wasn't easy, but then I met a coal miner named Tom in a bar, who was about 20 years older and told me I could come to stay in his place. I cleaned the place up for him and cooked meals for him. He found me a job as a waitress and said that it was my doing that he did not go to the bar any more. We got married and had three kids. We had a pretty good life, but then they closed the mine and Tom was out of work. He was busy with the union, demonstrated and all, but it didn't help. Then he went back to the bar and when he came home he was mean with the kids. One day he went after me with a log and hit me over the shoulder, causing a gash that needed suturing. I took the kids, ran to the shelter, and never returned. Then I swore I would never marry again. I stayed single, trying to raise the kids. Because I don't want to be on welfare, I have worked hard to make ends meet. The few men I got to know over 5 years all let me down. They wanted to use me and took advantage of the few things we had until I met Jerry. He had two kids of his own and was kind to them. His wife left him and moved in with a guy who did crack. He told me how awful he felt about it, and we sat together sharing our misery. When we decided to get married, we really wanted to make it work.

"It was difficult with the kids, but we held together. Jerry's little girl is very disturbed. She wets the bed, has nightmares, and doesn't pay attention in school. His older boy is hard to handle, too. He doesn't listen to me. If I punish him, he hates me and if I let him get away with things, my own kids get mad at me. It became such a drag that I did not feel like getting up any more. I was doing nothing and Jerry got upset with me, yelling at me and telling me that I was a bad mother. He was right—I was a bad mother and I couldn't stand the kids, the family, or anything. I cried a lot, until I thought to myself that I had a right to live a good life like everybody else. When I realized that, I felt a lot of energy and happiness. I went to town, made friends, bought myself nice clothes, and other stuff I don't remember. A voice kept talking to me, telling me that I was great, that I had to teach people about life and write my memoirs. For the first time, people noticed me, and I was very important. My name was even mentioned on TV. But Jerry couldn't stand it. He said it wasn't me and I made no sense. He was mad about all the money I spent and told me I had to care for the kids, but I had greater things on my mind. When I ran away, he sent the police after me to get me back and now I am here."

The nurse asked Barbara additional questions about her life process and her family to understand her needs and her struggle to meet them. Barbara was in a state of great confusion. The manic episode she had lived through had been an intense experience, the greatest high she had ever experienced in her life. She confessed to the nurse something she could never tell the doctor: She felt awakened by some great power that gave her incredible strength and ability and felt she was chosen to experience true life. How could the doctor deny her experience by calling it a chemical imbalance or even mental illness, which signified to her being crazy? She cried about being forced to swallow pills that would kill her off inside. She clung to the nurse in her desperation about losing her very existence. The nurse realized the immense significance of this experience in Barbara's vain struggle to find spirituality. Her coherence had been mutilated in a childhood devoid of affection, and she attempted to compensate with a pattern of being drawn to certain men who radiated warmth and acceptance. These men—her stepfather, the high school friend Tom, and Jerry—became her spiritual targets or reflections of the universal order. Barbara hoped to fill her void, to belong and become whole through a perfect congruence between her own self and these men. Unfortunately, the love objects were needy people themselves who had emotional wounds they tried to heal with Barbara's help, and they too needed more than what they could give.

The nurse wondered about the disasters that happened regularly each time these relationships deteriorated. Even though they looked like bolts from the blue, they were actually interwoven in the systemic family process. Upon further questioning, it turned out that even Tom's loss of his job developed disastrous dimensions only because the relationship had previously deteriorated and was tension ridden. The children's needs presented a burden, and Tom's and Barbara's differing opinions about discipline led to arguments with hurt feelings that could not be reconciled. Instead of pulling together to increase family cohesion in response to environmental and family demands, the couple drifted further apart to the point where the family system broke into pieces. These seemingly unrelated crises—her mother's divorce, the dead baby, Tom's unemployment, and her mental illness—served the purpose of ending the pain of failure and gave Barbara a chance to start anew and continue the succession of new family forms.

Assessment of the Individual

The nurse shared the systems diagram with Barbara and helped her to explore how her patterns may fit into the four process dimensions. Jointly, they discussed the patterns and the nurse arrived at the following insights.

System Maintenance. Up to the latest crisis, Barbara had seen her role as the organizer of the family. She had derived satisfaction from providing for the family's physical needs, housing, and safety. She contributed to the family income and mastered it alone for several years. She taught her children necessary lessons for life—how to be strong and fend for themselves. To the surprise of her partners who rescued her in a weak and helpless state, she developed tremendous efficiency, a strong will, and determination. Soon, Barbara's partners must have felt robbed of family responsibilities, useless, and only good enough to provide the necessary resources. Like her mother, Barbara fought against being held down and told what to do. It was through her authority and control of others that she maintained her self-image and reduced her anxiety. Thus, in her desperate attempt to break with the family's past, Barbara unknowingly adhered to long-learned patterns all the more. With each family collapse, Barbara pulled herself up and started over, feeling hurt but deriving satisfaction from her relentless drive and refusal to give up.

Coherence. Barbara, in her mode of surviving disasters, constituted the stability of the family, and family stability signified success and therefore served to uphold Barbara's personal coherence. However, the nature of family stability was mechanical rather than emotional. Like other women in her family, Barbara was driven by a mighty force derived from a self-image of being strong and able to cover up her innermost fears and desperate isolation. However, a counterforce, the craving for warmth and increasing anxiety, seemed to become the basic activator of each crisis, at the height of which Barbara let down her guard, revealed her impotence, lashed out in defense of her injured self, and followed her emotions. As a result, Barbara's coherence was shattered again and again as the family system went to pieces. Nevertheless, Barbara, the core of the family, regained her strength when the "offender" was ousted and a replacement was added to the system. The key to this family's curse has been Barbara's inability to grow and learn from the experiences.

Individuation. Although Barbara was successful in establishing a role in the world of work and in providing for the family, her childhood left her with a deficiency in forming human relationships. Like her mother, and possibly women of previous generations, Barbara tried to meet her strong need to be connected by attracting men who had an urge to rescue her. However, true individuation involves intimacy, or the giving up of oneself for the sake of the other. Thus, united in a system, a relationship can grow only through the exchange of energy and information and continuous readjustment to each other. Barbara, having learned to fight for survival and afraid of risking injury, could not let go of herself and trust another person. Instead, she used her controlling behavior to hold the relationship together. This invariably failed because her partners fought back by controlling her or withdrawing. Thus, each relationship evolved as a self-fulfilling prophesy.

System Change. Over the years, Barbara has reacted to her environment in a predictable fashion. Structural changes were cyclical as the family system expanded and returned to its core. Ironically, these changes served to protect Barbara's individual and family patterns from the need to change. This last time, however, something shifted in Barbara's life pattern. Barbara experienced what she believes was God's power. For the first time in her life, she let herself go and followed the voice, and for the first time in her life she experienced a true spiritual union, an intimacy with the universe. She made a system change in that she changed her self-perception from somebody weak but able to endure to a person inherently powerful and whole. Thus, she became a different person.

Assessment of Health

Figure 8.1 summarizes the changes in Barbara's life process. Before her illness (a), she sustained the stability of her life pattern with a controlling and rigid system maintenance. Coherence, inherently weak, was reinforced by her pride about survival. Because Barbara's pride was relative to the cyclical changes in her family pattern, personal coherence vacillated from a maximum after adding a new partner to a minimum just before separating from a partner. Individuation referred to work achievements, but growth through interpersonal relationships was lacking. The rigidity of the pattern blocked system change.

The manic episode (b) broke down system maintenance patterns and drove Barbara to experiment with new behaviors. The voices effected individuation through learning about the self and trusting her own abilities. Secondary to this experience, coherence was restored and Barbara's system changed. This new pattern is in danger of being destroyed, however, because Barbara is made to believe by the mental health system that she is sick.

The nurse realizes that her "disease" may in fact represent a first glimpse of health or a system change that could become permanent if it does not get killed off in its roots. New stability for Barbara can be procured if the family system grows and changes concurrently. Being the system's protagonist, Barbara needs to lead the way, allowing change in herself and letting others follow her tracks. Barbara could be empowered to arrive at a life process similar to the one pictured in Figure 8.1b (but with permanently drawn lines) if her symptoms are deemphasized or redefined as strengths.

The nurse sees individuation as the focal dimension and finds a need to start guidance at the interpersonal level. She hopes that growth within the marital relationship may allow the rest of the family to organize around it and give the children an opportunity to meet their developmental needs. In short, the challenging task consists of guiding Jerry and Barbara in laying the foundations for a successful stepfamily. To tackle this, the nurse needs more information about the family. She invites Jerry to a joint conference with Barbara. Together, they describe their present family as follows.

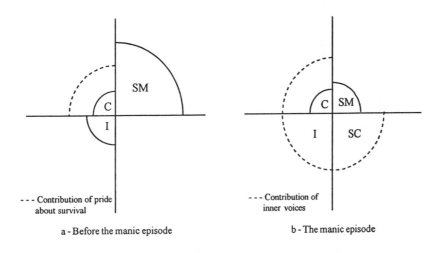

--- Contribution of pride
about survival

a - Before the manic episode

--- Contribution of
inner voices

b - The manic episode

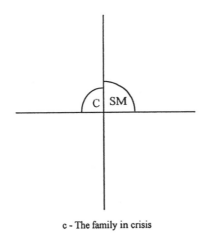

c - The family in crisis

Figure 8.1. Systemic Process of Barbara and Her Family

Assessment of the Family

System Maintenance. Jerry confirmed Barbara's difficulties of organizing the family and disciplining the children. He states that he had left it up to Barbara because she was good at it and he was not. He thought that raising the kids is the woman's job if he has to go out and earn the money. He is at a loss with his two kids. He goes in cycles of getting very upset with them, withdrawing privileges, and sending their friends away. Then he feels sorry and counteracts with too much generosity and sacrifice of his time and money. He understands that Barbara's children are jealous about this, especially because he has very little energy left to give them attention. They are doing better in school and don't need help with homework. Barbara states that her kids used to help her with chores, but now that they see that the others refuse, they do the same. What bothered Barbara most, however, was the hostility and anger in the family that got directed at her. No matter what she did, it was wrong. When she finally stopped doing anything, she got yelled at for that, too. System maintenance was in jeopardy due to these parenting problems and conflicts with disciplining the children.

Coherence. This dimension needed to be carefully evaluated because it is key to this family's survival. How much affection do Barbara and Jerry have for each other? Are they still committed to each other and the family? Jerry had been thinking of walking out but then hoped for help to come from somewhere. His last divorce was extremely painful and he wants no repetition. Barbara feels that she could make it if Jerry only had some understanding of her.

Individuation and System Change. Barbara's individuation is interpreted as a disease and has been discounted by the family and the health care system. Figure 8.1c shows the family in crisis, with system maintenance and coherence seriously reduced through system incongruence. The energy still available is spent on maintaining what is left of the system, leaving no room for growth of the family or its members.

Nursing Care

At this point, the nurse resists the traditional nursing approach, namely, to educate Barbara about manic depression and how Lithium would help her regain her chemical balance. Instead, she feels the need to make Barbara's last experience salient to the family. First, Jerry needs to understand Barbara's perspective of what had happened to her. The nurse states, "I have observed that Barbara has learned a lot about herself through this illness. For one thing, she has done things she has never trusted herself to be able to do: She has met new people, talked to them, and made them listen to her ideas. She has discovered some real leadership talent within herself. This is all new. Before, Barbara did not know that she could do these things. Barbara believes that God has given her this energy and revealed her talents, isn't this right? It seems to me that Barbara now is looking for opportunities to keep using these talents and become somebody she can be proud of." Barbara listens intently and nods. The nurse continues, "I understand that, for awhile, this experience was too much for her to handle and she had difficulties controlling her actions. But now, things look much better than they did in the past because Barbara recognizes her abilities. Jerry, you need to believe in her talents and your own, and then the two of you can run the family business and grow strong together. How does this sound to you?" Jerry seems reluctant to accept this view and persists that Barbara is very sick but admits that if she really believes she is strong enough to handle the family situation, the family would be better off. The nurse accepts the partial reconciliation of their differing perspectives and begins to focus on the vision of their future family process.

Targeting Individuation. Barbara and Jerry develop ideas about their roles as a couple and as parents and about ways to incorporate such changes into the family system. Then they talk about the needs of all the people in the family and how they could be met considering the resources and the available time. The nurse lets them develop their visions and observes that they get increasingly enthusiastic about it. She then summarizes the main points and suggests that they begin slowly with the changes and concentrate on one thing at a time.

Setting Goals, Learning Strategies. Together, the couple decides the most essential changes that are necessary: (a) They want time out as a couple. The decision is made to take Thursday evening off together and put Barbara's eldest girl in charge of the siblings. Rules and instructions for the children will be worked out. (b) They want each child to take responsibility for some duty of choice. This will be discussed, including who is to remind whom. Requests and gripes are to be addressed to Jerry in writing and will be dealt with weekly. The nurse is involved in constructing this plan but advises the couple against too-high expectations. Fully realizing the extent of emotional injury this family has suffered over time, she foresees significant resistance by the kids and suggests that to make this a success, they may want to see a family therapist for awhile. She asks them to think it over and invites the couple for another session with her in a week.

Evaluation

Barbara is discharged 2 days after the first interview. The couple reports some progress in that the kids seem willing to help out because Barbara had been sick. Jerry has assigned some tasks, but they may have been too much at once. Most did not get done. The couple did not go out together either, but Jerry states that they will make a serious effort next week and he thinks he will be able to trust Barbara's daughter to be in charge. Barbara has continued taking her medication "because the doctor said so." The nurse inquires how it makes her feel. Barbara says that it is like having no feelings. Everything is dull. Then she remarks that in some way it helps her not to feel hurt when the kids get mad at her. She can take things more calmly. Jerry thinks that maybe she needs this for the time being to keep her balance. The nurse wants to know what kind of feelings she can still experience. Does she feel love for Jerry or pride for handling a situation well? Barbara thinks for awhile and says, "A little—when I am away from the kids." The nurse concludes her contact with this family by bringing back the experience Barbara had with her illness and asks her to take some time for herself each day to think about herself, be accepting of herself, and give herself praise for doing well with the family. Jerry promises to help her think of these things. This is an important role for Jerry, and Barbara is delighted about getting such support.

Then Jerry says that he needs help too in handling his kids and wants Barbara's help. But she needs to keep a cool head for that. The nurse now gently introduces some pharmacological information about Lithium that is carefully attuned to Barbara's way of thinking. Ultimately, the couple decides that the medicine is needed right now. If the situation improves at home, Barbara will discuss the medical regime with her psychiatrist at that time. The nurse stresses the need for family therapy once more and equips the couple with the names and phone numbers of two agencies. When Barbara states she will call for an appointment, the nurse alerts them that she will call them in a week to see how they are doing and find out who the therapist is. She offers to talk with the therapist to help him or her understand the work they have done together and the goals they have set for their family. The couple agrees and signs a permit to release information.

This example depicts the complexity of family needs and necessary nursing skills. Traditionally, family nurses tend to act on what they know about difficulties encountered by new stepfamilies. Although the difficulties of creating stability within the partnership, family cohesion, family identity, and cooperation in the support and discipline of the children, as described in Chapter 3, are relevant here as well, these difficulties cannot be overcome without addressing Barbara's personal problems that have blocked system change within each previous family structure. The key problem recognized was Barbara's longing for spirituality, her inability to engage in individuation within the relationships with her partners, and her subsequent controlling behaviors triggered by her fears of losing the love objects she depended on. (See Chapter 9 for the discussion of such addictive dynamics.) Jerry's life process seemed driven by a need for a meek partner to be cared for to elevate his deficient self-concept. Confronted with Barbara's authoritarian behavior, he became fearful about losing his autonomy. Reacting to the anxiety, he attempted to control Barbara without success.

This process stands in stark contradiction to the qualities that Pill (1990) cited as key in successful stepfamilies: loose structure, space and personal freedom, and acceptance and recognition of each person's uniqueness. Barbara's rigid control and attempt to force the family to comply with her rules left little possibility for the examination of alternative attitudes, values, or opinions. Likewise, members who lacked autonomy felt misunderstood and rebelled overtly or with passive resistance and withdrew from family action. Barbara determined the family's identity and did not accommodate other members' visions. In this complex situation, the nurse recognized the enormous difficulties involved in helping Barbara and Jerry to change behaviors of a lifetime, and she assumed a family therapist would be best able to accomplish this challenge. Her care and liaison role between the family and the therapist was pivotal, however, in gaining their willingness to change and embark on a course toward congruence.

In addition to the guidance at the family level, the nurse fully acknowledges Barbara's incongruence that needs attention. The framework of systemic organization leads her to assume that a correction of the biological functions of the brain will be best supported by an optimal systemic life process of the family.

Finally, the example shows that the challenges of forming a new family must be evaluated at the family system level in terms of operations needed to succeed and achieve health. Likewise, at the individuals' level, ascribed family roles and the members' potential to support their own and the family's life process must be assessed. Consequently, the family system can grow only if the individuals within it are allowed to openly strive toward the goals they perceive as healthy.

Various family structures and the relative challenges of their concomitant processes were discussed in Chapter 3. Although change of family structure, and therefore change of process, is inherently difficult, nurses should refrain from automatically assuming that families are in crisis. It needs to be stressed again that nurses are most helpful if they view all families as systems in transformation. All these systems strive toward congruence within and with their environment by shifting roles, redefining family membership and responsibilities, and healing wounds within mutually supportive relationships. An assessment of the family process is indispensable to guide the nurse in the decision about the type of nursing care needed. Situations such as the one of Barbara's family require the nurse's support and guidance to enhance already existing or dormant family strengths while exploring the family behavioral repertoire and communication pattern and the need for additional strategies. Families are thus helped in their formidable task of restructuring system maintenance strategies in a way that will accommodate similarities and differences among family members and promote congruence with environmental systems. In Barbara's case, the nurse recognized the extent of the problems and advised continued psychiatric care and a referral to family therapy. But first, she initiated changes the family could make independently. At the same time, she warned them of difficulties. Her approach was one of empowerment through positive reinforcement of the efforts made. The family nurse's recognition of limitations of time and skills is of particular importance with complex cases such as the one in this chapter and the ones described in the remaining chapters of Part 3.

9

Crises With Addictions and Violence

The framework of systemic organization allowed the deduction that all family crises, irrespective of their origin, are developmental crises by their very definition. At this point, I propose a second hypothesis, namely, that developmental crises arise secondary to addictive processes within the families. The following will clarify this proposition.

According to the framework of systemic organization, congruence is a balance of systemic processes in which the target of spirituality is exceedingly important. Within this success-oriented culture, spirituality has become out of reach for many. To live up to society's expectations, people adhere to compulsive control and organization of their lives to the point of suppressing their need to belong and be appreciated. True belonging, inherent in the concept of spirituality, requires giving up self-interest and pride or backing off and accepting someone else's viewpoint. Such acts, however, are regarded as weakness and loss of stature. Consequently, human lives in this control-oriented society often become impoverished of spiritual values.

A multitude of social, psychological, or physical ailments in families and the community suggests that people suffer serious deficiencies in the spiritual realm. Triggered by spiritual needs, certain countermovements toward connectedness are evident. For example, an increasing number of individuals seek healing of emotional wounds within self-help groups available for all types of physical, social, and emotional problems. Furthermore, there is a surge toward religious fervor among people in need of a gratifying relationship with a superior being. The popularity of Eastern religions with practices that hold the promise of connectedness with the universe and the commercial success of courses that teach various techniques for the discovery of body and mind are other signs that people search for a renewal of their spirituality. Nevertheless, many individuals remain confused and caught by the mode of control or being controlled. They seek relief from anxiety, unhappiness, failure to relate to others, and mental and physical exhaustion through a misguided type of spirituality—an addiction.

Recently, a new understanding of addictions has emerged from social learning principles (Bandura, 1979) and from cognitive and experimental psychology (Marlatt & Gordon, 1985). This theoretical model, in contrast to the disease or morality models of addiction, views a great number of maladaptive behaviors, such as gambling, compulsive work, sex, overeating, pharmaceuticals, controlling jealousy, and addictive love (Peele & Brodsky, 1975), as learned habits that occur on a continuum of intensity. These habits are pursued for the purpose of immediate gratification, pleasure, or relief of tension. Although people recognize the often catastrophic effects of excessive habits, the habits per se are not necessarily considered maladaptive if practiced in moderation (Marlatt & Gordon, 1985). On the downside of this, habits generally considered good, such as working, loving, or taking pills for pain, can assume the harmful dimensions of an addiction if practiced in excess.

This model stands in concert with the framework of systemic organization, according to which individuals seek spiritual targets to lower anxiety or tension. Unable to pursue healthy relationships or other types of spirituality, individuals tend to seek relief by selecting targets that are harmful to their life process and replace individuation. As systems change through culture transformation, the environment is of major importance in influencing the choice of such targets. Culture determines which targets are acceptable, where behavioral limits are set, and what effects should be expected from a substance or interactional pattern (Marlatt & Rohsenow, 1980).

Findings of several research studies tend to support this phenomenon. For example, astonishing differences in drinking behaviors have been described in the book edited by Bennett and Ames (1985), suggesting that cultural paradigms that encourage heavy drinking may predict alcohol abuse better than individual needs or psychological characteristics of the alcoholics. Furthermore, a number of controlled studies examining the influence of culture on drug abuse behavior patterns showed that behavior differences were mainly attributed to social and environmental factors rather than race or ethnicity (Lillie-Blanton, Anthony, & Schuster, 1993). This suggests that the culture to which individuals are exposed daily promotes certain behavior patterns, including those that promise relief of tension.

Furthermore, attitudes shaped by the respective culture trigger individuals' expectations of desired effects (Marlatt & Rohsenow, 1980). Research that supports such dynamics includes a cross-cultural comparison showing that in some cultures drinking alcohol leads to passivity, whereas drinkers in other cultures become aggressive (Gelles & Loseke, 1993). The experiment of Lang (1981) also showed the power of culturally defined expectations. Subjects of that study, who were made to believe that they drank alcohol but had a nonalcoholic drink, acted as aggressive as those who actually did drink alcohol.

This discussion suggests that addictions are a complex pattern of compensation for lost control and of forming relationships of utmost dependency with culturally promoted targets in the attempt to find spirituality. Furthermore, addictions have been observed to inhibit the change of patterns, rendering families rigid and unable to grow and meet the members' developmental needs (Bepko & Krestan, 1985; Wegscheider, 1981). Thus, addiction encompasses the person's and the family's systemic process. The rigidity of the family process has been amply discussed by professionals involved in substance abuse therapy. As a result, most treatment approaches today include the family at least to some extent (Gacic, 1986; Vanicelli, 1987).

This broad understanding of addictions can easily be expanded to the highly publicized problem of domestic violence. Behavior patterns associated with drinking and violence are observed to have similar characteristics (Flanzer, 1993). In that sense, the framework of systemic organization leads to the proposition that both domestic violence and alcoholism, as well as all other types of behaviors ruled by preoccupation and obsession, can be conceptualized as addictions. Although the drink represents the spiritual target of the alcoholic, the perpetrator of violence strives to possess the love object, responding to an intense fear of losing it. Both the alcoholic and the violent abuser seek relief of systemic tension through their addictive behaviors. More will be explained with the help of illustrating cases.

Beforehand, it needs to be stated that addictions in families dictate all systemic processes and absorb all individuals, including the children. A natural tendency of family systems is to balance extremes with opposite extremes (Watzlawick, Beavin, & Jackson, 1967). This suggests that all individuals engaged in a relationship with an addicted family member will necessarily engage in complementary addictive behaviors themselves. These behaviors may involve the same addiction or another. Bepko and Krestan (1985) vividly describe this with case examples of alcoholic husbands who have overresponsible wives with a strong need to control others. Consequently, in a system ruled by addictive processes, the members are locked into roles that are difficult to change. The following three examples describe rigid addictive family roles and life processes that constitute desperate attempts to stabilize a system that would otherwise fall apart.

Example 1: Alcohol and Power

This is an urban family in the lower-socioeconomic bracket. Elsie, 33 years old, has two daughters, ages 14 and 15, from a first marriage and has been married to Darryl for a year. Her first marriage to an abusive alcoholic lasted 15 years and ended in divorce 2 years ago. Elsie had worked as a nurse's aide after dropping out of high school. Since the birth of her severely disabled elder daughter, Reina, Elsie has been the child's full-time caregiver supported by public assistance. Darryl is 36 years old and has a history of many short-term relationships without marital commitment. His work record reflects occasional low-paying jobs over brief periods. At the moment, he is enrolled in a government job-training program. Both Elsie and Darryl have histories of parental alcoholism. Whereas Elsie is firmly opposed to alcohol, Darryl frequently engages in binge drinking, denying that his drinking presents a problem.

Elsie's younger daughter, Terry, lives with her natural father, who has custody because she has previously refused to live with

Darryl. Terry, now extremely unhappy with her living situation and her alcoholic father, is pleading to come back to Elsie. Recently, she has attempted suicide twice. Reina, the elder daughter, is epileptic and severely cognitively impaired. She utters unintelligible sounds but is able to recognize people. She smiles and laughs with family members. Reina had been able to walk, but a recent surgery to correct her scoliosis left her paraplegic. She was discharged from the hospital 6 weeks ago and now has a large decubitus ulcer. Reina's increased care needs and Elsie's extreme anger at the medical system have subjected the family to tremendous tension. The nurse observes a crisis situation that threatens the fragile marital relationship.

Assessment of the Family

System Maintenance. Elsie is very well organized, even under high pressure. She is the decision maker in the family and performs most household tasks. She describes her strengths as being "able to hold onto money and get the bills paid." Elsie and Darryl's decision to get married was based on a mutual agreement. Darryl, who needed a place to live, was given housing and food for taking on the important function of protector, which provided Elsie with a feeling of safety. Darryl was successful in stopping the continued attempts of Elsie's ex-husband's intrusions to take her money and physically abuse her.

The demands of Reina's care and Terry's manipulative pleading to take her back into the family are more than Elsie can handle. Even more importantly, Elsie describes the family crisis as a loss of control over Darryl's drinking. The family is typical for its cycles of "wet" and "dry" patterns related to Darryl's drinking, as they are described in the literature (Liepman, Silva, & Nirenberg, 1989). The family process reveals an interpersonal struggle for control. Darryl's binge drinking and staying out all night triggers a chain of events. When Darryl returns, the dry period starts with Elsie's regaining her control. She yells at Darryl, withholds sex, or gives him the "silent treatment." Darryl, feeling guilty, apologizes and promises to prove himself by helping out in the house. Elsie assigns tasks to him and observes his performance carefully, criticizing and nagging whenever he fails to be perfect. Darryl, frustrated with Elsie's control, resists passively by "forgetting" tasks, thereby intensifying Elsie's nagging. Elsie, perceiving her loss of control, advances to more extreme measures. She contacts her ex-husband for comfort and to punish Darryl, whose jealousy, resentment, and anger are incited to the point where he enters his wet phase by storming out of the house to get thoroughly drunk.

Coherence. Elsie and Darryl are unhappy with their relationship because Darryl feels he's treated "like a child," and Elsie expresses unhappiness about the unfair division of labor. Nevertheless, Darryl and Elsie's marriage was never based on romantic love, and beneath all anger and resentment, there is a sense of gratitude and mutual respect. Furthermore, Darryl has warm feelings for Reina and a natural ability to understand her. Darryl amuses Reina, makes her laugh, and relates to her in a way nobody else can. Consequently, there is compatibility in the mutuality of emotional bonding with Reina but also within the before-mentioned agreement and their sexual relationship.

Individuation and System Change. This family is caught in a trap of uncontrollable behavior cycles typical of alcoholic systems (Steinglass, Bennett, Wolin, & Reiss, 1987). Energy is expended in an endless struggle for control, but the connectedness with environmental systems is seriously impaired and the system is unable to change. Neither Elsie nor Darryl has a significant role outside the family. Elsie's interactions with the health care system during Reina's hospitalization had deteriorated into altercations because the professionals accused Elsie of inadequate care and blamed her for the ulcer. They also refused to listen to her advice about Reina's nutritional preferences or comfort measures. Elsie's attempt to distance herself from her ex-husband is equally unsuccessful because she needs him as an actor to play out the control pattern.

Assessment of Family Health

Elsie has learned that unless she fights for control, she will be a victim of abuse. Consequently, she sees that a good husband should perform his role in such a way that she feels safe, gets help with her work, and is relieved of tension. Darryl craves affection, but all his life he has used alcohol to help him overcome the feeling of loneliness and lack of purpose that has haunted him since childhood. He has chosen his drink as his spiritual target, because it allows him a temporary illusion of coherence. Elsie and Darryl fall short in the process of spirituality. Because the family's connections to the environment are unsatisfactory, the entire responsibility for meeting the spiritual target is placed on the spousal relationship, which comprises extreme or addictive behaviors. Furthermore, the lack of success at achieving spirituality tilts the family process increasingly toward the control target. During Darryl's dry phase, there is a mutual dependency on each other, marked by testing or an expectation to deliver proof of commitment. Darryl is supposed to do household work to show gratitude, and Elsie is expected to love Darryl, even though he forgets his tasks. Transgressions trigger tremendous anxiety and anger that reinforce controlling maneuvers. During wet phases, Darryl, feeling devastated, switches his target of spirituality to alcohol, at which point Elsie finds herself in despair about having lost Darryl until he comes back and the cycle starts over.

Figure 9.1 depicts the dynamic shifts of the life process. System maintenance is strongest after a wet phase, when Elsie's control is effective and Darryl is willing to comply. Coherence then is equally optimal. System maintenance and coherence gradually decrease with Darryl's resistance to Elsie's control and reach their lowest point when Darryl leaves the house for the bar. Coherence increases when both realize their need for each other, and system maintenance jumps back to its optimum level when Darryl returns home. Individuation and system change are not possible because both are fully preoccupied with the patterns of mutual control.

Example 2: Jealousy, Love, and Violence

Susan has two children, a boy age 5 and a girl age 2. Susan was 16 when her son was born. At that time, she dropped out of school. The boy's father, a migrant worker, disappeared after he heard about the pregnancy. Susan lived in her parents' home, received public assistance, and did occasional work at a fast-food restaurant. Family life was marked by fights and violent accusations. A major issue was that her father demanded her money to buy crack cocaine and threatened to hurt her if she refused. Two years later, she found herself pregnant again. This time, the father of the unborn was a young man, Bill, who had secured a job as a

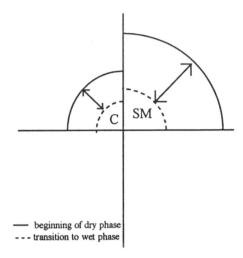

Figure 9.1. Systemic Process of Elsie and Darryl's Family

car mechanic, lived in a middle-class neighborhood, and was able to support a family. The two were married and enjoyed a happy first 6 months. After the delivery of the child, the relationship became increasingly problematic until Susan presented herself at a shelter for abused women after being beaten by her husband and threatened with a gun.

Assessment of the Family

System Maintenance. Susan saw her marriage as the solution to all of her problems. She desired structure and stability to serve as the foundation for raising her children. Susan has broken off all contact with her family. Contact with Bill's family is infrequent, except with a brother Bill trusts and visits occasionally. Bill's mother is widowed, with five of Bill's younger siblings still in the house. Bill's father died in a car accident when Bill was 14. At the time of their marriage, Bill got along well with Susan's little boy but never took responsibility for his care. Instead, he demanded Susan's time without considering the boy's needs. Susan has a good friend with a child of her own who often came to her rescue when Bill decided to go out and Susan had to be ready for him. Susan was allowed to drop off her son practically any time.

Her friend's house has been her boy's second home, even before Susan got married.

Bill's family role consists of work and financial matters, and Susan is responsible for household and children. Problems started with the birth of the new baby who was frequently colicky and irritable. Bill resented Susan rocking and cuddling the baby and demanded that she put the baby to bed and close the door to get Susan's undivided attention for himself. Then Bill started to discipline Susan's son for talking too loud and bothering them. Susan felt the need to protect the children from his rough treatment. She began leaving him out of her activities with the children and her girlfriend.

Coherence. When Susan distanced herself from Bill, not only by excluding him from an intimate relationship with the children but also by frequently refusing sexual contact, this caused a wave of jealousy. Bill forbade Susan's contact with her friend. After she escaped a few times against his advice, Bill began suspecting Susan of having a relationship with another man. His constant preoccupation with the thought of losing Susan to another man intensified his anxiety and anger. Bill resorted to bitter control. He brutally forced Susan to have sexual relations with him, thereby evoking repulsion and despair in Susan. Each sign of Susan's rebellion against Bill's control measures was punished with hurtful words and violent physical attacks.

Susan feels powerless and wonders what she has done to destroy the wonderful relationship they once had. Her feelings for Bill are ambivalent, torn between guilt about not responding to his needs and, at the same time, intense hatred. In moments of culminating desperation after being insulted and beaten, Susan breaks down into tears, sobbing uncontrollably. In those moments, Bill's dominance over her is broken, and Susan perceives an absurd sense of regained control as he bends down to her, seemingly destroyed by guilt. Bill declares his immense love for her and promises to never hurt her again if they could only start anew. Inebriated by a sudden feeling of oneness, they rise from their mutual hell and share with each other a brief euphoric moment of sexual togetherness. A few hours later, however, the illusion of true spirituality evaporates with the start of a new cycle of control.

Susan feels affection for her children; in fact, they give her the strength to continue her miserable existence. The young boy has become her major support and is always at her side. When she and Bill have altercations, the boy slips into his bedroom and Susan hears him crying faintly. Susan believes that he understands more about life and is more mature than most other children his age. Bill does not seem to notice him, which, Susan believes, is to the boy's advantage. On the other hand, Bill is keenly aware of the baby, his own daughter, who seems to remind him of his inadequacies as a father. He takes her crying personally, as if the baby is communicating her rejection to him. Once, Susan found Bill shaking the baby to make her be quiet. Susan ripped the baby out of his hands and has not left him alone with the children since.

Individuation. Bill goes to work every day, but his coworkers notice that he is preoccupied with jealousy. He calls Susan repeatedly and talks about his worries incessantly. He no longer goes out with his friends or spends time with his brother because he feels an urgent need to go home to check on Susan right after work. His process of individuation seems halted, because his thoughts are fixed by his obsession. Susan is a prisoner in her house. She is hesitant even to call her friend, because the calls show up on the telephone bill. Another reason for keeping away from people is their inability to understand her situation. They advise her to leave Bill but cannot see that she still loves him, because he is the only person she has ever known who has truly cared for her. He would not be jealous if he did not love her, and for those moments when he shows his true self, she wants to remain with him. In fact, she craves these moments of oneness, during which the heavens open and all anxiety disappears. If these moments have to be brought about through torture and pain, the pain may be worth it. Nevertheless, Susan has gone to the shelter for help, because she senses that Bill is out of control. She wants to find out how she could behave so that he trusts her more, and how she could prevent severe attacks. It is her challenge, her individuation, to learn how to understand and treat Bill. She figures it may have been the death of his father that made him insecure. Maybe someone can tell her what to do, because nothing seems to work.

Assessment of Family Health

Both Bill and Susan are deficient in personal coherence. They expected their relationship to provide them the sense of belonging (spirituality) they crave for. A healthy relationship requires mutual responding to each other's needs. Susan is able to give of herself. This may be a behavior learned from her abused mother. She gives her energy, time, and body to Bill out of a sense of obligation and harbors deep feelings of resentment about not receiving the understanding she deserves. Bill's attitude has been shaped by his family and the environment in which he grew up. He is convinced that Susan owes him the things he needs to be happy, because he got her out of her misery and keeps supporting her financially. Their personal needs are the foremost motivator in this relationship, and the struggle to meet them results in a battle for power and control that interferes with their pursuit of spirituality. Extreme control can be balanced only by extreme behaviors toward other targets. Their misguided spirituality is an addiction, a mutual craving to own their love object. As in alcoholic relationships, this couple lives through phases of control and abuse, comparable to the power struggle during the alcoholic's dry period, that is countered by moments of total submission to the addictive target, the love objects. The latter phases have a striking similarity with the uncontrolled drinking of the alcoholic's wet periods. As in alcoholism, the two patterns are cyclical. The key to health is individuation, which is hardly possible without a sound coherence. Susan's affection and concern for the children is a sign of health, because she has potential to grow within her role as a mother. However, there are indications that she may, like her own mother, use her children to meet her needs for support and affection, thereby inhibiting the children's developmental striving toward healthy growth and individuation. Bill is a good worker and generally gets along with his friends. He also gains strength through the relationship with his brother. Both of these sources of individuation harbor a potential for healing.

Figure 9.2 pictures the dynamic shifts of the life process. At the height of control and abuse, system maintenance is restricted to the care of the children, and coherence encompasses Susan's emotional bonding to the children. The relationship pattern of Susan and Bill is ruled by forces threatening to destroy family mainte-

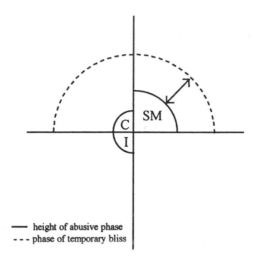

——— height of abusive phase
- - - phase of temporary bliss

Figure 9.2. Systemic Process of Susan and Bill's Family

nance and coherence. As the abusive patterns break down, a state of temporary bliss exists, which is marked by the broken lines in the diagram. This is followed by a shrinkage of both dimensions to the minimum marked by the solid line, as the abusive patterns take over again and grow in intensity.

Example 3: Success, Control, and Drugs

Charles, age 17, lives in an upper-middle-class neighborhood. His father is a general manager in a large automotive company, and his mother, aside from volunteering in several agencies for the poor, has been spending most of her energy raising the two boys in the family. Compared with his younger brother, Charles is small in stature, disinterested in sports, and much less popular among friends in school. Charles is the smarter of the two, however, especially in science. His parents have visions of him being a renowned chemist and have invested inordinate amounts of time and money in developing this potential. Charles has gone to numerous science and computer camps, has successfully competed in science fairs with his parents' strong support, and has been doing work in the science lab of his father's friend until recently.

   Problems with Charles started 6 months ago, when he began a relationship with a girl. Charles's parents never liked the girl and considered her a bad influence. Charles became very angry and rebellious with his parents, rejecting their advice and bluntly telling them to stay out of his life. Three months ago, Charles's father found some white powder in his room, which he took to his friend's lab. It turned out to be cocaine. That evening, Charles was confronted by his parents. It ended in a heated dispute with the father striking Charles, who stormed out of the house. The next day, Charles packed a few things, took $200 he found in his mother's dresser, and left without notice. The family initiated a nationwide police search that proved successful 6 weeks later. Charles, his girlfriend, and two other teens were found in another city and arrested for possession of cocaine. Charles's parents bailed him out and admitted him in a substance abuse treatment center for adolescents.

Assessment of Family Health

   System Maintenance. This family is extremely well organized and structured. Everyone is held to ascribed duties, and expectations of the family members' roles are clear. The house, meticulously clean inside and outside, is filled with expensive possessions. There is domestic help for heavy cleaning and yard work. Charles's mother cooks, bakes, washes the laundry, and keeps the house tidy in addition to doing volunteer duty. Her pastime activities include exercising daily, jogging, and gardening in the warm season. Charles's father often brings company-related people home to be entertained, and his wife organizes these events efficiently. Charles's younger brother is involved in football and swims in the summer. His mother takes him to practices and games and spends time with him supervising homework. The family takes regular trips to a nearby big city to see a musical or play and go shopping. They also have a yearly vacation that occasionally involves travel abroad.

   Coherence. Charles's mother comes from a close family. Her parents live nearby and are still independent and in good health. They visit often and are part of all birthday and holiday celebrations. Charles's mother has five siblings, each in a prestigious position or married to a wealthy husband. All but a sister live at great distances and visit their parents only once a year. The sister and her family are Charles's mother's closest allies. They live in the same suburb and their children are good friends. Charles's father grew up in a single-parent household after his parents' divorce when he was 5 years old. His mother recently died of cancer, and his sister is married to a Frenchman living overseas. She has not written since the mother's funeral. The nuclear family gives an outward appearance of harmony. The mother is very concerned about the family members' well-being to the point of being overbearing. Her relationship with her husband is cool and factual. She attempts to make up for the lack of warmth by being the children's confidante. She shares her own emotions with them openly, cries in front of them if she is disappointed with them, and expects them to be equally open with her. She also advises them about how they should behave around their father, thereby helping them to understand his problems. The father is perceived to be difficult by all. He values his work highly, is absent long hours, and is unavailable on many weekends. At home, he is impatient with the family if they do not live up to his expectations. He seems to regard his wife as a necessity to ease his hard life at work and to support him. He expresses his gratitude for that but does not seem to be concerned whether his wife is happy. He tells her about problems at work but has little inclination to listen to her "trivial" stories.

Charles's brother is his father's pride due to his athletic talents. They talk about sports together and their mutual aim is to get the boy on a good college football team. Charles, being the more sensitive of the two boys, is clearly his mother's favorite. Charles has worked hard in school to please his mother and earn her praise. His father, to the contrary, always criticizes him about something. After his mother refused to accept his girlfriend, Charles felt devastated. Being in love with this girl, he felt rejected by his family and, for the first time, hid his feelings from his mother. He lost his motivation in school and the urge to please his mother; he lost his sense of direction and his identity, which, he concluded, was his mother's and not his own. Out of this confusion arose the urge to find himself and be independent from all the things his parents forced him to be. That is when he started to associate with a group of friends who were dealing drugs and he convinced his girlfriend to help him with it.

Individuation and System Change. This family has been deficient in promoting a balanced growth of its members. All family members are required to fit in a prescribed mold. The father has been very successful in living up to the expectations of his company and society, because he sacrifices his family time and his free choice of actions. His behaviors take on the dimensions of a work addiction, because his spiritual targets have become the success and power he needs to maintain self-respect or coherence. Making these sacrifices, he feels entitled to support from the family, especially his wife. She has to pay for her luxuries by living her role, as he envisions it and the way the traditional family ideal prescribes it. Although she had the opportunity for individuation when the children were smaller, her experiences are not valued in the nuclear family now, especially because the children try to separate and find their own identity. Her parents and sister have played an important role over the years, listening to her concerns and helping her adjust to her husband's control without totally losing her sense of coherence. Nevertheless, she reacted to her impoverished lifestyle by clinging to Charles, the only sensitive family member. Parallel to her husband's work addiction, her relationship with Charles has assumed addictive proportions, in that she has not been able to adjust her interactional patterns to Charles's increasing developmental need for private space and differentiation. Charles's girlfriend constituted a severe threat to her, because she feared losing Charles. She therefore resorted to controlling him and, as a result, tragically lost him. Charles's brother, at least at the moment, experiences only minor problems because his interests are congruent with the mold into which he is supposed to fit. He has the father's support, but he, too, lacks the opportunity to acquire the skills of a loving relationship and healthy spirituality. Because his acceptance depends on performance, he becomes extremely vulnerable to the development of an addiction similar to his father's by embracing success as his own spiritual target.

Assessment of Family Health

Figure 9.3 summarizes the family process. Extensive system maintenance reflects the rigid patterns of control. Coherence is minimal, because two members, the father and the younger son,

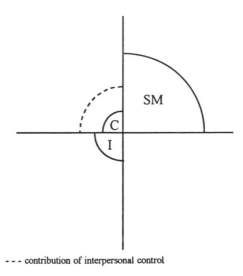

- - - contribution of interpersonal control

Figure 9.3. Systemic Process of Charles's Family

have little commitment to the family and focus their energies outward. The mother is left alone, because Charles is breaking out of the system. A large proportion of coherence is contributed by controlling patterns because individuals are obliged to live up to the family's reputation. Thus, this type of coherence constitutes a sense of belonging devoid of an emotional basis of commitment and love. Individuation is strictly related to work and educational activities. The members have difficulties in deriving satisfaction from human relationships. Nevertheless, the strengths of this family consist of its resources and education. Furthermore, the available extended family is supportive and models caring relationships. Charles's rebellion against his mother's stifling love would have been a sign of health if it had not been for the switch from one harmful spiritual target, his dependency on his mother, to a more detrimental one, cocaine. Nevertheless, his actions have led to a family crisis, which is needed for change, and Charles's treatment may constitute help for all as they realize their deficiencies.

The three examples show the pervasiveness of addictions in the family pattern. Although the examples span a range of socioeconomic status from poverty to wealth, they all bear witness to the broad conceptualization of addictions as behaviors executed in a desperate, obsessive attempt to gain congruence.

Cyclical Patterns of Addictions

Evidence cited in recent literature seems to support the cyclical pattern of addiction patterns, in that astonishing similarities between domestic violence and alcohol abuse cases have been observed by researchers in the field (Flanzer, 1993). Cyclical patterns have been explored extensively in alcoholism (Liepman et al., 1989) and are observed in two thirds of physical abuse cases (Walker, 1993). For example, Rosen and Stith (1993) describe a pattern of cyclic oscillations in power-submission and distance-closeness they call "seesaw coupling" (p. 428) that is similar to the example of Susan and Bill. The first two case examples illustrate such cycles. In both, they seem to emerge as homeostatic mechanisms or corrective actions employed by the addicted individuals and family system to balance extremes with their counterparts: extreme control with extreme submission, drinking with abstinence, distance with closeness, resentment with guilt, and hatred with love.

The development of addictive patterns is usually a prolonged process of reinforcing behaviors used to relieve tension (Steinglass et al., 1987). Cycles seem to develop at the point where the behaviors reach extreme levels. As they surpass accepted norms, they evoke negative reactions in family members, friends, and the community, thereby inducing guilt in the addicted individual and a temporary reversal of the behavior. If guilt is the key to the development of cycles, one would expect highly tolerated addictions, such as fanatic religious practices, hypochondriasis, or abuse of prescription drugs, to progress in a linear, increasingly intensive fashion. The third example bears witness to this hypothesis. A high cultural tolerance for work addiction in this society seems to explain why the patterns in Charles's family showed no cyclical fluctuation. Over the years, no one felt guilty about or reacted negatively to the father's excessive work engagement. In fact, Charles's father was not aware of his exhaustive work habits, and his wife dutifully tolerated the restrictions on personal freedom and growth until the emotional demands on Charles surpassed the threshold of tolerance.

Etiology of Addictions

The second feature that violence and substance abuse are believed to have in common is generational transmission. Little is known, however, about the nature of the process. Transmission research in alcoholism has focused mainly on biological variables. Although strong evidence shows that genetic factors influence the development of alcoholism, such factors contribute little to generational transmission (Steinglass et al., 1987). This leaves room for the alternative explanation, namely, the process of social learning (Bandura, 1979). This theory has been extremely popular in the early child abuse literature. Research in delinquency, aggressiveness, homicides, and family violence also presents considerable evidence that violence breeds violence (Widom, 1989). Recently, however, Kaufman and Zigler (1987), among others, noted many weaknesses of research methodology and claimed that the transmission hypothesis had been overstated, thereby unnecessarily raising the fears of members from abusive families and their spouses about their future.

The framework of systemic organization may be useful in providing guidance, because it promotes a balance between the transmission of family cultural patterns, including addictions, and their transformation through individuation. Consequently, according to this framework, individuals are not simply victims of the family life process but are empowered to change their own patterns and those of the family through system change. Although biological factors are an integral part of the person's systemic process, they interact intimately with the mind and the environment. Biological processes elicit perceptions and behaviors and are hardly distinguishable within the person's systemic process and struggle to overcome incongruence and tension. Consequently, an addiction, according to the framework of systemic organization, signifies a systemic process that lacks health rather than being a disease. In contrast, the medical conceptualization of addiction as a biological disease tends to negate the strengths and abilities of the individual and carries the potential to be counterproductive if it excuses the afflicted person from engaging in individuation.

The Life Process With Addiction

On the individual level, addicted persons are in need of establishing a sound coherence. Their deficiency in coherence may have existed since childhood and may be reinforced by the addiction. Addicted individuals respond to a strong need to belong but are unable to maintain mutually satisfying relationships. Instead, they adhere to targets that inadvertently control their lives. Realizing the loss of control over their lives, they compensate by assuming power in greatly diverse manners. Elsie and Bill openly control their love objects, whereas Darryl, Susan, and Charles respond with covert, sometimes subtle, countercontrol. Charles's father displaces his need for control onto all other family members, and Charles's mother counteracts her fear of isolation through the emotional control of Charles.

The defense of their coherence and a shift toward control for the purpose of maintaining the system are common to all, but the methods of doing so differ. Maintenance of a healthy coherence is a lifelong process and requires a basic self-acceptance, a sense of direction, and a meaning for life. Coherence and individuation are closely tied together within the process of spirituality. A healthy sense of self arises from nurturing relationships through individuation, and the use of a person's potential and interchange with the environment are possible only if the person feels confident due to a sound sense of coherence. Healthy coherence differs from an ego built predominantly through control processes. Such an ego is vulnerable, in that it needs constant maintenance by controlling or outdoing others. Thus, it becomes easily deflated if it does not accomplish its high-reaching aspirations.

The childhood of all the persons in the examples seems to have robbed them of the opportunity to develop a sound coherence. Instead, they struggle to maintain their wounded ego. Although the mothers of Elsie, Susan, and Charles have been socialized to submit to the control of a seemingly powerful male, they yearn for true spirituality in a relationship and resort to various types of control measures because they fall short of achieving mutuality in their relationships. Darryl has failed to live up to the expectations of society and has resigned, seeking comfort by selecting alcohol as a spiritual partner. Bill, lacking sound coherence, ascribes to the superior societal image of masculinity, according to which he expects to earn power by owning Susan. Consequently, he lashes out in the fear of losing her, because his image is threatened. In contrast, Charles's father, who has reached his high professional goals, finds himself emotionally isolated despite his power. Striving to gain coherence, he increasingly assumes power in the family.

Nursing Care

The key to the nursing of addicted persons is the guidance in establishing reciprocal relationships and growth through individuation. It follows that the rehabilitation process is interpersonal. The framework of systemic organization often leads to nursing approaches that constitute aberrations from the conventional mode. Theory-based nursing interventions are outlined next. They refer to the case examples cited earlier.

Breaking the Wet-Dry Cycles. The case of Elsie and Darryl is described in greater detail elsewhere (Friedemann & Youngblood, 1992). The couple attended 10 sessions with a mental health nurse associated with the visiting nurse agency in charge of Reina, the disabled child. Coherence was identified by the couple as the dimension most in need of attention and Darryl's drinking was deemphasized by the nurse. Using the steps of the ADD HEALTH model described in Chapter 2, Elsie and Darryl were first encouraged to identify behaviors they had practiced in the past to show each other's love. Examples they listed were going shopping together, hugging, cooking a good meal for Darryl, and making Reina laugh. They were then asked to use these behaviors at home. The nurse encouraged direct communication and praised their efforts. Next, they defined their ideal family together, in which they would enjoy sharing space and time with each other and engage jointly in Reina's caregiving. They also decided to stay firm on setting limits for Terry, who was allowed to call but could not join them during this vulnerable stage of family development. After gaining some confidence in their interactional patterns, they were ready to confront their control conflict.

The nurse presented to them the behavior cycles they had previously described, using a technique called *behavior-loop mapping* (Liepman et al., 1989). The visual representation pictured in Figure 9.4 helped them understand their responses and allowed them to use their own creativity in finding alternative behaviors. To break the cycle of control, they needed to overcome their addiction through spirituality or a mutually satisfying relationship. As the alternative loop shows, it was first decided that Elsie should refrain from telling Darryl what to do, and both were to hug each other each time they were helpful. This resulted in Darryl's doing a few minor repairs around the house and helping Elsie clean up the kitchen. Darryl's help gave them time to go out together during the week. They used the time to talk about how they were doing together and show each other appreciation. When Darryl did not do a promised task, Elsie was to ask him whether he wanted to do something else instead and let him decide.

As Steinglass et al. (1987) noted, alcoholic families differ greatly in the way they react to drinking behaviors. In this case, Darryl did not want to stop drinking, because sobriety would make him feel like a misfit within his own family. Elsie respected this but asked him to refrain from binge drinking. It was not easy for Darryl, because pressure from Reina's condition mounted. He relapsed twice during the course of treatment. The nurse then worked predominantly with Elsie, helping her to acknowledge Darryl's difficulties and not take his behavior as a personal affront. As her reactions mellowed, Darryl's need to drink excessively diminished, and Elsie was able to redefine his drinking as a social activity that did not greatly threaten their family togetherness. At the same time, Elsie was making plans for completing high school requirements and subsequently starting a 2-year college program in nursing. Even though her education was put on hold until Reina's condition improved, Elsie upheld her courage by reminding herself of these plans.

Breaking the Cycles of Violence. The ideal care for Susan and Bill would take a similar direction. In reality, however, the conventional approach differs significantly. In the shelter, Susan is counseled on an

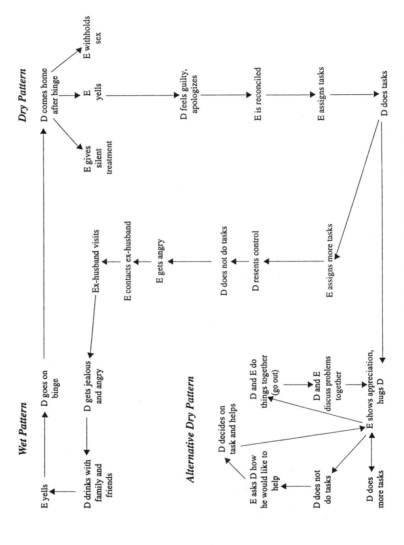

Figure 9.4. Behavior Loops for Elsie and Darryl

individual basis. Her need for individuation is addressed in terms of self-development, and she is urged to set the goal of separating from Bill and becoming self-reliant. However, clinical experience with female victims, as well as research, has shown that the majority of women do not leave their partners (Serra, 1993). Numerous theories are used to explain the phenomenon, from masochism (Snell, Rosenwald, & Robey, 1964) and social learning (Bandura, 1979) to female socialization toward dependence (Pagalow, 1981) to learned helplessness (Seligman, 1975) and Walker's cycle of violence (Walker, 1979, 1984). This cycle has three phases—tension building, battering, and loving remorse—as was demonstrated by the case of Susan and Bill. Key to repeating the cycle is said to be the woman's delusion that she can control her partner's behavior (Serra, 1993). In contrast, Bowker (1993) alerts us to the fact that such control may not be delusional, because many women attempt to maintain and improve their relationships and eventually succeed in living without violence. Women who were battered, sometimes over many years, have been observed to keep working hard to free themselves of their dependency by seeking personal growth through individuation, whether or not they separate from the partner.

Nursing with the framework of systemic organization accentuates and supports the family's striving toward health. At the same time, health is not necessarily defined as the separation of the partners. Susan is asked to define health for herself as she starts to understand her life process, her strong need to belong, and her willingness to sacrifice her autonomy and self-determination in exchange for some moments of passionate love.

Bill needs care as well, because he is a victim of his own impulses. In fact, he may need more guidance than Susan. Bill needs to redefine his world and his role within it. Only through understanding his own dependency and his urge to kindle his vulnerable ego by possessing Susan can he recognize that his individuation process needs to join Susan's to gain congruence and family coherence. Bill also needs to rethink the concept of family. So far, he has seen his role only in relation to Susan, demanding from her reciprocity that she cannot deliver without neglecting the children. Depending on her loyalty toward the children, Susan may decide to terminate the relationship if Bill is unwilling to develop his role as a father and support her with her responsibilities. For now, however, she wants to do her best to make the relationship work.

The nurse's task with this family is difficult. Although Elsie and Darryl in the first example show a remarkable readiness to work on their relationship together, the situation of Susan and Bill presents a much greater challenge. The nurse in this case is a highly skilled mental health practitioner who works for a community center and does consulting in Susan's shelter. When Susan decides to leave the shelter to go home and try to make peace with Bill, she sees her role as mediator. Her goal is to get Bill involved in an ongoing abusers' group.

On the basis of the literature and Susan's story, the nurse suspects that Bill is suspicious and tends to externalize the blame. He is likely to feel victimized by the professionals in Susan's shelter because he suspects that they side with Susan and blame him for the crisis. Although he feels guilty about hurting Susan, he rationalizes that his reactions are justified. At work, he finds reasonable support in his thinking in that some of his coworkers empathize with his jealousy and encourage him to crack down on Susan to show that he is the man. Another compounding factor is the restraining order issued by the police as a result of the last life-threatening assault. Bill is angry and feels that he has been treated unjustly, because he "would never have pulled the trigger."

On the telephone, the nurse practitioner introduces herself as the person working with Susan to make things better in the family. Bill asks her with irritation in his voice to make his commonsense rules clear to Susan. He would never hurt her again if she follows his rules. The nurse acknowledges his wishes as legitimate but not realistic. She then speaks for Susan, starting with the positives. "Susan loves you," she says, "more than anybody else. She is very grateful to you for giving her a home and helping her raise the children. She recognizes you as a very caring and warm person when you are your true self. She loves the way you comfort her when she cries, the way you tell her that you love her, and she believes that you really want to support her." Bill, now very attentive, seems surprised. "Susan never tells me this," Bill responds. The nurse answers, "Susan is not sure how to talk to you. You have two personalities. The mean and jealous one she is afraid of. You accuse her of dating other men and cheating on you, and when she tells you it's not true you get very upset and tell her she is lying.

You check on her and she can't please you. Susan came to me asking me for help for you, not for herself. She asks me to help you see that she has been faithful to you, so you could love her again."

After this conversation, Bill agrees to a visit in the nurse's office at the community center. During that session with Bill, the nurse stresses the need for a good family, which means sharing and working together. Bill is willing to listen to an explanation of the framework of systemic organization and helps the nurse to define family coherence, and the nurse consistently reflects on how Susan or the children would react to his suggestions. The outcome is Bill's understanding that Susan wants his help with the children and asks him to share playtime and fun with them as well. Bill realizes that Susan will be more ready to dedicate herself to him if he grants her space and an opportunity to do things important to her. Seeing more clearly where the shortcomings are in the family process, Bill becomes less resistant and finally agrees to make contact with the leader of a local all-male abusers' group. His greatest need is to feel connected to people of his kind who understand his strong emotions and help him to accept himself. The nurse then works with Susan on family matters, taking a close look at control issues and finding strategies to break the cycle of violence similar to Elsie and Darryl's in the first example. It is hoped that Bill will join them after some time passes and some changes become evident.

Regulating Closeness and Distance. The case of Charles bears many similarities as well. As in Susan and Bill's case, the nurse needs to overcome resistance, mainly from the father, who strongly believes in the perfection of his lifestyle. He will feel upset about being drawn into some therapy, because it is difficult for him to see a connection between his son's irresponsible behavior and the family. The nurse practitioner at the rehabilitation center may be best advised to start the nursing process by initially including the mother only, because she seems to be particularly hurt by the crisis. The focus is on her relationship with Charles, and both parties need to gain understanding of their personal life process with the help of the system diagram. On the basis of her understanding of Charles's needs, the mother may redefine Charles's rebellion as an attempt to gain independence and therefore as a necessary but misguided step in his development. Furthermore, she will recognize her own difficulty in letting Charles grow up. The nurse assures her that this difficulty is encountered by many mothers, and her reaction to Charles's girlfriend was not unusual. Then, in support of Charles, the nurse assures him that feeling hurt was a very natural reaction, but his decision to do drugs was not based on sound judgment. Charles then opens up and describes how he was teased about being "the professor" and felt left out in school until some classmates dared him to try cocaine. Charles surprised them with his readiness to participate and he earned their respect for his fearlessness. For the first time, Charles felt part of a peer group and he was elated.

This family has many strengths to make the future work for them. Charles is intelligent and basically understands his foolishness. His young age and searching nature make him open to new strategies with family and peers. Furthermore, he still envisions his future as a chemist. Charles's mother has excellent cognitive resources and some insight into family patterns. Her extended family serves as a significant support. The position of Charles's father as decision maker is accepted to a certain extent by all members. This acceptance renders setting limits for Charles reasonably promising. Recognizing this, the nurse invites the father under the pretext of needing his guidance to establish rules for Charles. She thereby involves him in the process of modifying family system maintenance, allowing the father to take the leading role but advocating for other members' rights for space and individuation. This includes Charles's brother. The session leaves an impression on Charles's father, because it becomes apparent to him that he has failed to respect the needs of his family.

The following session is spent discussing the couple's relationship, accentuating the mother's developmental need to find new meaning in her life, because her parenting duties must evolve as the children grow and need more freedom to move independently. The mother is given the opportunity to describe her volunteering activities and interests to her husband, and the nurse expresses admiration for her dedication and energy spent on the various social projects. Again, the father is surprised to get to know his wife from a perspective he did not know existed. The remaining sessions include the entire family and have the purpose of reinforcing what was said and finding strategies to increase family coherence. Merely by bringing these members together on a path of mutual understanding, the father experiences individuation and increases his sensitivity to the needs of others. When Charles returns home, the family starts to accept the father as a role model, and he senses that he is needed to help Charles find his way.

Summary

These suggested approaches are merely examples. Nurses can decide on various ways to go, depending on the families' and their own resources. Perhaps the most important step of the treatment consists of rendering the family ready to accept help. If this is accomplished, it remains up to the nurse to continue the nursing process or to refer the family to therapy, a support group, or a helping agency.

The reader may have noticed that the treatment issue with addicted families has a certain commonality with other cases cited in previous chapters. First, all are crises that affect the family as well as each individual. Furthermore, all of these crises, whether they are related to structural changes, unmet developmental tasks, or addictions, are developmental crises in the sense of inhibiting the ability of family members to grow and meet their ongoing developmental needs. Finally, it needs to be mentioned that behaviors described in prior examples, if not representing blatant addictions, border on obsessions that have a striking similarity with addictive patterns.

In the first developmental crisis described in Chapter 7, Kristen searches for a spiritual target. Her lack of mutuality in her relationship with Carl renders her need for success at work extreme, which makes it proportionately difficult to assume the new task of mothering a baby. In the second example, Sandy sacrifices herself to perfection in motherhood and social activities to an extent that borders on addiction. Elizabeth, in the third example, once addicted to alcohol, now becomes a martyr. She shifts her irresponsible behavior to patterns of dutiful caregiving, addictive in the sense that it robs her of enjoyment from life and freedom to grow. Her target of spirituality is the view of herself as a good person and a way to heaven. Frank and Dorothy, in the fourth example, adhere to their work and family roles to the point that their flexibility to make a change in the system is lost. They too are unable to grow in their relationship and target spirituality in caring for each other. This requires them to take turns in being sick and being cared for.

Among the examples of crises related to structural changes, Barbara is not unlike Susan in that she seeks spirituality with love objects and is unable to maintain a mutually gratifying relationship. She differs in that she can replace the object of love, if the relationship turns sour, and feels pride in surviving each new disaster.

In short, it seems most advantageous to get away from labeling problems as addictions to truly understand individuals and families, because labels include a number of predetermined judgments and stereotypes. Instead, nurses should build on the strengths of individuals and families. They need to examine the entire systemic process, including the intensity by which all types of behaviors are pursued. Furthermore, the target at which these behaviors are directed needs to be examined as well as the counterreactions they elicit in family members or contacts in the community.

10

Research With the
Family Life Process and Crisis

The main body of the literature on crises in families and addictions reviewed for this chapter is based on quantitative research designs. Most are correlational, some are predictive, and others present elaborate structural linear models. Conceptual thinking about crises and addictions in families that underlies these studies is strongly influenced by stress and coping models, crisis theory, biomedical theories, and others that are shared among a number of disciplines, including nursing. The theories have in common a relatively simplistic understanding of persons and groups of persons as being hit by some type of stressor, a sudden change, or an addiction, generally considered a disease, that overtaxes the person's or the family's resources and consequently produces a specific outcome. Not surprisingly, relationships between stressors and outcomes are generally weak and often lack consistency between similar studies. For example, Fiese (1993) points out that clinical reports about parental alcohol abuse cite many adverse effects on children, and the relative research studies fall miserably short in producing clear scientific evidence. The most promising predictors of the children's mental health are family process variables such as conflict (Werner, 1986), family crises (Miller & Jang, 1977), or family rituals (Fiese, 1993; Wolin & Bennett, 1984).

This seems to support the proposition that the same stressor can have varying effects on family members, depending on their general family functioning process. As researchers realized the importance of family processes in terms of the well-being of individuals, a surge occurred in family research as investigators attempted to insert family typology as a covariant in the coping process. A well-known example of a theoretical framework serving as a basis for many studies is the expanded T-Double ABCX Model (McCubbin & McCubbin, 1987). Family typologies recently defined, however, have been chosen rather arbitrarily. They are based on results of stress and coping research and variables deemed to be important for system functioning but lack a firm conceptual basis.

Although the linear model approach may sound more logical and promising than others, it also harbors serious problems in terms of its usage with the framework of systemic organization: (a) It is linear and defies systems principles. Looking at the family as a variable, it offers no provision for exploring continuously evolving processes. (b) It claims to explore an objective truth, but each person's view of the family is highly subjective. (c) It offers no solution to the unit of analysis problem. (d) It focuses on central tendencies but neglects the diversity among families. (e) It does not explore change over time. Each of these problems is briefly summarized.

Systemic research defies the linear causality assumption underlying the quantitative research paradigm. Systemic processes are assumed to be circular and nonrecursive in that variable A changes variable B and many others, all of which change variable A via feedback loops. Variable A, then, together with the other changed variables, keeps changing B. In this process, both the original independent variable A and the dependent variable B take turns in becoming alternately causative agents or outcomes, depending on the perspective taken in examining the process. Consequently, there are no true independent variables, but all are dependent on the process and truly variable as the process changes over time. As the system evolves and culture is transformed, a snapshot taken of the process at any one point in time by a cross-sectional study will not reveal the true and entire nature of the process.

The second major issue is subjectivity. The framework of systemic organization assumes that every truth is subjective, meaning that individuals experience their life process as well as the family's in their own unique way. Their individuation throughout life has led them to a private understanding about who they are and how they should execute their roles as individuals and family members. Furthermore, defining family roles, rights, and responsibilities invariably sets expectations about the role of others whose supportive involvement is needed in the family process. It follows that if all members create the family subjectively in relation to their own needs and role perceptions, the family truth is where the various perceptions meet each other.

Because such truths are constantly shifting, adjusting, and changing in the search for congruence, there cannot be one objective truth, but ironically, objective truth is what empirical research operating under the logical positivist paradigm claims to discover (Dzurec & Abraham, 1993). Paper-and-pencil tools as well as structured observations with trained observers yield data that are highly subjected to the respondents' or observers' perceptions. Quantitative data interpretation relies on probability and inference to arrive at generalizable norms claimed to be reality. By judging certain attributes or behaviors as good or normal without exploring the system's motivation or interchange among members and with its environment, the reality thus created expresses an artificial objectivity that has little to do with the system's actual life process.

As the family typology is introduced into models representing the phenomena of interest, models of coping have become unusually cumbersome, complex, and difficult to test. The family can be viewed as a screen that promotes, inhibits, or channels certain responses to the stressor. It can be envisioned as a stressor, further complicating an individual's coping, or it can be an outcome or a result of the individual members' behaviors and actions. Irrespective of its position, it is considered to be one or several variables to be operationalized at the family system level. Consequently, entangled in the complexity of systems and the interface of the individuals and the family is the third issue that has long pertained to family research, namely, problems with keeping the unit of analysis or system level consistent throughout the design. Difficulties arise with the operationalization of variables at the family level. Consequently, concepts such as family coping, family well-being, family conflict, or family stress lack clarity or logic, especially if they represent the sum or average of individual responses.

Furthermore, family process needs to be evaluated by individuals, and because responses are likely to diverge, many questions have arisen. Debates are ongoing over the use of one versus multiple respondents and how to analyze data from multiple individuals. Such issues and validity questions related to the assessment of families from individual responses are discussed extensively elsewhere (i.e., Draper & Marcos, 1990; Feetham, Meister, Bell, & Gilliss, 1993). The difficulties cannot be resolved by the use of the framework of systemic organization. Although the researcher's task consists of exploring processes instead of linear relationships, the issue of interface between individuals and the family system persists and needs to be carefully evaluated when proposing innovative designs, including triangulation methods.

The fourth issue refers to the diversity of families. The framework of systemic organization urges an evaluation of the systemic process of each family, because variations in family reactions to change and tension are extensive, even if the situational context is held stable. What truly matters for knowledge building about families is not commonalities but differences, or the family factors responsible for such differences. The majority of research studies are strictly based on averages, thereby discounting diversity, and may be minimally meaningful in terms of building family knowledge. Much remains to be learned about how families differ and which factors differentiate family processes that predict the outcome of crisis or the pursuit of congruence.

The last problem is lack of knowledge about change. Longitudinal studies are rare and when they are conducted, they usually represent the family process frozen at various points in time. This allows a look at differences but explains little about how the differences occurred. Differently stated, quantitative longitudinal designs examine alterations in variable A or variable B without understanding the life process in which both variables play a role or the particular role they play in bringing about change of the system.

Chapter 6 has outlined what the tasks may be for nurse researchers in exploring and operationalizing the moving patterns of space, time, and energy. Creativity in research methods was suggested, including the integration of the qualitative and quantitative paradigm and other types of triangulation.

The preceding discussion suggests that the search for objective truth may be futile. Therefore, the question now involves the utility of research methods in the discovery of subjective truths for the purpose of testing the midrange theories cited earlier. Lowenberg (1993) states that through a hermeneutic perspective, reality is envisioned as a "buzzing chaos" (p. 65), a conceptualization in tune with this framework. In assessing such reality, the shortcomings of quantitative designs outlined earlier are plentiful. Qualitative research methods also have inherent difficulties. Although qualitative research explores the lived experience, the question arises whether the perceptive reality pertains to the respondent, the researcher, or both. For example, in searching for understanding of addictive patterns, methods of Heideggerian hermeneutics seem ideal (Woolfolk, Sass, & Messer, 1988), and the tool for uncovering the patterns could be unstructured interviews (Diekelmann, Allen, & Tanner, 1989). Sandelowski (1993), however, describes this research process as an artful endeavor resulting in an interpretive product that does not represent the respondent's unique worldview, but instead a constructed reality that combines both the researcher's and respondent's perspectives.

Such a reality seems to be the product of an individuation and system change process in which data evolve and gain meaning as they touch and fuse with the researcher's own life process and value system. Consequently, what is measured is the evolving interpersonal process within a small segment of time, in which the subject's and researcher's realities are united and become inseparable. This very phenomenon renders qualitative research unreplicable (Sandelowski, 1993).

Qualitative methods that start the exploratory process with a tentative conceptualization of the process based on working hypotheses or midrange theories (Cronbach, 1975) are grouped under the category of analytic induction by Polit and Hungler (1991) and seem particularly useful in working with the framework of systemic organization. For example, ethnographers examine conceptual structures or frames for coherence by focusing on differences or breakdowns with each case. Inconsistencies with the hypothesized process must be resolved by modifying the frame to create a new fit. Consequently, the conceptual frame or schema is continuously corrected until it accommodates all case variations (Agar, 1986).

Although ethnography is ideal for testing theories, researchers using it and similar methods have been engaged for years in a heated debate about validity. It revolves around inside (emic) or outside (etic) realities as well as generalizability. The emic view reflecting the realities of the participants should be the focus; however, the researcher's etic view as an outsider is needed for interpretation and theory building. As individuation occurs, the separation of the two views is as difficult as with other methods. Here, too, the researcher becomes part of the process to be studied, grows with it, and influences its course at least to some extent.

This shows clearly that there is no perfect method available to research proposition statements and test this theory. One suggestion is to take research findings as not more than an educated guess and gain theoretical support through various research methods. The advantages of triangulation in overcoming weaknesses and enhancing validity have been discussed in Chapter 6. It is also advised to explore processes longitudinally.

The following is an example of a design for a study with the purpose of exploring the theory-based statement that blockage of individuation eventually leads to crisis. A researcher might examine specific processes of families who find themselves in a difficult situation, such as adjustment to a divorce or to retirement. The researcher would expect some of these families to do well, whereas others end up in crisis. If the process leads to health, individuation behaviors should be observed and members should report learning and personal growth. Friedemann's (1991a) screening tool, the Assessment of Strategies in Families (ASF), may be of some use. The tool is theory-based and evaluates individuation in terms of the family members' motivation and openness to interact with the environment, assuming that by doing so they would learn and grow in the process.

Like all others, this tool is subjective, meaning that the subjects' perception about their individuation may differ considerably from their actual behaviors. In assessing crisis, however, such subjectivity may be advantageous. The crisis process seems to be heavily driven by perception. In fact, a crisis may develop because family members perceive that they have lost control and the opportunity to grow, irrespective of their potential abilities they could put to use. In measuring individuation repeatedly over time, the researcher would expect that a decrease in scores may be related to the development of a family crisis that could be measured with the help of a family conflict or crisis instrument.

The inclusion of several family members would give the researcher additional information about the relative importance of individual perceptions for the evolution of the process. It might answer questions such as the following: Is family crisis more likely if the mothers' individuation score decreases more than the fathers'? Is a crisis most likely, if all members' individuation scores decrease? How strongly are the children's individuation scores related to the crisis outcome?

Because all of the above quantitative measures are based on averages, much information specific to each family's process is not available. The study might be enhanced by method triangulation to validate quantitative indicators and gain insight into diverse ways of functioning. The researcher may decide on a series of semistructured qualitative interviews to be taped and later transcribed. Because the family process is likely to be influenced by the interference of the researcher who joins the family system (sensitization), it is not advisable to reuse the subjects of the quantitative study. In such interviews, a wide range of individuation behaviors and underlying attitudes and values can be explored, and the perspectives of various family members should be included. If repeated interviews are too time-consuming or costly, progress over time and shifts in perception as reported in retrospect can be recorded and documented in a case study format. Commonalities and differences in the families' individuation behaviors, or lack thereof, and factors presumably important in supporting individuation are described and organized according to themes.

Secondary studies could be added to enhance knowledge of the process. For example, the researcher may be interested in the validity of the quantitative measure and use method triangulation to test it. Several subjects who previously completed the ASF could also be interviewed with regard to their perception of individual and family individuation, but subjects who were previously interviewed could be asked to fill out the ASF. Different sequencing of the methods and comparison of ASF scores and interview responses of both groups will indicate if the subjects were sensitized by either method.

Next, the results achieved quantitatively and qualitatively are compared and the findings are logically integrated by adhering closely to the theory. For that purpose, the researcher may decide to list all statements describing individuation of family members and the family's adjustment to their differences for each subject family. The list could then be compared with the score for individuation on the ASF assessment tool. To demonstrate coherence in the measure and validity of the tool, the researcher expects families with high scores to comment heavily on individuation, and those with low scores are expected to have commented about the lack thereof or not mentioned the topic.

As previously stated, in analyzing such complex information, the researcher should not lose sight of possible changes that may have been induced through the research and interviewing process. Instead of treating such change as an obstacle to objectivity, this additional dimension could be used to generate knowledge about the families' ability to change toward health or nursing. Because the framework of systemic organization defines nursing as taking part in the family's life process and offering support by helping the family to see clearly, the very process of nursing differs little from interactive interviewing that takes place in qualitative research. In fact, researchers who carefully avoid any type of controlling suggestions or offering of solutions or normative interventions may become the most effective helpers, because they do not elicit resistive countermoves from the family. Collins, Given, and Berry (1989) reported that 52% of their subjects who answered open-ended questions were aware of at least one effect on their awareness, perception, or coping. It seems safe to assume that extensive nonstructured interviews may elicit even more pronounced changes.

To examine whether this holds true, a nurse researcher can add a few questions to inquire about the subjects' perception of personal and family growth as they see it related to the research process and their reasoning about why it happened. Such information would provide clarity about nursing and the individuation process in line with the framework of systemic organization. The comparison of various cases could demonstrate how certain families benefit while others fail to do so.

In addition, comparative methodological triangulation can be employed if the researcher is interested in the individuation process that accompanies various research methods. For example, the question may refer to what aspect of interaction with the research process is therapeutic: Communication with the researcher, responding to a questionnaire, or simply learning through the life process. A sample of subjects exposed to the same stressor for a similar length of time could be collected to find an answer. Of those participants, families who were interviewed could be compared to others who were not and those who had filled out a paper-and-pencil tool of the same topic.

All of these research suggestions were derived secondary to the initial propositional statement. The examples employ various methods combined in such a way that shortcomings can be minimized and the meaning of findings can be enhanced. Earlier mentioned cautions about various designs and paradigms of research are applicable here as well. Furthermore, the theoretical fit of instruments is of major importance in quantitative designs. Instruments should be retested and possibly adapted for their use with a particular population to gain conceptual validity. Rigor is also needed in qualitative research in a way that it does not unnecessarily compromise the flexibility needed to create meaningful portraits of human experience (Sandelowski, 1993).

The above design uses triangulation to address completeness by focusing on various perspectives of the same phenomenon (Fielding & Fielding, 1986). Triangulation is also used for confirmation of the results and concurrent validation of the individuation dimension of the ASF by examining the similarity or divergence of the two different measures. The essence of designing research plans that even remotely hint at the complexity of family process is to purposefully specify what the various research methods are to accomplish and how they are to contribute to a fuller understanding of the phenomenon and the testing of the theory. Such designs are rare but seem to constitute a worthwhile goal for which to strive.

PART

4

Families in Crisis:
Crises With Disease and Death

Introduction

The content of this part involves the life process of families who are forced to change their patterns as a result of a serious illness of a family member. The chapters draw heavily from the content of the previous chapters in that a disease, or pathology in medical terms, demands a change of family life patterns and may become a contributing factor in the development of a crisis if the family process fails to meet its members' developmental needs. Table P4.1 summarizes the concepts of the framework of systemic organization relative to health and their relationship to each other. The table clarifies the differences between theory-based nursing and medicine. Because nurses work within the medical system, they base their definition of disease or illness on symptoms of pathology. This is compatible with the framework of systemic organization, but, in addition to offering physical care, nurses must address health in terms of the life process of the patient and family, which differs significantly from medical explanations. Of importance is the subjective experience of the disease and its interpretation. The integration of the broad concept of health into the thought process of the nurse is imperative for theory-based interpretations of the disease, the understanding of patients' and families' reactions to it, and the development of appropriate nursing actions.

It needs to be restated that a newly diseased family member represents a change from within the system that requires a response no different from responses to structural, developmental, and behavioral changes discussed earlier. Thus, disease does not cause a family crisis but may become a factor in unfolding a developmental crisis from within the system. As previously explained, such developmental crises are exacerbated by a family process already deficient in meeting its targets. Such families burdened with additional demands for change due to the disease are likely to accelerate their destructive course by blocking individuation and personal growth of family members.

The assumption of system connectedness complicates matters by suggesting that the occurrence of changes in body functioning may be a far more complex phenomenon than is portrayed by the medical model. Ancient religions and health philosophies of civilizations in the East and West have unanimously accepted the interdependence of humans and their environment as well as the patterns of nature and

TABLE P4.1 Summary of Health Concepts

Framework of Systemic Organization

Health

- Global subjective experience of the degree of congruence within the system and with the environment
- Ranges from low health to high health
- Every system has health—no health is impossible.

Body and emotions belong to one unified being and cannot be separated.

- Interpretation of sensations and feelings related to health result in well-being if health is high; anxiety if health is low
- Other negative emotions (i.e., guilt, hostility, depression) are secondary to anxiety.
- Well-being and anxiety are dynamic and fluctuate. It is significant to estimate their ratio over time.

Disease/illness

- Signifies a cluster of somatic symptoms (i.e., pain, nausea, fever, cardiac arrhythmia, diarrhea) and *wellness* is the absence of disease/illness.
- Symptoms of pathology may be signs of health if they are congruent with human development (old age, disability), serve as indicators of system incongruence, and lead to change
- The symptoms may be a hindrance to health if they increase anxiety and anxiety becomes a self-reinforcing agent

---

Medical model

Physical disease/illness and *health* are antithetical and present a continuum.

Emotional/mental illness and *emotional/mental health* are antithetical and present a continuum. *Body and emotions are separate entities.*

---

the elements as the key to health. Although modern science has reduced the explanation of pathology to a linear causal and mechanistic course with a predictable outcome, the competing explanation of health has persisted throughout the centuries. Documentation of the persistent use of folk medicinal practices, even in industrialized nations, and the rebirth of interest in Eastern philosophies, as well as ancient Western healing principles such as homeopathy, speak to an inherent knowing that health involves congruence and thus a process of balancing forces within and without.

Rogers (1970) has articulated this basic principle in terms of nursing, and Margret Newman (1979) has followed suit. Both theorists purport that there is an overlaid pattern "reflected in the energy exchange within man and between man and the environment" (Newman, 1983, p. 163). Like Newman's framework, the framework of systemic organization views disease as a manifestation of the person's basic pattern. If the systemic life process fails to reach congruence, recovery from the disease requires not simply the control of physical symptoms but a rearrangement of the life process that accepts and incorporates the symptoms as manifestations of a process striving for health. The disease therefore has the potential to trigger a search for meaning and reevaluation of values and beliefs by way of individuation that may steer the person toward congruence and health, reduced anxiety, and well-being.

Ironically, only through acceptance and recognition of the disease's function within the individual's and the family's life process can energy be freed to regain congruence and peace of mind. This occurs irrespective of whether or not the symptoms persist. Persons who encounter health in such a way will report that they are healthy despite chronic debility (Newman, 1983). In fact, this type of individuation seems to be the essence of maintaining health while aging and preparing for death. Ideally, families accept disease as a natural phenomenon to be expected within each generation's life span and as an opportunity to learn about one's own true nature.

Disease affects families and their members as much as the afflicted individuals. Some families are instrumental in enhancing individuation in such situations, but others contribute to the development of a crisis due to their persistence on control. In this culture, when disease occurs, the first way to control entails an alliance with a physician who will treat or cure the disease. Most families ascribe to the medical model and are apt to advocate such an approach, sometimes by methods of extreme coercion, in cases where afflicted individuals are reluctant to follow suit.

Conducting a battle against pathologies may not be sufficient, however. A serious illness, which presents a threat to the stability of patient and family and the realization that the illusion of infallible health can no longer be maintained, may demand a transformation of basic beliefs about the power of medicine and human resilience. Thus, the prevention or resolution of a disease-related crisis occurs by educating families about the broad meaning of health and signifies growth through individuation and system change.

Nurses have many opportunities to observe families change and grow as they reorient themselves within an illness situation. In fact, work with these families is usually rewarding and growth-promoting for the nurses involved. The teaching of caregiving skills, rehabilitation, and tertiary prevention is easier if the family is open to experience a new meaning of health and the nurse is welcomed into the system. In contrast, families on the verge of a crisis or in crisis present a challenge. Because these family members express their fear of change through avoidance, hostility, or dependence, nurses tend to feel powerless and helpless. The content of this part offers the framework for the analysis of family situations and the testing of the nurse's self-awareness in interacting with the family. Nurses are guided to distinguish between troubled families and those who need minimal assistance. Case examples illustrate ways to assess and comprehend health quickly. This will allow informed decision making and channeling of time and energy competently to those families who need them most.

This part is divided into several chapters. Chapter 11 focuses on the interaction of families with acute care institutions and the family's adjustment to a sudden illness or accident. Death of a family member is the topic of Chapter 12, with particular emphasis on the nursing process that facilitates system change and growth. The theme of Chapter 13 is family caregiving to a chronically ill member, a process built into system maintenance and family coherence. Included here is a discussion of the nurse's role in facilitating decisions related to institutionalization. The same theme is examined in Chapter 14, as the family struggles to support a member with a mental illness. These clinically oriented chapters are followed by a summarizing discussion of research of the family process in the case of disease.

11

Families and the Acute Care System

In industrialized countries, the majority of people are born and die in health care institutions. Although this alone attests to the significance of such institutions to society, the health care system pursues the remarkable goal of restoring people's physical health, productivity, and self-sufficiency and prevents or minimizes impairment or limitations. To achieve that, people are required to submit to the control of the medical system and endure diagnostic tests, surgeries, and intensive medical and psychiatric treatments. Hospitals, clinics, rehabilitation centers, or home care agencies are systems that function like all social systems. They constitute the environment for clients of all ages and their families as well as for the health care personnel who serve the institutions as subsystems in specific roles.

Entry into the health care system as a result of an acute illness can be a traumatic experience. Often, individuals have denied their symptoms and discomfort over extended time periods and finally come to the realization that they do not go away without intervention. If their cognitive facilities remain intact, afflicted persons may experience severe anxiety upon realizing that it is no longer reasonable to deny their vulnerability and eventual death. The disease threatens their personal coherence as well as their ability to reach the goals of stability, control, and, consequently, congruence.

Clients plagued by anxiety may find little relief in a hospital bed as the disease becomes the center of attention. Within the medical model, the disease is considered separate from personhood and the experiences connected to it. Medical personnel and society in general see in the disease an enemy whom they are destined to fight. This puts the clients immediately in the position of victims and a burden to the family and society.

As they enter the acute care system, clients are temporarily relieved of their obligation to perform family and community roles and are expected to become helpless patients. The relief of obligations, however, is tied to a loss of autonomy, identity, and status as clients submit to the medical authorities. Although the transformation occurs without great difficulties in "ideal patients" who expect assistance and are willing to become dependent, many others are observed to experience difficulties and react with hostility, resignation, extreme dependency, passive resistance, or denial.

The framework of systemic organization leads to the prediction that persons will respond to anxiety and incongruence the way they usually do in threatening situations. Consequently, persons who respond to demands for change by denial may, during the course of their hospitalization, find extraordinary means to maintain their system. They avoid acknowledging all or part of the meaning of their illness (Hackett & Cassem, 1982). In severe cases, they may construct a reality in concert with their idea of a life they perceive to deserve. Clinicians tell of individuals who resort to delusions, confusion, or even hallucinations ordinarily employed by psychotic persons in the attempt to maintain an illusory stability that provides comfort.

In marked contrast to denial is the reaction called sensitization. Marsden and Dracup (1991) studied patients after myocardial infarctions. Sensitized clients focused heavily on their symptoms and exhibited extraordinary vigilance toward anything that might harm their bodies. Such control, however, is ineffective in lowering anxiety (Cromwell, Butterfield, Brayfield, & Curry, 1977). Similarly, clients who naturally depend on the help of others may become resigned and childlike in their dependency on the nurse and medical staff. Persons most difficult to handle, however, have a pattern of responding to threats with aggression, hostility, or exertion of control over others, including toward the nurse. Health professionals tend to reinforce the alienating patterns of the patients in that they withdraw physically and/or emotionally, thereby further increasing the patients' incongruence and anxiety. This leaves the patients labeled, alone, and without a person who truly understands their suffering.

The situation is complicated by the hospital unit, which constitutes not only the clients' environment but also the family's. Family members are to follow strict regulations, depend on hospital staff for information and guidance, and subordinate the family patterns to those of the hospital. Plagued by anxiety about the condition of their sick member and the threat of death, they feel helpless and powerless if the institution ignores their needs and fails to provide assurance and comfort. Families experience reactions similar to the afflicted member's. They may respond to their anxiety through heavy involvement and oversolicitousness that, if not dampened, may present a serious threat to the recovery of the patient (Marsden & Dracup, 1991). If families are to be truly supportive of a life process that leads the afflicted member to health, they need to understand their role and feel supported by the health care environment.

Family support in most hospitals, however, is insufficiently anchored in institutional policies and practices. Much depends on the nurses' creativity in accommodating family needs. Family-centered care is often endangered in systems that struggle for economic survival by discharging patients early (McShane, 1991). In today's hospitals, a smaller number of professional nurses deal with ever-increasing acuity and complexity of their patients' conditions. Nevertheless, strides toward family-centered care have been made, especially in pediatrics.

Research began with Molter's (1979) classic study and has expanded ever since. These studies illuminate family needs for information, access to the patient, and guidance in interacting with the system. For example, Hardgrove and Roberts (1989) advocate changes in the health care environment to facilitate staff-family interactions in pediatric units. They describe architectural designs and family-directed policies, such as open visiting hours, rooming-in for parents, sibling visitation, participation in care, and temporary family housing. Summarizing the literature about pediatric units, De Chesney (1986) describes family needs. Translated into the terms of systemic organization framework, De Chesney (1986) deduces the common needs of all families for flexibility and growth through individuation and for the maintenance of coherence. The fulfillment of both needs prevents crisis and occurs in as many different ways as there are different families. This suggests that family interventions need to be equally varied and based on each family's unique life pattern.

Studies of family stressors and needs have been executed in adult critical care units as well. Families were found to be concerned about the survival or future quality of life of their loved one, finances, and transportation (Bedsworth & Molen, 1982; Hodovanic, Reardon, Reese, & Wedges, 1984). On the basis of a secondary data analysis of 27 studies of family needs measured with the Critical Care Family Needs Inventory developed by Molter and Leske (1983), the researchers arrived at three categories of needs or primary concerns to families with members in critical care units. They were (a) assurance needs involving honest answers and mechanisms to encourage hope and decrease uncertainty, (b) proximity needs or being with the patient, and (c) needs for information. These needs suggest that families in the critical care situation focused predominantly on the patient, rather than on themselves (Lynn-McHale & Smith, 1991). Research done in the 1980s purports that the majority of such family needs were met by critical care nurses (Boumann, 1984; Lynn-McHale & Bellinger, 1988; Rodgers, 1983), whereas the families' own emotional needs tended to be neglected (Lynn-McHale & Smith, 1991).

Although the focus on the patients' illness seems natural in the early phase of hospitalization, nurses are advised to support the family's integrity and assess the system maintenance process systematically from the very beginning (Lynn-McHale & Smith, 1991). Expanding on this, Trygar-Artinian (1991) describes the process of creating a shared understanding between nurse and family that leads to secondary psychological benefits for the nurse through individuation, the process explained in Chapter 2.

Although many positive strides toward the care of families occur, progress has been strewn with problems. Since the 1970s, many publications have addressed the interaction between client, family, and the health care system (Shapiro, 1983; Young, 1983). Ragiel (1984) described family care in today's hospitals as a tripartite construct combining providers, patient and family, and a process in which control is pursued and information serves as the key to power for health care providers. Furthermore, a great discrepancy has been observed between families and providers in their perception of the hospitalization experience (Norris & Grove, 1986). Consequently, if the systemic interaction between providers and families truly targets control and there is little consensus about the role each party is to play, one may safely assume that families are viewed as uncooperative intruders if they disagree with the hospital's ways of maintaining control. Treated as such, families become seriously distressed (Oberst & James, 1985). Nurses are caught between the provider's paradigm of power and domination and the ethics of caring. They may feel compelled to assist bewildered families but perceive themselves unqualified to provide the care families need (Smith, Kupferschmid, Dawson, & Briones, 1991).

According to the framework of systemic organization, families, like the clients, interact with the health care system in many different ways. A healthy process of caring for families needs to be directed toward spirituality or connecting with the family, rather than control, and toward growth, rather than rigid maintenance of mechanisms to protect the institution against family interference. In a hospital environment that puts increasing emphasis on technology, power, control, and money, the inclusion of families in the care process may serve as an antidote to dehumanization (Kupferschmid, Briones, Dawson, & Drongowski, 1991; Naisbett, 1982).

Although nurses are not usually in a position to directly influence the overall systemic process of the large bureaucratic organization of the hospital, they have excellent opportunities to meet families at the subsystem level: the unit, where care is given. They feel their way into the family process; offer understanding, acceptance, and assurance; and serve as a family-hospital liaison by encouraging both family and health care professionals to articulate their needs and discuss solutions.

The following case example illustrates nursing care that focuses on congruence between client, family, nurse, and the hospital. All systems involved must adjust to each other (spirituality) to approach congruence without sacrificing the stability they need to maintain coherence. The example is described in considerable detail to lead the reader through the nursing process. Consequently, it represents a model for care also applicable to the other cases described in this chapter.

Ralph, age 55, is presently in the intensive care unit (ICU) of a large university hospital. He was admitted three days ago following an episode of severe rectal bleeding. During emergency surgery a cancerous tumor was found in the rectum, part of the colon was removed, and a colostomy was performed. Ralph was in critical condition after the surgery because he had a reaction to a blood transfusion. Now stabilized, he is very weak, drowsy from pain medications, and unable to carry long conversations.

When Ralph was informed about the colostomy and his diagnosis by the doctor, he showed no emotions and asked no questions. While taking care of the colostomy, his nurse encourages him to ask questions but realizes that he is not yet ready to face the problem. Consequently, he does not push Ralph. Ralph seems to trust his nurse and hesitantly tells him that he is worried about his wife, Betty. Would he be so kind to inform her about his disease? The nurse has previously talked with Betty, told her about the ICU routine, and attempted to make her as comfortable as possible. Ralph's request seems an opportunity, however, to gain better understanding about the care needed by Ralph and his family. In a conference with Betty he collects data about Ralph and the family system systematically, following the assessment outline presented in Tables 2.1 and 2.2 (see Chapter 2), highlighting what is important. The aim of the first assessment is to contrast Ralph's previous patterns with his present needs for care and his future potential.

Assessment of the Individual

System Maintenance. Ralph's need for care has been assessed previously and is periodically adjusted as his condition improves. Presently, his physical care is extensive and Ralph's participation is restricted to brushing his teeth, washing his face and arms, deep breathing and coughing, and minimal participation in a range of motion exercises. Even that seems to exhaust him and causes increased pain.

Ralph owns a painting company that has contracts with various apartment complexes and employs six painters and a secretary. Ralph does the administrative work but goes out to paint frequently when help is needed. Time for recreational activities has been scarce, but recently, business has been slow, causing a strain on finances. Ralph worries about the future, but Betty reports that he has always worried even when there was nothing to worry about. He gets himself all worked up about problems with his painters but does not talk about things. Betty knows about tension at work from his gloomy mood but is unable to get the details from Ralph.

Work is Ralph's life. He stays in the office all day, comes home to eat, then spends the evening with the newspaper and TV. He sleeps about 6 hours. Ralph has never participated much in family life. On weekends, he rarely leaves the house. He may wash his car or fix something but shows no interest in recreational or cultural events and does not read. Ralph has not been to a church service since his childhood. He has one friend who comes by occasionally to share a glass of beer. The family used to rent a cabin in the woods for their vacation, and Ralph found fishing in a nearby stream to be relaxing. After the children were grown, he saw no use in it any more. Betty reports that Ralph has been rather unhappy and moody but was not sure why he was frustrated with his life.

Coherence. Ralph is a loner and does not communicate his emotions. He takes no initiative in trying something new but may tag along if his wife takes the lead. Ralph had worked to fulfill a dream. He saved money to buy property on which he wanted to build a home. Betty reports that he truly blossomed while he was making plans. But then, it turned out that there was a requirement to build a connection to the sewer system that was exorbitantly expensive. Betty discouraged Ralph from pursuing the planning any further because she was not keen on living there anyway. She thinks that Ralph's recent mood may have been connected to this disappointment, because he seems to have even less energy and frequently sits in the armchair daydreaming.

Ralph and Betty feel close. Betty knows that she is the only person Ralph really trusts and she has accepted him the way he is. They do not talk much, but it does not seem to matter. Through Betty, Ralph gains access to family and friends because they respect the fact that Betty and Ralph are a unit not to be separated. Ralph's pride is his work and his role as provider for the family. Consequently, his pride related to his children is based on their success at work. Other values, human and family values, belong to the realm of his wife. It seems that both acknowledge and accept the fact that they complement and need each other to be full human beings.

Individuation. Ralph individuates in interaction with his wife. Betty does much emotional work for him. She makes him aware of other perspectives of evaluating situations when he is upset and frustrated. She models a positive and accepting attitude that permits the discovery of aesthetic beauty in life. Despite her vitality and intelligence, Betty admits that she too needs Ralph, who often keeps cool when she becomes emotional about family squabbles or finances. Work is generally fulfilling for Ralph, especially if he succeeds in satisfying his customers. The couple never discusses religious or philosophical matters. Betty does not know whether Ralph believes in God but feels that he seeks his answer through her. She knows that, like her, he is terrified about losing her and their mutual wish is to be united after death.

System Change. Ralph has difficulties healing his wounds. He has never fully reconciled himself with his difficult childhood. He expects high standards from people, including his children, and gets angry if they do not live up to them. Ralph poorly expresses anger and frustration and Betty tries to assist him. She knows how to dilute his bitterness about people but feels that she has been less than successful in helping him deal with the disappointment about the planned construction of a home. Betty suspects that he attempted to prove his worth with this project and is unable to change his attitude and values about this. She is afraid that his cancer may be related to Ralph's frustration and the belief that there is nothing left to live for.

Assessment of Individual Health

Betty is a most valuable source of data, because she seems to know Ralph better than he does. In discussing the systemic diagram, Betty and the nurse arrive at the illustration represented by Figure 11.1a: Ralph strongly emphasizes stability through work and the relationship with Betty. He tends to accentuate control by pressuring people to abide by his standards. Any change is a serious threat to him. When Betty sees a need for change, she tends to pull him in the direction of spirituality, by showing him love and affection within their relationship, and opens him up to evaluate the situation in a more flexible way. Through Betty, Ralph gains access to the family, nature, and the beauty of life. Thus, Ralph can remain coherent through a sense of pride in his

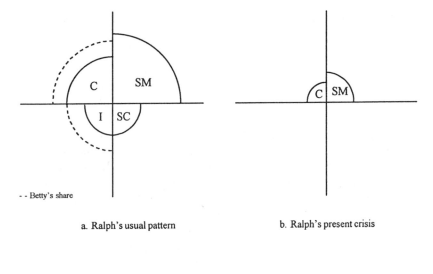

a. Ralph's usual pattern   b. Ralph's present crisis

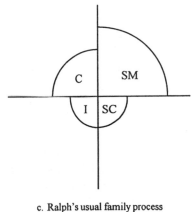

c. Ralph's usual family process

Figure 11.1. Systemic Process of Ralph

achievements and connectedness within the spousal relationship. The relationship constitutes an environment in which Ralph can individuate. Nevertheless, due to Ralph's strong need to maintain his usual life pattern and avoid change if at all possible, individuation tends be a labored process, a struggle that sometimes involves hurt feelings. This focus on system maintenance has been ingrained in Ralph's chaotic childhood, in which stability was lacking, and has served as a useful way to maintain his self-worth and coherence.

In his new situation, Ralph is confronted with the task of system change. To accomplish that, he needs to enter a process of individuation in which he has to confront his vulnerability and acknowledge ways of gaining self-worth other than earning money and building a new home. The one way to arrive at this will be through Ralph's realization of what he means to his wife simply by being who he is. This assessment stands in stark contrast to the usual way of evaluating and treating clients such as Ralph in hospital units. Ralph appears overly dependent and weak in relation to societal values, such as the virtue of fighting against the odds. Ralph needs to learn to be a man and a warrior to tackle this "thing." The systemic diagram, however, shows that it is the so-called dependence that works in his favor and is a true strength. The nurse realizes that Ralph can be helped only through the relationship with his wife on the level of the interactional system and possibly within his family system. Consequently, to gain a fuller understanding, the nurse must proceed by assessing the family and its interactions. Family data are collected systematically during a meeting with Betty and the two sons, following Table 2.2 in Chapter 2.

Assessment of the Family

System Maintenance. The couple has two sons, ages 27 and 20. The elder son is married and has two small children. The younger son is a student at a community college and lives at home. Betty's mother also lives in the same town and is rather independent despite her age of 85 years. Two of Betty's sisters live within 2 hours' driving distance. The family gets together at least once every year on a holiday. Other persons of importance are Ralph's previously mentioned close friend and his wife, who is Betty's friend, as well as two women friends who have kept in contact with Betty since they were schoolmates.

The family lives in a modest home in a semirural area. Betty has been a mother and homemaker all her life and now feels responsible for her grandchildren. She organizes visits and gives advice with family problems. Ralph participates in family visits as a quiet observer. When asked for advice, he will answer. Sometimes, he gets irritable about the children's activity level and makes some sarcastic remark, to which Betty quickly responds in a reconciliatory way by telling Ralph that this is just how children are. Every day the young son spends his free time with a girlfriend. He hardly takes part in the usual rhythm of the family. He comes home late, rarely eats with the parents, and brings his girlfriend to eat over without previous announcement. Betty seems to understand his need for space and adjusts by always cooking something extra, just in case. She also refrains from asking him about feelings or daily experiences, because he is closed up like his father. Ralph and his son have occasional differences of opinion that prompt them to argue. In such situations, Betty intervenes by setting them both straight.

Generally, the family is content with their daily life. In earlier years, Betty had resented Ralph's lack of involvement with the children and failure to take the initiative for the planning of family activities. She does no longer expect these things but instead feels grateful for Ralph's affection. Their sexual life seems gratifying as well, as Betty states that Ralph is tender, considerate of her feelings, and has never laid eyes on another woman. Recently, Betty has difficulties dealing with Ralph's sour mood, which she hoped would dissipate eventually. She cannot understand why Ralph cannot pull out of it and experiences problems with self-control. When she gets irritated, she gets tempted to let him have it also.

Coherence. Ralph has the effect of a foreign body among the younger members of the family. It is well known what topics are of interest to him and those are the only ones addressed in his presence. Ralph's children were always expected to behave in ways that please Ralph, and today they resent that they were never allowed to really be themselves. Family interactions are warmer and more relaxed in his absence. Betty masters tensions with a sense of humor. Ralph has the best relationship with his younger son.

Values that are stressed in the family are commitment to work, thoroughness, and industriousness, all purported by Ralph. Furthermore, it is undesirable to argue and fight and whoever loses self-control is considered weak. One tolerates inconveniences without protest, because they are part of life. Introduced by Betty is the belief that wishes and emotions should not be unloaded onto others and that it is everyone's duty to be content and in good spirits. To the nurse's question whether this might not lead to a certain pressure to act happy to satisfy the family, Betty states that she never thought of that possibility but wants to think about it.

Individuation. Individuation of the couple has been discussed previously. The younger members have always felt free to pursue the interests of their choice as long as they worked hard and applied themselves. The few friends of the family have similar attitudes and values and bring little incentive to explore new ideas. Betty, however, likes to read books that are meaningful and make her think about life. She is also excited to hear about her elder son's experiences with a political office he has taken on in his township and discuss his ideas.

System Change. Despite Ralph's resistance, the family has found ways to introduce change. The elder son acts as consultant to Betty in situations in which she sees a need for change, but the younger son takes his father's side in promoting no change. This grouping seems to promote an equilibrium in the power structure and can be seen as positive, even though change becomes more difficult. Betty and the elder son usually circumvent the two and plan a strategy of influencing Ralph to loosen his resistance without noticing and making him believe that he has initiated the change. Ralph and the younger son become agreeable when they notice positive effects of the change. The present situation is a threat to all. The children and grandmother are worried about Betty even more than about Ralph, wondering whether she will hold up under the pressure of this illness.

Assessment of Family Health

The family process has worked for years and Betty sees no need for change. Control needs to be achieved to regain congruence. System maintenance entails an adjustment of behavioral rules and family roles to the situation as well as a compromise of individual wishes. Betty is the key to controlling the family operation, decision making, planning care, and coordinating the tasks. Financial planning, so far Ralph's function, is now in Betty's hands as well. With Ralph being absent, shifts in family operation can take place. The roles of the other family members are supportive and serve family coherence more than system maintenance. Coherence has always been compromised because the family is divided into two camps but the division serves the purpose of support while the family struggles to gain individuation. Incentives for new attitudes and values come from Betty and the elder son. Most of these are countered by Ralph and the younger son, but some leave an impact and encourage Betty to continue. Figure 11.1c shows that processes of all dimensions are present. The family members are fairly satisfied with their family and evaluate their congruence and family health as sufficient. Consequently, together with the nurse, they decide to use the existing family processes in enhancing Ralph's systemic process.

Nursing Care

The nurse asks Betty and her sons to think about Ralph's systemic process by using the diagram showing Ralph's usual pattern in Figure 11.1a and his crisis in Figure 11.1b. They discuss how Ralph could be supported in finding coherence in accepting that he means a lot to the family. The nurse promises Betty to help her discuss the situation with Ralph on her next visit. After the conference, he informs Ralph that Betty is very worried about him because he means a lot to her. At home, Betty prompts the younger son to write a short letter. Ralph receives the letter 2 days later and is happy to learn that his son misses him.

When Betty visits again, Ralph is feeling better and is ready to be transferred to a step-down unit. The nurse joins the two as promised. Betty starts by telling Ralph that although she was discussing the family with the nurse, she started realizing how devastated Ralph must have felt as the plans for building a home fell through. As Ralph appears to contemplate the situation, Betty adds that she is aware of the fact that he had intended to build the home to please her. She does not feel that he is at fault for not succeeding. Instead, she suggests that the two of them need a new start after this difficult time. Betty continues by stating that she has been terribly worried about losing him and asks Ralph whether he does not agree that they are very lucky. The fact that they have detected the cancer before it was too late and that Ralph and she can now continue on together is more important than money or a new home. Ralph replies that he had actually thought about this and is glad that the house was not built, because she now has the money available just in case he should die. Betty, touched by his concern for her, starts to cry. The nurse leaves the room as the two hold hands.

Evaluation

The nurse is astonished how little he needed to contribute to the process. His assumption that the family was strong enough to find its own solution was right. He has helped the family to resolve the crisis by suggesting to explore its life process. The solution has not occurred as expected. Surprisingly, Ralph had taken steps toward his own individuation by shifting priorities and recognizing how much his family cares. He can now contribute by caring for them, thereby gaining back his coherence through spirituality. His disease has brought his personal crisis to a culmination, whereby he was jolted into understanding that his life process was in need of change. His connectedness with Betty gave him the strength to search for options. The solution appeared to him natural and simple, and he wondered why he could not think of this before. He feels free of guilt and is ready to look at life as something to be enjoyed.

Suddenly, Ralph is ready to move on. In the step-down unit he wants to see his colostomy and shows interest in its function. He lets Betty see it as well and they both learn about colostomy care and make plans for his discharge. Their sense of being in this together gives them the strength to accept the uncertainty of the diagnosis.

This example describes a family in crisis. Difficulties had persisted for some time. For years, Ralph's rigidity had been a problem for the family. Although Betty was extraordinarily accommodating, she felt at a loss as Ralph reacted to his disappointment about the building project with anger and depression without being able to accept it. Instead of acknowledging that the unsuccessful venture was just a misfortune and that there is more to life (system change), he persisted in the value of being obligated to provide and secure a new home for Betty (system maintenance), which generated the belief that he was miserably failing. As in any crisis, Ralph ceased to grow and perceive alternative options. This developmental crisis was carried over to the family level. Betty's ingenious methods of making Ralph examine his values and individuate failed miserably. Family life patterns experienced tension and incongruence that again affected Ralph and created a vicious cycle. Whether Ralph's incongruence weakened his immune system and allowed the cancer to develop cannot be determined. However, it became clear to the nurse that his surgery was not the only thing needed by Ralph to regain health.

The nursing process according to the framework of systemic organization differs from conventional approaches. Nurses are usually trained to think in a linear fashion. Had the nurse in the example been less insightful, he would have assessed Ralph as being in denial and in need of accepting his diagnosis. He would have given Ralph information about his surgery, his progress, and his prognosis, trying hard to get Ralph to look at his future as being hopeful. He would have given Betty information as well and encouraged her to cheer up Ralph. All these approaches would have been based on the situation of the disease taken out of the context of Ralph's real-life situation. Ralph was not a good patient. Hospital expectations wanted him to be more assertive, self-directed, and in charge of his own care much sooner. Responding to those values, the nurse would have coerced him into self-care without addressing the motives for his lack of initiative. Ralph's response would have been frustration about being misunderstood and a still stronger sense of worthlessness. Increased anger might have made Betty's communication with him difficult as well.

Instead of assuming that there is a general approach to each disease entity, the nurse entered into the situation without preconceived opinions. He encouraged Ralph's self-care, not in terms of making him participate in his own hygiene, but by letting him take charge of directing his own healing. Obviously, Ralph had no knowledge about medical treatments or a desire to influence them, but he sensed the nurse's genuine interest in going along with him without pushing him. Trust in his nurse gave him the courage to bring up his major concern, his wife. What followed was a response to the situation as it unfolded gradually.

There are many possibilities to employ the framework of systemic organization in acute care. Mirr (1991) stresses that families in crisis are particularly open to influence by the nurse, but Simpson (1991) warns that no intervention serves for all families. What is helpful to some may be upsetting to others, depending on their perception of the situation. Consequently, there is a need for aesthetic knowledge or knowledge revealed as a result of experiencing the client's situation subjectively, as it was first described by Caper (1978). According to Bournaki and Germain (1993), the process of gaining this knowledge is the art of nursing. The knowledge unfolds as the nurse immerses herself or himself in the situation and then ponders the meaning and interprets it by drawing from assessment data and his or her own life experience. The nurse uses intuition in detecting the essential, trusts his or her own experience of the situation, and expresses it to the family. Consistent with the process of individuation leading to spirituality and with the nursing process described in Chapter 2, "the nurse transcends her or his own existing aesthetic knowledge, and new knowledge emerges in the art/act" (Bournaki & Germain, 1993, p. 85). Although it may be difficult for novices to have intuition and trust it, the framework of systemic organization may be a useful teaching tool to increase awareness of the uniqueness of the situation of clients and their family and gradually increase self-confidence.

With expertise, time is no hindering factor, as aesthetic knowledge is gained almost instantly by responding to subtle cues. By the use of aesthetic knowledge, nurses actually save time in that they elicit the right questions and focus the assessment on essentials without going astray. Nursing based on human values and the need for spirituality in the life process is all the more important, because families are faced with difficult decisions referring to treatment and care, finances, and ethical issues. They need access to a nurse they can trust, information and help with thinking through such decisions, and sorting out their emotions (Mirr, 1991). Caine (1991) suggests that technical practice can be transformed into caring practice through which nurses make a difference in the lives of families and patients and gain the insight that their caring can make the difference. Such is the process of individuation.

In summary, nursing care is a combination of acts directed to assist the life processes of patient and family. Clearly, Ralph's need was great in the area of system maintenance. The nurse cannot neglect to make plans for discharge, teaching Ralph and Betty necessary procedures and setting up a support system at home to meet Ralph's physical needs. Although these nursing acts promote the reestablishment of stability and control for Ralph and the family, a need for growth and spirituality was found essential in building the foundation for a healthy family process. In fact, without strong coherence and a new way of prioritizing the various facets of life through individuation, the relationship between Betty and Ralph would have been strained and the quality of caregiving at home jeopardized. The example describes a crisis resolution that is likely to promote new resources to be built in the family's system maintenance for use in future times.

The nurse's contribution to the solution appeared minor, because the family process seemed to have just waited for the push to start moving. Although this may be true, the key to expert nursing is the art of perceiving when the time is ripe to make the move. Ralph's subtle, unexpected move instantly revealed to the nurse the urgency of the issue. How easy it is to pass over such a subtle clue! Thus, the major barrier to excellence in nursing care is not the availability of time but a lack of the nurse's aesthetic knowledge. Aesthetic knowledge is demonstrated by the ability to let the personal systemic pattern be touched by the client's rhythm and pattern and to find harmony between the two.

12

Families and the Crisis of Death

The process of spirituality described earlier is the essence of nursing in the endstage of a human life, more so than in any other situation. There is a dire need for superior nursing care in all stages of life, but even more so in the last months of a person's life, in which physical processes deteriorate and many serious symptoms present grave difficulties to patient and family.

It is estimated that in addition to the patient, between 1 and 7 million family members are deeply affected every year by the transformation of their family system due to death. Yet this nation still slumbers in intense denial of the finality of human existence and steers its resources toward research and advanced technology to prolong life. Expertise in nursing care preparing the client for death has almost vanished (Lillard & Marietta, 1989).

Referring to the situation in hospitals during the 1960s, Glaser and Strauss (1965) described the "social death" of clients that occurred before the actual cessation of life, because clients in the endstage were geographically moved from the center of activities and avoided by nurses who were afraid to communicate with them out of fear that the topic of death might be raised. This process of isolation was intensified by family members who pretended against the patient's better knowledge that everything would be fine and thus inhibited any productive

214

communication and release of emotions. Today, expert care is delivered in hospice settings and other specialized units with highly qualified staff. Yet the majority of people still die in general hospital units and, what is worse, in nursing homes under the care of nonprofessional staff. One observes an alarming trend of endstage clients being transferred to less expensive facilities, only to die a few days later. As long as success in nursing is defined as cure of the disease along the paradigm patterned and controlled by medicine, nurses find little satisfaction in assisting dying patients. They feel helpless if they cannot improve the patient's physical condition, even more so if they work in a nursing home, in which an atmosphere of despair by far outweighs the spirit of hope.

Nurses who enjoy working with the dying client are considered odd by many others who wonder how long it will take them to burn out. Nevertheless, nurses who love their work with the terminally ill do exist. These individuals experience personal growth instead of burnout. Key to their thriving are acceptance and understanding of death as a natural human process and a focus on life and living opportunities as targets for spirituality.

Fear of death is central to all people. Rollo May (1977) suggested that fear of death can never be conquered directly, because humans do not simply have the fear—their fear is built into their very existence and presents itself as the driving force in everyday life. A parallel to this, within the framework of systemic organization, is the concept of ultimate congruence that can never be reached, because the human system is finite, whereas universal order is not. Thus, the human body is a hindrance to achieving a permanent union with universal order and the incongruence remains a source of anxiety.

Stephen Levine (1989), who has taught workshops together with Kübler-Ross and has embraced Buddhist principles in his quest for answers, explains that the agony of death involves mainly the vanishing of our image of who we are. He explains that this image is a mind structure often called identity, ego, or self- or body image. It constitutes a person's coherence, as the framework of systemic organization defines it, and is developed over a lifetime and believed to be real. Based on the illusion that the human physical existence is the only reality, the defense of this mind structure becomes the ulterior motive of the human life process and necessitates the denial of physical vulnerability and death. However, this mind structure has to be dissolved to gain victory over death. Individuals who are able to remain healthy when shaken by symptoms of failing physical processes are seen to prepare for death as their thoughts, feelings, and experiences with which they have defined themselves disappear in vastness, thereby revealing the nature of the true self experienced as a phenomenon of the flow of lasting energy. Consequently, death experienced as life loses its sting, and the separateness of the imagined self dissolves into a oneness with an all-encompassing reality to be revealed (Levine, 1989).

Other writers similarly describe death as a process of transition (Benoliel, 1987; Parks, 1975). For example, Parks (1975) explains that in the process of dying, a certain set of values and beliefs is exchanged for another. This carries an astonishing resemblance to the system change process that I have described. If one assumes there is an immortal spirit in each person, the framework of systemic organization points to the proposition that death constitutes the ultimate system change and challenge through which individuals become liberated from the barriers imposed by the value and belief structure that is bound to Earth and underlies their life process. Through death, the human system can shed its physical limitations and open up its structure to expand its process and find ultimate congruence that allows the flow of its energy to become one with the universal order.

It is difficult to visualize the process of overcoming the fear of death in any other way than through spirituality or religion in its ancient sense. As Beck (1989) explains, the original meaning of religion is derived from the Latin verb *religare,* which means to bind back or to bind man and the gods. Thus, it seems to express the human longing to be part of a greater order to which one is allowed to return after death. Nurses experienced in working with the dying report that they observe a power of healing before death, as the suffering clients suddenly become calm and serene in awaiting their end. This seems to mark the end of an individuation process triggered by a long chain of losses and the breakage point at which vanity and self-deception are irreversibly shattered. Painful crises and reconciliation with many losses seem to be necessary constituents of this maturation process through which individuals experience gradual system change, and their coherence gradually takes on a fluid structure without boundaries.

To be able to experience the agony of the dying without being deeply disconcerted, nurses need to reconcile themselves with their own death. Such nurses acknowledge their anxieties as they arise inevitably in proportion to their sense of helplessness. They focus away from the client's rapid disintegration to the mystery of life. They discover life in the process of dying and health in the midst of physical deterioration. The discovery is not a philosophical abstraction but an intense personal experience, an individuation process that unfolds within a spiritual systemic union with a dying client. Consequently, the individuation and growth experienced by their clients become their own and enrich their own existence. In fact, nurses are given the opportunity to break their denial of death and prepare themselves for their own final transition if they accept the wisdom of their clients in guiding them through their own gradual system change. Nurses courageous enough to embark on such a journey, while working in an environment without hope for cure, will not only sustain their energy but experience a healing force that will enrich their daily lives. The following example illustrates the above.

Harry F., comatose, was transferred to a single room to die. He is 46 years old, tall, and rather emaciated. Long strands of his gray hair are spread over the pillow. He was admitted with severe internal injuries after attempting to end his life under a train. Two days ago, his condition seemed to improve, but now he suffers from septicemia, a high fever, and periodic convulsions. This last accident was his third attempt to commit suicide. Harry had been depressed for years; his medical history cites two psychiatric hospitalizations. Harry was a drifter without family or reliable contacts. Nothing more about his life is known.

The nurse has concluded her a.m. care. Harry's respirations are labored with intermittent accelerations and periods of apnea lasting a seemingly eternal 2 to 3 seconds. The nurse notices gurgling sounds from his trachea; his face is tense, almost contorted, and his mouth is wide open. The nurse senses an almost irresistible urge to run, but at the same time, something within her holds her back and leaves her dazzled. Her anxiety is acute; she feels her coronary arteries pulsate and her hands are icy. Harry's breath resounds in the hollow room, and with each pause it threatens to give up. The nurse cannot tolerate the sound of it and starts to talk while she watches him intensely. "Mr. F., why is it that you die here all by yourself? Where is your family? I can't leave you here all alone." After a sudden twitch of his arms and hands, Harry suddenly relaxes and his breath sounds more shallow and even. The nurse grasps his hand—as cold as hers. "I'll stay with you, don't be afraid, your pain will be over soon." At this time, thoughts are rushing through her mind: *Strange, I don't know this man, but it feels like he is a friend. He wants to tell me something—I shouldn't be afraid. Weird, why am I not afraid any more? I wish I knew about his life. I wonder if he thinks about it? Maybe he is happy to die. Did he really never have anybody who loved him? He cannot be such a bad person to deserve that. Or was he some kind of genius or prophet misunderstood and despised by people?* The nurse looks at him intensely and feels far removed; she doesn't know where. Outside, she hears the chirping of a bird and she feels Harry's hand twitch again. She thinks, *What is it he wants to tell me? If I had to die like him, I would miss my life—all my friends. He wants to keep me here. This is like the "Princess and the Frog"; the ugly frog, in whom there is some hidden beauty. Mr. F., you will soon wake up in your wonderful kingdom.* Without realizing it, she bends down and kisses him softly on the cheek. Harry releases a deep sigh and pulls back his hand. His breath stops and his muscles relax. "Have a good journey, Mr. F.," the nurse says and a tear rolls down her face.

This nurse experienced the healing power of death and was personally touched by it. The 10 minutes in Harry's room have made her a different person. Something happened to her, because she allowed herself to experience it and, as a result, her fear of death disappeared temporarily. The process that Jean Watson (1985) calls *presencing* may have occurred here in that the nurse has allowed herself to experience the diffusion of boundaries between herself and the client, which gave rise to a deep meaning difficult to express in words. Possibly, Harry granted her a glimpse of universal order. In-depth conversations with dying clients, as Kübler-Ross (1969) describes them, may be possible only in ideal situations. This example shows, however, that a systemic connection can take place without words. Individuation occurred as the nurse observed Harry's subtle responses and her own and became aware of the life energy radiated by the dying person that touched her own self. The physical cues made the nurse believe that individuation took place in Harry's system as well and that she may have been part of it. It made her wonder if she had replaced the family he had lost years ago. She realized that one of the noblest roles a nurse can assume is that of a "sister" or "mother," or a "brother" or "father," for clients who need this type of human congruence as a bridge to connect with the universal order.

Death is not always a beautiful experience. Staff in the emergency room are fully aware of its cruelty. On many occasions, patients have no time to prepare for death; on others, the heroic procedures employed by the hospital staff to maintain the patients' lives prevent them from getting ready to die. Other patients are unwilling to let go of life and suffer immense anger and pain to the very end. However, no one is equipped to fully understand death and no one can tell what system change takes place in the last moment of life.

Surviving family members resort to explanations that offer comfort to them through religious beliefs or personal philosophies. If nurses are to be helpful to grieving families, they must attempt access to the unique world of these families—their thoughts and their explanations—and guide the families to find meaning congruent with their life process. Effective nurses are keenly vigilant of their own reactions to the situation, intercept the interference of personal beliefs and values, and refrain from offering solutions that are not in tune with the families' perceptions.

Maureen stands at the bed of her dead child, 9-year-old Amanda, in a children's hospital at a large medical center. Motionless, Maureen looks like a ghost, her skin almost transparent. During the past 2 months, she has spent every afternoon in the hospital, slept there often, and went to work in the local bank every morning. She needs her part-time income to survive, because her husband had left her for a better life with another woman. Maureen reported that he had suffered great pains about Amanda's illness and was looking for a way out. Amanda's leukemia was diagnosed 3 years ago. It was not a typical case, and Amanda's body responded poorly to chemotherapy. Now Amanda has given up the fight. She was astonishingly mature for her age, tolerated her pains, and tried to console Maureen. Just before she died, she said, "It won't hurt anymore. Soon, you will come to visit me and we'll play together like before. Don't be sad, it will be all right." Maureen had been so strong, and the nurse admired her. Now, she appears dangerously fragile, and immense pain is reflected by her posture and facial features. The nurse has learned several facts about Maureen that she now recapitulates silently.

Assessment of the Individual

System Maintenance. Maureen structures her life and plans her activities very carefully. She is physically healthy and proud that she hardly ever has to see a doctor. She has complained of problems, however, of not being able to go to sleep or waking up from bad dreams. Despite being tired, she does high-quality work at the bank and has never let her problems interfere with her performance. Work is Maureen's life. She is highly regarded because she is willing to do more than the usual assignments, taking work home if there is a need. Her simple apartment is always clean and orderly. Maureen has not taken a vacation for 4 years and hardly knows how to relax. She does not have time for reading books or attending shows or concerts—activities she used to enjoy in the past.

Coherence and Individuation. Religion has not been very important in Maureen's life. It seems, however, that her relationship with Amanda had taken on a spiritual quality. Maureen seemed to have found in Amanda those parts of herself that she had neglected: spontaneity, beauty, purity, and artistic expression. Complemented by Amanda, Maureen felt whole. As she suffered with Amanda, she felt alive and human, but she came across rather detached and cold with other people, even her extended family. Once, Maureen admitted to the nurse that she felt kind of afraid and alone, because there was so much cruelty around her, and she always had to fight to keep above water.

Assessment of Individual Health

For obvious reasons, it is inappropriate for the nurse to discuss the systemic diagram with Maureen during this time of crisis. Consequently, nursing actions are planned on the basis of previously assessed data and knowledge about death and grieving. The nurse has no knowledge about Maureen's ability to make necessary system changes. The assessment data, however, help her to deduce some hypotheses in relation to Maureen's life process: It seems that Maureen uses much energy to suppress anxiety by controlling and regulating her life. She adheres to structure out of fear of losing integrity. Because stability is of such great importance, the likelihood that system change is difficult for Maureen is great. Work tends to stabilize Maureen's life. In fact, one could imagine a desperate crisis if the opportunity to work was lost. The nurse visualizes bottomless despair, because Maureen has lost that which allows her to be fully human and supplements her congruence. The path to healing will be the search for a new kind of individuation, but how can she do that?

Figure 12.1 shows Maureen's diagram before Amanda's death, as the nurse envisions it. Predominant is system maintenance. Coherence is nourished by achievement at work and supplemented by her emotional bond with Amanda, providing her access to the wonders of life and her own spiritual being. Individuation and system change occurred mainly through the relationship with Amanda. The question arises whether Amanda is truly dead for Maureen. Could she not continue to serve as a source of inspiration and individuation in the time to come?

Assessment of the Family

In the search for an answer, the nurse recalls what she knows about Maureen's family: The members in Maureen's family are equally structured, industrious, disciplined, and emotionally rather detached. They share the values of independence, competence, and the need to excel that constitute the basis of family coherence. Maureen has been considered a misfit ever since she married a musician. But she was not alone. Her rebellious younger brother was ostracized when he persisted on an acting career and was engaged in homosexual relationships. His creative talents were never recognized. Maureen, however, has kept up communication because she feels drawn to him as the most sensitive member of her family. Thus, he has visited with her during Amanda's illness. Maureen has told of occasions when he was able to distract Amanda when she was in pain and make her laugh. Her brother had many of the same characteristics as her ex-husband. Like him, he can create a world of dreams, immerse himself in it, and forget the other reality. Maureen has often

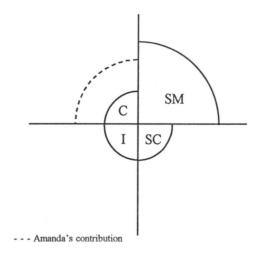

- - - Amanda's contribution

Figure 12.1. Systemic Process of Maureen

envied both men for this ability she could have used so well. She has never worked through her pain about the divorce and still misses her husband.

Maureen's parents set the tone in the family, and according to them, Maureen has invoked her own misery. There was little compassion about her difficult times. Maureen feels cheated, misunderstood, and mistreated. The capacity of individuation within the family of origin is very limited. Maureen and her brother, however, have formed a viable subsystem in which growth is possible. It is ruled by a set of values separate from the rest of their family that provides them with a distinct identity. This identity has also been shared with Amanda, and Amanda has contributed by seeing in Maureen's brother a substitute father. Could it not be possible to let Amanda live on as a link that unites the two and gives them a shared purpose?

Nursing Care

As the nurse contemplates what she knows about Maureen, it occurs to her that at the moment, Maureen needs a chance to free that part within herself that feels and can grow, the part that causes excruciating pain but at the same time has the capacity to connect and find comfort. Realizing her own fear and the danger that her fear may inhibit a free flow of systemic energy, she recognizes the need for an environment in which Maureen and the nurse could find each other. She invites Maureen for a short walk along the wooded path on the hospital premises. That would give the staff a chance to dress Amanda and make her look pretty for Maureen to say good-bye before she is taken away.

Maureen follows the nurse, hardly realizing where she is going. The two walk silently, until they reach the trees. Suddenly, a little mouse scurries across their path. "Did you see the mouse? Amanda would have been so excited; she was crazy about little animals," Maureen exclaims. "I know," states the nurse quietly, "I brought her a little stuffed bunny and a dog to cuddle with in the unit, and she was so happy. It must really hurt to think of these things right now." Maureen looks pitifully lost and starts to cry softly. Looking at her, the nurse is compelled to hug her. Maureen in turn clings to her sobbing, her body contracting in rhythmical contortions. After some time, Maureen relaxes, and they sit down on a large tree stump. Wiping her own tears, the nurse remarks, "I will miss Amanda, too. She was such a happy child who could cheer us all up." "Now, her pains are gone. She was looking forward to that," Maureen replies. Then they talk for awhile. Maureen confesses that she made Amanda's life difficult by arguing with her ex-husband, but then adds that Amanda was always understanding and did not hold anything against her. The nurse confirms this and tells Maureen how much she has admired her motherly dedication and her insightful communication with the child.

Back in the hospital, Maureen says good-bye to Amanda. She feels exhausted but relieved. The nurse remarks that she does not think that Maureen should go home alone and asks her if she knows somebody who could stay with her for a day or two. Maureen replies that this is unnecessary. Thinking about her brother's role in the family system, the nurse wonders if Maureen has told him about Amanda's death. When Maureen answers negatively, the nurse offers to call him and Maureen accepts. On the phone, her brother asks to talk to Maureen, and the two have a lengthy conversation between tears. Then, Maureen reports to the nurse that her brother will pick her up at the hospital and spend the night with her.

Nursing care has helped Maureen to initiate the process of system change by allowing her to experience grief and thereby recognize the loss as reality. Maureen realizes that Amanda has become a part of herself and that she can help her see herself as a whole person even now. The sense of purpose Maureen has gained through Amanda is not actually lost but lives on as long as Amanda is remembered, and Maureen's brother can help to keep the remembrance alive. The system change needed involves an incorporation of those things that Maureen learned and experienced within the spiritual union with Amanda permanently into her coherence, thereby freeing energy previously used to maintain the union and invest it in new individuation. This is a lengthy process marked by periods of insight and growth and recurrent setbacks. Often, the energy of a tight bond is difficult to set free, because the surviving person clings to the "ghost" of the deceased to bring back what was lost, a process that reduces pain initially but eliminates the potential for growth and healing over time.

Healthy grief is difficult to describe, because it becomes part of a person's life process and, accordingly, follows a highly individualistic path. Davies, Chekryn-Reimer, and Martens (1990), who studied the experience of families with a member dying of cancer, conceptualized their adjustment to the death as a transition that is described as "fading away." Families mentioned themes relative to three basic tasks within the adjustment process: acknowledging the ending, getting through a neutral zone, and setting out on a new beginning. This suggests that, like the dying member, families experience system change in which the crisis makes evident the need to redefine roles and family coherence. The old orientation has to give way to preparing for the future. As the death occurs, the families enter a confusing reality of pain and emptiness, within which they struggle to find meaning as a basis for change. Finally, a new beginning arises slowly, as the remembrance of the dead member's physical existence "fades away" and allows something positive to emerge from the experience. In an expanded study, the same authors also describe guidelines for nurses but stress the fact that families differ greatly in the methods and the time frame they use in adjusting. Some families have difficulties for many years and others never overcome them. Consequently, it is misleading to portray normative behaviors or grieving periods. The success of the grieving process at a given time, however, can be estimated from the intensity and frequency of anxiety and pain family members still experience. One needs to keep in mind, however, that painful memories are integrated in each person's life process and become reactivated periodically, depending on mood and external circumstances, and it may take a long time for these memories to fade away. Nevertheless, when grief consumes individuation and growth over an extended period of time, a chronic crisis situation will have destructive effects on the system.

Good nursing care throughout the process of dying has the potential to assist the family in using strategies that promote growth and prevent destruction. The findings of several studies of families in the hospital setting suggest that family members prefer to focus all of their attention on the maintenance of the patient's system and expect the nurse to do likewise (Hull, 1989; McGinnis, 1986; Molter, 1979). Rando (1984) suggests that families are in the best position to prevent their ill member's social death by giving the afflicted person opportunities to be useful and appreciated to the very end. Nurses offer information about the patient and the process of dying to enhance system maintenance: information about expected physical symptoms, psychosocial needs, and ways to preserve the patient's dignity.

In a highly technical environment, family members may feel anxious, intimidated, and on the verge of losing self-control. Sharing feelings with the nurse and individuation seem difficult. Hull (1991) stresses a sensitive approach that refrains from pressuring families to ventilate feelings but instead respects the need to maintain composure. Without a preestablished base of trust, loss of composure may signify loss of dignity to most people. In contrast to an acute care setting, nurses involved with families over a longer time period, in their homes or through a hospice program, are viewed differently. Nurses are welcomed as consultants if they assist the families in remaining in charge of the family process and the care they provide. Family members expect such nurses to ease their burden and consequently rate their effective support as important as professional competence and the provision of information (Hull, 1991).

In anticipation of death, nurses are advised to explore the families' readiness for change. By discussing previous losses with the family, they help them foresee changes without destroying hope. Nurses allow families to verbalize or otherwise express their fears and plan with them a course of action tailored to their unique needs and abilities to make changes (Chekryn-Reimer, Davies, & Martens, 1991). Consequently, the stage is set to start the healing process immediately after the death. Families who trust their nurses may want to use them as resources for information about their own adjustment process as they search for meaning and attempt to "normalize" the experience (Chekryn-Reimer et al., 1991).

Crises of death are resolved like other serious disruptions. In healthy families, members are observed to assist each other through words and gestures in strengthening their own coherence and finding acceptable solutions. In distinguishing between healthy families and those who need assistance, it is of prime importance that nurses notice signs indicating that family members are distancing themselves instead of pulling together and that individuation is impaired. Such cues suggest that the system's coherence may be in disarray. Nurses need to focus their attention on persons who are anxious, depressed, or angry about their situation; dwell on injustice and unfairness; or blame themselves or others for their pain. Nurses seek to gain the trust of such clients and encourage them to search for a new purpose and new ways of interpreting their situation.

Nevertheless, even excellent nursing care is often rejected by families who are not ready to make changes, and empathic patience is not always rewarded with trust and willingness to be helped. Ultimately, it is the clients' own responsibility to break down the defenses that uphold a no longer functional stability.

In summary, nursing care of families suffering a death involves understanding the very special way the family moves in its life process and guiding the individuals in their search for a new congruence. As nurses open up their own system and enter into a union with their clients, changes can take place and growth occurs in both nurses and clients. In a highly technical environment, such care may be difficult but is sorely needed. Nurses should realize that an open heart may actually keep time commitments to a minimum in that an atmosphere of trust facilitates the family's cooperation in the nursing process. Furthermore, nurses do what is ethically right, gain satisfaction from their actions, and strengthen their own coherence.

13

Families With Chronically Ill Members

This chapter focuses on the process of system change induced or in-fluenced by a chronic condition that imposes limitations on the func-tioning of one or more family members. For the theoretical description of this phenomenon, several issues of importance are described. The first involves the long-term developmental nature of the change pro-cess, in which afflicted individuals, primary caregivers, and families are engaged. The second issue concerns the needs and expectations of individuals and families that may differ significantly with those of health care professionals. This is closely related to the final issue dis-cussed here, namely, the gradual substitution of informal care through outside resources, formal programs, and, ultimately, institutionaliza-tion, a process that often threatens the autonomy of patient and family.

The Process of Acceptance

The onset of a chronic condition may be abrupt as in the case of an acute illness or an accidental injury of a family member or the birth of a child afflicted with a congenital defect. In contrast, conditions such as hypertension, multiple sclerosis, some cancers, or AIDS may have an insidious onset that delays their diagnosis. Typically, at some point in time, however, the afflicted individual is subjected to a battery of diagnostic procedures and suffers the shock of a diagnosis that signifies a projection of that person's future chances or lack thereof. Experiences of patients and reactions of families to the shock of a sudden illness were described in Chapter 11. If the diagnosis spells out future difficulties and limitations, however, the initial acute phase marks only the beginning of a long chain of losses (Lego, 1994). These losses concern the level of physical functioning and, perhaps more important, the emotional well-being or coherence of the person. Even under the best possible circumstances, such as a total remission of a cancer, people of all ages have reported persistent psychological problems based on uncertainty and fear of symptom recurrence that have an impact on normal psychosocial development and the quality of life (Fritz & Williams, 1988; Greenberg, Kazak, & Meadows, 1989).

Most researchers and clinical experts in the field explain the patient's adjustment to chronic illness in terms of a coping process. From this perspective, they view loss-related difficulties as stress, a negative force to which the individual is subjected. From the medical perspective, a successful outcome of the coping process signifies survival or stabilization of symptoms. A large number of studies on coping with chronic illnesses focus on such outcomes. For example, cancer patients have been found to survive longer if they actively dealt with their disease and expressed their anger (Cohen, 1984) or if they refused to succumb and denied their symptoms (Pettingale, Morris, Greer, & Haybittle, 1985). In contrast, patients with poorer chances of survival suffered from resignation and hopelessness (Lewis & Bloom, 1979) or from insecurity and self-pity (Borysenko, 1984). These studies do not present any information about the quality of life of the survivors or the health of their systemic process. The medical and stress-coping models generally assume that patients should fight their disease as long as possible. This view tends to disregard the full complexity of the experience by omitting aspects, such as pain, grief, or healing (Brown & Powell-Cope, 1993), or the acceptance of the condition.

Acceptance of illness, seemingly the opposite of the previously described struggle against disease, has been found crucial in promoting mental health (Pruchno & Resch, 1989). Most stress-coping researchers have conceptualized acceptance of illness as just another coping mechanism and thus have failed to reconcile its apparent contradiction with symptom control. A reconciliation of the two poles is possible using the framework of systemic organization.

Within this framework, the person who wants to find health has to become cognizant of the organic dysfunction by experiencing discomfort or illness. Eisenberg (1977) clarified the terms by explaining that patients suffer and experience their illness, whereas the physician diagnoses the disease. That is, when experiencing illness, the person grows by owning, living, and taking on full responsibility for health (Kotarba, 1983). Because health involves the subjective experience of the total life process, it includes illness. Consequently, a successful outcome of the struggle with chronic illness signifies the management of life with illness that results in congruence, low anxiety, and therefore quality of life (Ragsdale, Kotarba, & Morrow, 1992).

Managing the symptoms and accepting the discomfort and losses are not contradictions. Instead, the two processes are directed toward two different targets, spirituality and control, that are pursued at the same time. The afflicted person needs to regain coherence through an individuation process that leads to system change or a redefinition of values and self-concept. Stated differently, acceptance occurs through activation of the target of spirituality that results in subsequent shifts within the control target and movement toward a new balance. Spiritual well-being, according to Vaughan (1986), becomes evident through a sense of inner peace, appreciation of life, and compassion for others, and it is expressed through actions and emotions (Stoll, 1989).

The emotional aspects of acceptance seem to be embedded in the search for meaning. Although perception and appraisal of stressful events are integral parts of coping models (Lazarus & Folkman, 1984a; Silver & Wortman, 1980), in a holistic view, meaning is derived from connectedness and a sense of belonging. For example, Andrews, Williams, and Neil (1993, p. 197) describe the relationship of HIV-positive mothers to their children in terms of an "engagement with the world," and a sense of purpose through finding a balance between attachment and loss, hope and despair, and engagement and withdrawal. This vividly describes the dynamic nature of the person's constant spiritual struggle to find connectedness and growth, an ongoing developmental process of learning, self-reflection, and redefinition of the self.

Actions related to acceptance of the illness seem to be those that Ragsdale et al. (1992), in their phenomenological study of persons with AIDS, found to be the management of practical problems associated with the illness. Although these behaviors strive toward the target of control, the same behaviors provide the average person in this achievement-oriented society with a sense of accomplishment and pride that supports coherence and self-worth.

Without acceptance, the chronically ill person views the disease as an enemy to be fought with bitterness, hatred, and anger. Because of the futility of the struggle, emotional energy is drained and depleted, leaving the person exhausted and unable to find enjoyment in life. This leads to the second issue mentioned at the beginning of this chapter—the expectations of the health care system that often stand in contrast to the client's needs for healing.

Differing Expectations

Within the health care system, the afflicted person is not encouraged to own the health problem. Instead, the patients are excused from performing their roles as before and expected to follow the physician's regime to recover with minimal disability (Wynne, Shields, & Sirkin, 1992). Hofland (1988) describes the patients' loss of autonomy in a highly technical health care system, in which they are threatened to be left to their own devices if they do not cooperate. Physicians who define the patients' best interest take on a strongly paternalistic role that leaves patients without a chance for an open challenge (Cicirelli, 1992).

The issue of poor patient compliance with the prescribed regime has plagued the health care system for years. Grappling with the complexity of the issue, theoretical models such as the Fishbein Model (Ajzen & Fishbein, 1980) have incorporated attitudinal and social predictors of compliance. Although suggesting some linear causal relationships, research findings based on such models provide little insight into the diversity of patients' attitudes or the processes of maintaining or changing them. Furthermore, little is known about how families could become systems of support if they hinder acceptance or progress. Again, key to these basic questions seems to be the systemic process.

On the basis of the assumption that a threat to a system's process will trigger intensified striving toward the same targets (more of the same behaviors) (Kantor & Lehr, 1975), compliant patients ascribe to the same values as the health care professionals who care for them. They agree with the goals set for them and take on the responsibility to contribute to their rehabilitation by teaming up with health care professionals in their fight against the disease and the minimization of symptoms. Despite their drastically different understanding of illness, nurses who work with the framework of systemic organization do not take an opposing stance to convert the patients' value system. Instead, they support their clients' life process as long as it leads to health but watch it for incongruence and sources of anxiety. If problems occur, nurses offer assistance and help the clients to examine the values and the need for system change.

In contrast to cooperative clients, noncompliant patients have differing expectations about their recovery. The conflict exists between expectations imposed by the health professionals and the patients' own need to find systemic congruence that relates to their specific life process. For example, the futility of prescribing strict diets to persons who are addicted to overeating is well documented. These persons misdirect their attempt to find connectedness or spirituality to food and eating, because they seek relief from the pain of feeling isolated. The removal of their target of addiction creates a void in their life process that cannot be tolerated over time without being replaced (see Part 3 of this book). A similar conflict may hold true for cardiac patients who have maintained their coherence solely by power and influence within their position at work. Feeling weak, sick, and unable to work after a myocardial infarction is likely to present a devastating blow to their self-image. If the patients have never learned to build coherence and self-worth through another type of connectedness, for example, mutually respecting and giving human relationships or a relationship with nature, system change will be difficult. These persons are in danger of engaging in self-destructive denial of their physical limitations to revert to their old lifestyle and exercise of power for the purpose of gratification.

Nursing of noncompliant clients is difficult. In many instances, systemic needs to return to the old lifestyle and the concomitant lack of acceptance of the illness are stronger than the threat of debility or death. Without consideration of the person's entire life process, excessive behaviors or addictions included, the effect of health teaching is minimal. Likewise, the power of threatening descriptions of future disasters due to noncompliance is short-lived at best. Bribing the patient with rewards seems equally ineffective. Although the provision of information is a necessary prerequisite for change, change is no certain consequence. In fact, patients may refuse, ignore, or "forget" information, and they have a legal right to refuse treatment whether or not they have rationally contemplated their decision.

All of this points again to the complexity of the patient's systemic process. If information can become an agent of recovery through individuation and system change, the nurse must first gain a basic understanding of the patient's system maintenance, coherence, and the underlying values and beliefs. Furthermore, the function of the patient's family in the recovery process needs to be explored to engage the system in a supportive and reinforcing manner.

The three themes of this chapter—long-term change and development, the clash between expectations and the caregiving career, and the complementary nature of informal and formal caregiving—become especially vivid at the level of the family. The following example highlights the themes as well as the interface of the afflicted individual's life process and that of her family.

Edith, 80 years old, recently entered a nursing home. Three years ago she had a stroke that left her with hemiplegia and mild aphasia. Edith has never been married. Until she retired, she was a primary school teacher and actively involved in various social programs in her community. After retirement, she continued working for the Council on Education, serving as an adviser in issues of child socialization and early education. Removed from city traffic, she owned a condominium on the third floor of a large building, where she had a lovely view of a nearby mountain range. When her sister's husband died 10 years ago, her sister, Anna, moved in with her because the two women had always felt very close. Anna, too, had led a very active life until recently.

As Edith recovered from the stroke, she participated in an intensive rehabilitation program in a nursing home. She was an ideal patient with an incredible determination to learn walking with a cane and gain back her ability to speak fluently. Her days in the rehabilitation program were busy with physiotherapy, occupational therapy, and recreational activities. Edith got much encouragement from the staff who made her feel proud of her accomplishments. She learned to stand up and sit down, put on most of her clothing, shower independently, and walk from one end of the hall to the other. Speech therapy helped her to substitute certain words and make herself understood. When the time came for discharge, Anna was willing to help Edith with her daily activities, and Anna's daughter took over the heavy household chores for the two women.

Initially, Edith was elated to be back home. Soon enough, however, she realized that she was a burden to the others, having to ask for help to complete even simple tasks. She was increasingly bothered by her niece, who lovingly attended to her needs before she even had a chance to voice them. On occasion, Edith responded gruffly and noticed immediately that she hurt her niece's feelings. Feeling guilty, she was quiet about it but was unable to shake off her anger about her helpless situation. During times when Edith was home alone, she fully visualized the losses she had never dealt with before, and she realized how unrealistic it was to expect to return to her old lifestyle. Instead of being active and going places, she now was trapped in her condominium without being able to master the stairs to the front door. Reading was most difficult, and when she tried to write a note, she noticed that the words did not look right. Edith's anger grew stronger and was now directed at her condition. Anna and her daughter suffered from Edith's moods, her many complaints and demands, nagging about little things, and lack of gratitude for their help. Then, Edith started to refuse to practice walking, bathing, or even eating. One day, the niece, unable to tolerate the tension, exploded with anger and shouted that she could not stand this behavior, that Edith should shape up or she would leave. At night, Edith swallowed a handful of sleeping pills. Anna discovered the empty bottle and called the ambulance just in time.

After spending a few days in the hospital, Edith found herself in a new nursing home. A psychiatric evaluation has led to the diagnosis of reactive depression. Anna informs the nurse of the earlier events, and Edith adds some details to it from her perspective. To gain full understanding of the extent of Edith's losses, the nurse has to examine Edith's life process before and after her stroke and connect this information with Edith's potential of regaining certain functions. The synthesis of his assessment reads as follows.

Assessment of the Individual

System Maintenance. Edith's system maintenance has suffered a serious blow, because everyday activities such as hygiene, housework, family recreation, and, above all, functions in the community can no longer be executed or need assistance. The changes are difficult to tolerate, because Edith has always placed great emphasis on the target of control. Her work in the community has sustained her coherence and served as a source for individuation. Edith's remaining strengths are keen thought processes and intelligence, excellent vision and hearing, speech and reading sufficient for basic communication, and walking with a cane with good potential for improvement of agility and endurance. These strengths have not been used to their full potential.

Coherence. Edith's condition has left a profound impact on her coherence. Only with a shattered feeling of self-worth is a person able to attempt suicide. In her desperation, Edith has misinterpreted her family's loving assistance as a crippling interference to her attempts at regaining independence. This perception may have been realistic to a certain extent, but after each angry outbreak, when the family members withdrew temporarily, Edith realized how heavily she depended on them. At the moment of her niece's outrage, Edith experienced sudden intense anxiety about being deserted and cut off from family, friends, and environment and basically from her own self, which she did not seem to recognize any more.

Individuation. No individuation is possible as long as Edith remains depressed and unable to absorb her losses. The aging process normally requires a slow shift toward the spirituality target, a move that Edith has avoided by pushing herself to remain "young" and active. Her handicap has the potential to serve as a painful but necessary trigger to induce the unavoidable and necessary developmental process of aging. In that sense, her handicap signifies health if Edith learns to redefine her self-image and priorities in life. She has to rediscover herself as a whole being to regain confidence and happiness.

System Change. System change can occur through the individuation process described earlier. System change implies new values, changed attitudes, and patterns of behavior. What exactly needs to change has to be determined by Edith. The nurse, however, can point out her many resources and encourage attempts at a change. The cooperation and support of the family members are of great help in the process.

Nursing Care

The nurse realizes that Edith's family is still in shock as a result of the crisis. Edith's admission to this nursing home has not been easy. Anna and the niece were forced to admit that they failed to master the situation, and they feel strong guilt about it. The niece, above all, is obsessed with the thought of having caused Edith's mental breakdown. Reacting to their helplessness, they try to assume control in the nursing home by ensuring that Edith is cared for exactly "the right way." Both try to discuss Edith's care with the nursing staff and give them instructions and advice. Unfortunately, however, the staff is too busy to take notice of their needs and avoid the two women so they will not be bothered by their constant vigilance. Visiting has become very stressful, because Edith hardly talks to them and the sight of many other suffering residents intensifies their emotional burden. To their great relief, the nurse invites them to a mutual discussion of the situation.

Assessment of Health and Goal Setting

At first, the focus is on adjusting nursing home routines to Edith's usual daily patterns. Soon, however, the topic shifts to interpersonal problems, and the nurse lets them ventilate feelings and pain. She then assures them that they did not cause the situation but that their reactions arose from the situation and were human and understandable. The three women then explore with the systemic diagram Edith's need for system change, and the nurse urges Anna and her daughter to be patient and give Edith time to come to grips with her debility.

Figure 13.1 shows a simplified version of Edith's systemic diagrams. Before her stroke (a), the major emphasis was on system maintenance in the form of hard work and commitment to community work. Her involvement allowed a sound coherence and growth through individuation. System change was adequate, because she adjusted to her retirement and new roles in the community. There was no urgent need to make basic changes in her value system. With the crisis (b), Edith lost control over self-care as well as activities that promote growth. Unable to maintain coherence, her systemic process was blocked and a developmental crisis occurred. Her continued focus on system maintenance and a desperate attempt to gain back her old life prevented her from recognizing an opportunity for individuation and system change through mastering her losses. Figure 13.1c shows the desired outcome of the crisis. Edith's coherence needs to be replenished through a reevaluation of her achievements relative to the losses and limitations. To accomplish system change, Edith needs continued understanding and support of the family. System change can start in the nursing home by setting goals and planning strategies that can preserve Edith's autonomy as the situation allows it. Spirituality needs to be weighted more heavily because strong coherence and individuation are prerequisites for system change.

Assessment of the Family

The nurse draws Figure 13.2, a representation of what their well-organized and healthy family may have looked like before Edith's stroke (a) and after the sudden developmental crisis (b) that reduced individuation to a minimum and inhibited system change. The emotionally troubled family has lost the capacity to grow, but it maintains its old organizational patterns and performs the tasks as usual in a rote manner. On the basis of the joint assessment, everyone agrees that the family has lost coherence, because it experiences interpersonal friction and is adjusting poorly to the situation. A crisis resolution implies renewed togetherness and mutual support through which coherence may gain strength while anxiety and guilt are reduced. As new solutions for the reorganization of the family appear and better meet the needs of its members, the goal to reinstate the original family process (a) can be accomplished with the help of modified caregiving strategies and new attitudes.

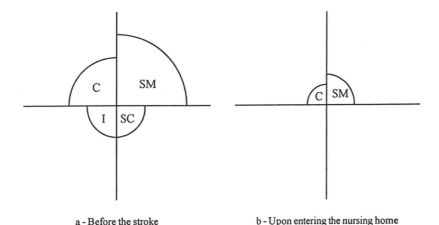

a - Before the stroke   b - Upon entering the nursing home

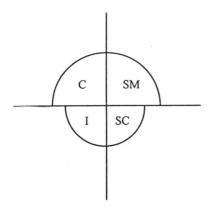

c - Future potential

Figure 13.1. Systemic Process of Edith

Nursing Care

Nursing care of Edith involves patience in establishing trust and new hope to help her overcome her depression. The nurse uses strategies, such as continuous emphasis on abilities and strengths, pointing out progress and helping Edith to get acquainted with another woman who works on overcoming a similar handicap. At

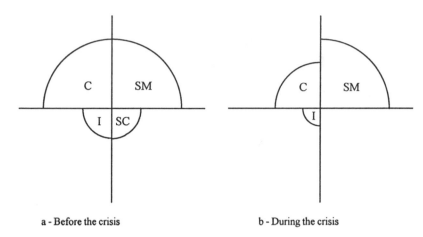

a - Before the crisis   b - During the crisis

Figure 13.2. Systemic Process of Edith's Family

the point when Edith shows renewed hope and motivation, work with the family centers on discharge planning, specifically the decision to take Edith home or keep her in a nursing home, and making projections about the family's involvement in the care and support of Edith. Anna feels that she would like another chance if she could get some help in handling the caregiving situation. The nurse then guides both women in analyzing the family's system maintenance, all persons' activities of daily living, and the necessary caregiving tasks. It appears that Edith's biggest disappointment was her inability to master the stairs and leave the house. With the help of a physical therapist, the projection is made that Edith can learn to walk the stairs and have enough strength for a short walk outside. This will also allow Anna to take Edith by car to senior citizens' meetings or to church. The goal is set for working hard on this skill during the remaining time in the nursing home.

Before preparing the two women for their caregiving tasks, the nurse gives them opportunities to express feelings and anxiety about future crises. Then they discuss with Edith how her autonomy can be preserved, how she can use her skills to be helpful and productive, and what activities she can or wants to do on her own. The importance of continuously communicating personal needs to one another and voicing frustrations openly but in a loving manner is stressed throughout.

Although the example focuses on Edith's need for development and growth, in which the illness becomes the agent of change, the role of the family in support of this process becomes equally evident. Caregiving and the family process, deeply affected by a new type of relationship with Edith, have also become a major constituent of the two women's life processes and have continuous repercussions on Edith. Anna and her daughter identify very strongly with Edith's helplessness and feel a calling to serve her.

The literature cites similar examples of illness becoming a major focus in the family process. Thus, findings of chronic pain research imply that pain and suffering may become a necessity for the sustenance of some family systems as the symptoms become chronic and often involve multiple family members (Gentry, Shows, & Thomas, 1974; Mohamed, Weisz, & Waring, 1978; Violon & Guirgea, 1984) who all use pain as a spiritual target through which they find family closeness. In Edith's example, however, chronicity was not encouraged within the system. Instead, the family members' perception of Edith's helplessness was vehemently rejected by Edith, who values independence, thereby creating a conflict. In its function of balancing forces, the conflict promoted health.

Long-Term Caregiving

Caregiving values and behaviors are integral components of the family's system maintenance and coherence. In fact, they are difficult to separate from everyday system maintenance and coherence activities. Consequently, Montgomery and Kosloski (1994) report serious difficulties in using caregiving tasks as predictors of burden, because spouses who now give care have done so all their lives by performing tasks such as cooking, making doctor's appointments, prescribing home remedies, and encouraging, entertaining, and cheering up their loved one.

Informal family caregiving is a societal expectation and families who fulfill these expectations are offered some assistance by external care systems. Healthy caregiving occurs in the presence of family health, defined as reasonable congruence between the members, the internal process of the family, external systems of care, and societal values.

Consequently, caregiving operates well when family values are in agreement with medical and societal expectations. This was shown by a recent study of chronically ill children. Family members who reported strict compliance with their child's treatment experienced individual and family health evidenced by family cohesion, personal growth, and better physical health of the child compared with families who were less compliant. In those systems, individuals were less committed to family coherence and felt that the illness hindered the pursuit of their valued lifestyle (Patterson, Budd, Goetz, & Warwick, 1993).

Conflicts between societal expectations and personal values occur frequently, leading to social distance and the perception of caregiving burden (Sayles-Cross, 1993). Udelman and Udelman (1980) observed many families who were unable to remain integrated and became disorganized either temporarily or permanently. Likewise, Rosman (1988) reports a splintering effect of chronic illness on some families. Little is known, however, about the interpersonal process leading to such results. In concordance with the dynamics of crisis outlined in Part 3 of this book, experts seem to suspect that families who disintegrate when exposed to chronic illness do so as a result of exacerbation of already existing conflicts (Hough, Lewis, & Woods, 1991). In contrast, well-functioning family systems draw together (Masters, Cerreto, & Mendlowitz, 1983; Rait & Lederberg, 1989) and experience confidence in caring, mutual appreciation, open communication, and a common meaning of the experience (Hough et al., 1991). The key to health seems to be the relationship between the caregiver(s) and the person in need of care. The relationship thrives if its systemic process promotes individuation and growth for all involved. The long-term struggle of maintaining health within the caregiver-patient relationship despite progressive losses with increasing debility of the chronically ill person will be discussed in relation to caring for patients with dementia in the last part of Chapter 14.

The health of the caregiving system and the quality of caregiving are neither dichotomous nor uniform over time. The experience of Anna and her daughter is typical for caregivers who reach the limit of their capacity for compassion. Hours of relative harmony are followed by periods of self-pity and anger about losses. The family process is marked by dynamics of ambivalence and oscillations, because family members attach and withdraw (Lego, 1994), defend their rights, sacrifice their freedom, attack each other, and pull back with remorse. Edith's family was reasonably congruent at the onset of Edith's illness, and the longing for togetherness and interpersonal harmony persisted throughout the crisis as Anna and her daughter strongly supported each other.

As in Edith's family, crisis can occur even in a previously healthy system. Caregiving is generally described as a crisis. Brody (1985) described it as normative family stress. Caregiving of family members is based on a high sense of responsibility anchored in the family value system (Wolfson, Handfield-Jones, Glass, McClaran, & Keyserlingk, 1993) and has multiple costs (Sayles-Cross, 1993). Caregiving as a complex, interpersonal process is highly affected by the values underlying system maintenance, specifically, the perception of family and gender roles influenced by cultural scripts. Thus, spouses feel particularly committed to caregiving (Montgomery & Kosloski, 1994), and if there is no spouse, caregiving is most often provided by the eldest daughter (Tennstedt & McKinlay, 1989). An example of ethnic influence is the extraordinary sense of responsibility for caregiving anchored in a high commitment toward one's kin in the African American community (Stack, 1990). The great complexity of family situations and diversity of family patterns explain why uniform gender roles or cultural patterns of caregiving cannot easily be defined (Nelson, 1993) and why the perception of burden differs greatly among caregivers with similarly extensive caregiving tasks (Sloman & Konstantareas, 1990).

Transition to Formal Care

Although the caregiving situation affects the whole family system, the responsibility for the care often rests with one person. Thus, the majority of the literature focuses on the primary caregiver. Recently, caregivers have been viewed following a predictable course, starting with informal caring, gradual substitution of formal care for informal care, and eventual institutionalization of the patient (Montgomery & Kosloski, 1994). This speaks to a horizontal development of the caregiver role and the family process in addition to the short-term oscillations described earlier. Historically, no-cost informal care has been considered a family obligation. Recently, there has been a fear among policymakers that families tend to relinquish their duties and leave them up to formal programs and institutions. This, however, has not been substantiated by research. Although caregiving has become increasingly difficult for many families who also have to engage in gainful employment for reasons of survival, families generally take their obligations toward ailing members seriously. Substitution of informal care occurs mainly as a result of a transition, such as a loss or the aging of a primary caregiver, increasing disability, and the greater need for care of the patient (Tennstedt, Crawford, & McKinlay, 1993).

The mere availability of formal programs and institutions does not imply their use. In fact, families fail to seek out services even if they are recommended by professionals (Lawton, Brody, & Saperstein, 1989; Montgomery, 1987). For example, Montgomery and Borgatta (1985) reported that one third of eligible families who were offered educational and respite services free of charge refused to use them. Resource use has been described as hierarchical, depending on availability. Spouses and adult children are preferred as caregivers (Stoller & Earl, 1983). If children are unavailable, other relatives may take over responsibilities (Cantor, 1979). Help from friends and neighbors is less common in this culture (Stoller & Earl, 1983) but has been mentioned as a distinguishing feature in African American families (Conway, 1985; Hatch, 1991; Krause, 1988). At the bottom of the hierarchy are formal services used only in emergencies or when everything else fails.

In the earlier example, Edith's family resorted to nursing home care as a result of their crises and inability to handle the situation. This is not unusual. The last step of substitution is often accompanied by much pain and severe guilt on the part of the family (Stevens, Walsh, & Baldwin, 1993). Wilson (1989) describes this endstage of caregiving as turning responsibilities over to professionals. In many instances, the process is gradual and progressive as caregiving demands become greater, allowing time for preparation. It is easy to recognize that in Edith's family, the problem must have been greatly magnified by the sudden change and lack of a gradual adjustment.

After institutionalization, most families remain involved with their loved ones. They may experience a certain sense of relief about giving up difficult caregiving tasks, but their report of stress is no less than before (Cohn & Jay, 1988; Moss & Kurland, 1979). Families are requested to adjust to still another system, the nursing home, and the role they are to take is unclear to them (Bowers, 1988; Brody, 1985). According to the framework of systemic organization, families will first attempt to maintain their systemic process and expand their family into the nursing home.

Having lost direct control over the physical caregiving process, family members, as in the case of Anna and her daughter, often attempt to control the staff by instructing them and watching carefully whether they follow their directions. Bowers (1988) called these behaviors "protective caring." If negative responses are encountered from the staff, families, to protect their coherence, tend to become increasingly demanding and critical of the nursing staff (Smith & Bengston, 1979).

In summary, findings of a recent study show the relevance of system congruence for family health in that the major difficulties reported by families concerned lack of cooperation of the resident or other relatives (family coherence) and of the nursing home staff (congruence with the environment) (Pruchno & Kleban, 1993).

All of this seems to indicate that families need to be helped, not only to maintain control but to be involved in care and build alliances with the staff (Stevens et al., 1993), a goal that targets spirituality. Edith's nurse exemplifies such care in detail. The framework of systemic organization, supported by research cited earlier, has still further implications for nursing. The diversity of family process demands from the nurse an insightful and nonjudgmental approach geared to the specific needs of the family. To maintain the system by giving hands-on care may not be the aim of all families, and not all families want to make decisions about nursing care. In some cases, families decide to leave the responsibility to the nurses and take a well-deserved break after years of caring. In others, the unwillingness to be involved may be based on a history of emotional distance, long-standing interpersonal difficulties, and old wounds that have never been healed. Consequently, it is imperative that nurses refrain from labeling families as noncaring, mean, or overinvolved because they do not fit in their expected norm for families.

If families are to be partners of nurses, their roles in the partnership system can have many different features and have to be defined clearly. Therefore, nurses assess the family members no differently from clients and apply the nursing process to them as if they were their clients by using the process described in Chapter 2. As they guide family members toward their desired systemic targets to find new congruence and health in interacting with the resident and the nursing home system, nurses will discover happier families and residents, a better climate in the unit, and personal growth related to meaningful interactions.

14

Families With Chronic Mental Illness/Developmental Disabilities

Disabilities that encompass the mental, cognitive, or emotional realm are widespread and deeply affect not only the afflicted individuals but their families and society as a whole. Although certain reactions to the illness and caregiving problems are comparable to the ones of families who care for physically disabled members, others are unique. This discussion involves the nursing process related to three categories of chronic conditions, namely, developmental disabilities, mental/emotional illnesses, and dementias. The categories vary in etiology, symptoms, and course of the condition. Consequently, the family's initial reactions and long-term adjustments differ accordingly. Over time, individuals with a developmental disability are in need of support to develop their potential. A health care/special education program is recommended that uses an interactive approach between the family and the professionals who represent the various disciplines (Green, 1990). After the initial shock, grief, and disappointment upon diagnosis, the family is expected to support the developmental process of their child while attending to often severe physical problems and limitations that may manifest themselves concurrently. Guidance is required in choosing services from various agencies that best respond to the needs of the families to render this difficult task successful:

programs that are flexible, individualized, and responsive to change over time (Hobbs et al., 1984).

Mentally ill patients, in conjunction with the pharmacological maintenance, need rehabilitation with a focus on optimal economic and social functions to become members of society who contribute in their special way despite limitations. Families involved with mental illness deal with uncertainty, loss, and faltering expectations and are often required to accept a supporting and monitoring role with their afflicted family member as a lifelong duty (Hatfield, 1990).

Dementias, as a rule, affect older families who experience a slow "death" of the patient's personality and skills. Their challenge consists of adjusting to an ever-changing relationship with the afflicted person and finding ways to maintain the loved one's identity and dignity (Jones & Martinson, 1992; Orona, 1990).

Despite these differences, nursing of families with the framework of systemic organization is similar in all categories in that the nurse provides the support to a life process through which individuals derive satisfaction, meaning, and congruence. This is rooted in an image of humanity that acknowledges an innate need to belong and be accepted (spirituality) as well as an always present potential for growth. Furthermore, the theory of systemic organization is based on the assumption that individuals whose physical, cognitive, or emotional responses are compromised will develop often remarkable skills and creativity in enhancing their remaining abilities through which they stay whole despite their deficiencies. Such abilities are beautifully described in the clinical tales of Oliver Sacks (1987). It follows that, ideally, nursing and the rehabilitative process are keenly sensitive to nurturing and encouraging creative powers of the patients while helping them to move closer to society's expectations. Nothing expresses the true art of nursing better than the enormously difficult task of finding a balance between human wholeness and functional expectations and leading the patient and family accordingly. Because the behaviors of individuals with mental, cognitive, or emotional debilities are often gross aberrations, nursing care demands a highly perceptive, judgment-free examination of the benefits of such patterns to the patient's unique life process. The focus is on abilities instead of limitations and on human dignity and worth rather than on social and economic inadequacies. In family work, Carl Dunst's model for working with families who have developmentally disabled children advocates a partnership through which families become empowered to use their own resources (Dunst, Trivette, & Deal, 1988). The model has become widely accepted in social work and can be applied to the nursing of families with this framework as well.

It is easy to recognize that client- and family-driven nursing care are not always in tune with the usual rehabilitative process. Rehabilitation follows the medical model and the goal of normalization to a great extent. The process stresses the control of pathologies and defects and pursues corrective action and patient training toward an optimally productive lifestyle defined by society norms. This determines the definition of success or failure and leads to a clear distinction between educable versus uneducable persons, the latter of which are in greatest danger of being failed by the system. The families of the educable are expected to follow the advice of professionals with minimal input. Therefore, even in the most promising situations, the danger exists that the client's unique abilities are overlooked if they do not serve an obvious, socially useful purpose. The remainder of this chapter serves to illuminate ways to use this framework to minimize such danger.

Families With Developmental Disabilities

The trend toward normalization seems to be in tune with today's health care model and people's expectations. In terms of the framework of systemic organization, it signifies a pull toward the target of control that carries within it the inherent danger of compromising spirituality and congruence of the child, family, and professional team. Mainstreaming, a manifestation of normalization, has strong support from many parents who insist that their sometimes severely handicapped children be given the opportunity to be taught in classrooms together with nondisabled children. The issue has been controversial, according to Marcia Reback (1994), Chair of the Task Force on Special Education of the American Federation of Teachers. The line between usefulness and abuse of mainstreaming is a fine one and can be drawn only by responding to the child's unique life process and potential strengths. However, mainstreaming often nurtures the families' emotional needs. Perhaps it rekindles and justifies the parents' strong desire to have a normal child. Perhaps mothers and fathers who object to special education classrooms, even if necessary resources are unavailable in the regular classroom situation, cling to the illusion of an intact child. The controversy of mainstreaming illuminates the issue of keeping separate the needs of the child and those of the family and the challenge of reconciling the two sets of needs, if they differ significantly. Generally, in a society that values intellectual achievement very highly, parents have difficulties terminating their grief about the loss of a cognitively intact child. Thus, to find a solution, the family necessarily becomes a client of the health care team.

According to this framework, parents who have accepted their situation fully focus on the part of their child that is intact and strive to enhance it. At the same time, they respect limitations and avoid pushing skills that are beyond the child's capabilities. Basically, such parents provide support for the sake of the child, who is considered whole in a special way. They describe a personal growth process (individuation) occurring concurrently with their grief work. Their child takes on significance in revealing to them aspects of life that are truly meaningful, aspects they would have overlooked under regular circumstances. Nevertheless, these parents will vacillate between periods of self-pity and grief and times of feeling fulfilled and fortunate. Grief never totally dissolves, even in the best of parents. It is cyclical and keeps returning as the child encounters various life situations and goes through developmental changes (Olshansky, 1962; Seligman & Darling, 1989). Nevertheless, healthy parents have learned to acknowledge their grief as part of their emotional being to prevent being overtaken by it and have learned to see the light beyond. The struggle is lifelong and is easier at some times and harder at others. Other changes and incongruencies in the general life process of each family member and the family system are intimately interwoven and have a serious potential to disturb a sometimes fragile congruence.

The involvement of nurses with such families may be short-term only. They may witness the birth of a disabled child, may be involved in the testing and diagnosing of disabilities, may take care of physical problems during times of corrective surgery interventions or other hospitalizations, or they may engage in teaching family members physical care management. In terms of their long-term responsibilities, however, nurses need to provide families with continuity and support over time.

The solution is seen in family-centered case management programs that provide considerable relief, even though professionals report having to stretch the system to the limits to truly serve the families (Knoll, 1994). Families have long suffered from a fragmented health care system that responds well to emergencies but neglects to provide continuity. Beyond health care needs, families require help with educational, psychological, social, or financial problems that may cut across several government agencies. Within effective interdisciplinary programs, nurses work as team members. A comprehensive understanding of the family's situation can be considerably enhanced by various professionals evaluating strengths and problems from their own perspective. Communication and joint planning by the team are paramount to arriving at a unified approach and avoiding mixed messages to the family. Although nurses need to function within a role designated by the team, they can contribute much to the team's comprehension of the family's struggle and to the team members' growth if they use the framework of systemic organization and gain with it a broad overall understanding of the family's life process.

Catherine is 17 years old and has been lovingly cared for by her family since birth. She is mildly spastic and her mental functioning is severely compromised. If people speak to her, she smiles. She whines when she is uncomfortable and makes various kinds of noises that express excitement in handling objects or hearing music. Catherine has no speech and does not discriminate between people, a fact that is particularly difficult for her dedicated mother. Nevertheless, both parents are deeply involved with Catherine, watch her patterns of activity, and help each other guess what she might feel, perceive, or think. They provide stimulation that seems to make her happy, such as music, a stroll to the duck pond, and other activities. Catherine attends a special educational program. Due to the hard work of the parents with the visiting nurse, Catherine has responded to bowel and bladder training and can be kept clean thanks to a meticulous routine. She sits freely and can roll over on the floor. With a physical therapy program, she has arrived at a point where she can be pulled up to a standing position and carry her weight with her own legs to take a few steps if she is held under her arms and kept in balance. This progress was a tremendous relief for her mother, because the transfer from bed to wheelchair and toileting have become easier.

Three weeks ago, Catherine had surgery on her knee to stretch the tendons for better extension of the leg. As a program team member, the nurse has visited postoperatively and has left her card with the family. All went well, but yesterday, the mother called the nurse in despair. For several days now, Catherine starts crying unexpectedly when she is handled and sometimes when she sits on the floor. Her mother states between sobs, "It is so hard that she cannot tell me what hurts. I have tried everything, but she tries to hit me. She is so unhappy. I don't know what to do."

During a joint visit by the nurse and the physical therapist, measures are devised to improve leg circulation by looser bandaging, massaging, positioning, and foot exercises. Then, the nurse takes the mother aside for a private talk, because she senses that the crisis is based on other problems as well. As a result of an intensive conversation, the nurse is able to report to the team the following.

Catherine's mother is extremely worried about the family's future. She is torn between an obligation and a strong wish to get out of the situation. For some time, she has had a feeling of burnout. She does not receive the rewards she expects through her care. She feels down and less able to cheer up Catherine. Then, she notices that Catherine responds to others more positively than to her. The fact that Catherine is just as happy with other people makes her feel useless, and a desire to get away to take on a job outside the house becomes strong. This, in turn, creates more guilt, and she thinks of herself as a victim as well as a failure. In the past, while caring for Catherine, she has succeeded in nourishing her own coherence. Through her expertise, she has felt competent and able to take charge. As a result of Catherine's recent crying outbursts and her inability to calm her down, however, she suddenly feels overwhelmed. Helplessness has quietly and increasingly gotten a hold of her and seems to overpower her. Although the individuation process had been at a minimum for some time, at the present, she can no longer see beyond the crisis, and her confusion obliterates the path to solutions. Her husband is of no support either. He does not understand why she suddenly cannot handle the situation and tells her in no uncertain terms that Catherine needs her and taking a job would be detrimental for Catherine and the family.

The team, on the basis of the nurse's description, decides to help Catherine's mother and father to jointly examine options for Catherine's ongoing care as an adult. The aim is to explore with the parents growth-promoting activities. The social worker is put in charge of the situation, and the team stresses the importance of giving much support to Catherine's mother by acknowledging her expertise in caring for Catherine and at the same time supporting her in her desire to lead a life of her own. The team approach seems successful. When the physical therapist inquires the next day, Catherine's mother reports progress. Catherine's pain seems to have improved. She has cried only once. The nurse calls the mother the same day and tells her that she has shared her concerns with the team and that the social worker will visit with the family for a talk about Catherine's future.

The social worker's visit results in a plan to enroll Catherine in an all-day treatment program that would give her mother an opportunity to accept employment. Catherine's father seems to have a better understanding of his wife's needs and offers to drive Catherine to the program every day. Catherine's mother shares the employment ads in the local newspaper with the social worker and shows her two to which she plans to respond.

The framework of systemic organization is suitable for interdisciplinary work. Generally, teams that are concerned with complex family problems operate with an open systems framework. Therefore, the terms, explanation of processes, and derived strategies are salient to professionals of various disciplines. This example shows how a nurse can guide the team to a successful intervention. The needs of Catherine's mother came into focus as a result of the nurse's keen perception. Although she might have been able to negotiate a solution independently, she was also aware of the team's understanding of her role limits. It was important for the whole team to be informed, plan jointly, and back up the action of the person delegated the responsibility of negotiation for future work with the family. The example also shows that even exemplary parents who are well adjusted to their situation may encounter difficult times in which the demands of caregiving and changes of their developmental needs induce incongruence. They become overwhelmed, unable to individuate, and slide into crisis.

The nursing approach described in Chapter 11 also applies to working with families interfacing with various health care settings when a child is born, when diagnosis of a severe deficit occurs, or when the child is hospitalized for a physical problem. Insightful planning and interventions in such short-term situations will be invaluable to families if nurses succeed to quickly communicate unique family strengths and possible incongruencies to the case manager who maintains contact with the family over time. Other issues relevant to families with members who have developmental disabilities are also faced by families with mentally ill members and are discussed in the next section.

Families With Mental Illness

Explanations of the etiology of mental illnesses follow a trend similar to those referring to developmental disabilities. Increasingly, causative factors of mental illness are thought to be of a biological nature. The trend stands in contrast to historically held beliefs that have shaped treatment methods and public policy over time. The family has long been thought of as a system that either fosters or damages the health of its members. The persistence of this assumption is revealed by a review of family studies documented in the 1980s showing that the body of health-related articles still speaks to the negative effects of the family system on its members (Berardo, 1990; Ross, Mirowski, & Goldstein, 1990).

Like physical health, mental health in individuals is often believed to be rooted in the family. In fact, traditional family therapy has gained its reputation through work with families of the mentally ill. The term *psychosomatic family,* coined by Minuchin and his associates (Minuchin et al., 1975), has exerted a significant influence on family science over time.

The debate about the etiology of eating disorders is of interest here. Although eating disorders seem to have a strong genetic component (Strober, Lampert, Morrell, Burroughs, & Jacobs, 1990), sociological and family factors seem to be equally relevant, even though their interaction is poorly understood (Killian, 1994). Much has been written about the destructive dynamics of anorexic families (i.e., Calam, Waller, Slade, & Newton, 1990; Heron & Leheup, 1984; Humphrey, 1986; Kog & Vandereycken, 1985, 1989), but the alternative explanation arising from an open systems view came into discussion only recently. Kent and Clopton (1992) suggested that the family dynamics observed by researchers of eating disorders may not be inherent characteristics of the families but may be associated with the families' attempt to control the afflicted member's symptoms and reactions to the treatment of the condition.

Today, renowned family therapists continue to work under the assumption that symptoms of mental illness can be reversed by interfering with destructive family dynamics, so-called *psychotic family games* (Selvini-Palazzoli, Cirillo, Selvini, & Sorrentino, 1989). Nevertheless, research has recently shifted to an open systems perspective that allows a broader interpretation of the phenomenon. If the afflicted individual's condition is a biological dysfunction, it may be plausible that family dynamics specific to a variety of mental illnesses may actually be an adaptation to the symptoms of the individual (Sloman & Konstantareas, 1990). For example, the findings of a study of autism have attested to significant changes in family interaction patterns over time (Tinbergen & Tinbergen, 1972). The same shift is seen in research on expressed emotions (EE). Traditionally, researchers have supported the view that emotional overinvolvement in the family is distressing to the patient and a cause for repeated relapse (Vaughn & Leff, 1976). Recent research, however, has explored EE as an interpersonal phenomenon, and findings report that patient and family members are equally affected by the expression of emotion as they mutually respond to each other's mood states (Florin, Nostadt, Reck, Franzen, & Jenkins, 1992; Hahlweg et al., 1989). Even though families may not be the initiators of problems, these research findings suggest that family reactions and interactions may be predictive of the patients' long-term adjustment. Consequently, the family system may have an active role in the maintenance of the symptomatology.

In summary, the literature of today bears witness to several stances: the family process as a contributing factor to the etiology of the mental illness as a sustaining mechanism and as an adaptive outcome in response to the symptoms. As a result, numerous writers advocate the need for multidimensional models in dealing with families (Engel, 1982; Griffith, Griffith, & Slovik, 1989; Sloman & Konstantareas, 1990).

Families themselves seem to prefer biochemical explanations of mental illness, because they free them from the historically perpetuated induction of guilt and social stigma. Nevertheless, families remain confused about their responses to symptoms of the afflicted member that are hard to control and vary with the general family climate (Sloman & Konstantareas, 1990). For example, biological symptoms, such as the inability to concentrate or complete a task, may evoke reactions of impatience in family members and anger about laziness (Johnson, 1987), and these reactions may be strongest if the family also struggles with other conflicts and crises.

The framework of systemic organization does not speak against the possibility of genetic factors. In fact, the interplay of biological and interpersonal factors is clearly visible as in the example of a schizophrenic family member's biological inability to connect on a social/emotional level, which evokes unusual patterns of relating, while the family struggles with explanations and justification of its reactions to the outside world (Moltz, 1993). Consequently, this framework is in tune with Engel (1980, 1982) and explains the phenomenon as a continuous interaction of systems at all levels and their continuous change over time.

Consequently, the manifestations of the patient's condition are intimately interwoven with the processes of the family and the larger environment, people of contact, and messages received from the society. Inherent in the family system as conceptualized within this framework lies a core conflict typical of many cases, namely, the dispute about control at the expense of mutuality and connectedness (spirituality). This conflict is illustrated by the following example.

Tim is being discharged from the psychiatric hospital. It was his fourth admission after being in remission for 6 months. His mother, fearing for her life, had called the police when she woke up one night and saw Tim standing at the head of her bed with a kitchen knife in one hand and caressing the blade with the other while his eyes seemed to stare into space.

Once, Tim had been a high achiever in school but was never popular among his schoolmates. His disease first occurred at age 19 after a college exam and shortly after the breakup of a brief relationship with a girl. At that time, Tim was tormented by anxiety about being followed by the police. Voices told him to undress and hide under his bed for safety. He remained under the bed for hours, shivering from anxiety and cold. He insisted on remaining in his hiding place, refusing to accept food or drink.

After the initial hospitalization, Tom was prescribed psychotropic medication. Nevertheless, acute episodes recurred. With each subsequent exacerbation, his aggressive impulses seemed to intensify, which put his family in a state of increasing apprehension. During acute episodes of his illness, Tim feels possessed by the tormenting voices. In fact, he even loses his sense of who he is, as if his body has dissolved in space. Completely lacking control and stability, he experiences change that seems like a wild metamorphosis, through which his shape and consistency become fluid, allowing him to turn into one thing or another in rapid succession. The experience is highly spiritual and feels like a deadly grip by a power that possesses him, molds him, and threatens to destroy him.

Now, back in his home, Tim attempts with desperate intensity to regain stability and control by avoiding any type of growth-promoting challenges. Tim's anxiety remains overwhelming, and he clings to his mother, hoping that her coherence will nourish his own. Tim is referred to a mental health team whose task is to specify a long-range treatment plan. His psychiatric nurse summarizes the assessment.

Assessment of the Individuum

System Maintenance. In times of remission, Tim wants to control his daily rhythm. He feels pressured by any type of interference and reacts with counterpressure. Therefore, he resists his mother, who insists that he get up in the morning, by sleeping particularly long and watching TV until late at night. Likewise, he is stubborn in his refusal to help around the house. Tim refuses to eat with the family but instead takes from the refrigerator what he likes, mainly sweets. He takes his medications without regularity. He may go for days without it and then suddenly swallow several tablets at once. Tim's contact with people outside the family is minimal. For entertainment, he walks to a nearby mall to buy cigarettes and a magazine and in the hope of seeing a beautiful young woman. He has been obsessed with the idea of becoming a famous bass guitar player since the time when, after a rock concert he attended, the bass player gave him a signed photograph. He has bought every existing record and tape of the band and has bought himself a guitar. When he is at home alone, he experiments with the instrument, bringing forth some rudimentary tunes. The few music lessons his family allowed him to take were a failure, because Tim did not have the concentration needed for disciplined practice. The failure triggered one of his hospitalizations. It is easy to recognize that the activities listed here under system maintenance are also meant to serve Tim's coherence.

Coherence. Tim's self-esteem was deficient even before the outbreak of the disease. As a child, he was overprotected by his mother and considered strange by his schoolmates. He was useful to a few whom he helped with homework, but he lived in constant fear of others who derived pleasure in teasing and terrorizing him. Although Tim was able to maintain some coherence through achieving good grades, his disease seems to have shattered it all. Presently, his self-worth is based on the illusion of becoming a famous bass guitar player. In contrast to this delusion of grandeur, Tim is plagued by anxiety, does not dare speak to people, and has to be accompanied by his mother to get a haircut or buy clothes. He treats his mother as his "servant." In reality, however, she represents to him a substitute for his lost self. He clings to her, only to push her away as soon as she expects him to be independent.

Individuation and System Change. A growth process is hardly possible in Tim's present life pattern. A certain degree of coherence or self-confidence is a necessity for any person to venture out and explore systems in the environment. Tim's anxiety increased as soon as he left the protective hospital environment. Tim sees himself as totally incompetent and without abilities; he feels exhausted, listless, and weak. The only relief comes through an escape into a dream world. Through fantasies, he gains powers; in fact, the powers become extraordinary and greater than other people's. This feeling of omnipotence, however, is taken away from Tim by the medications. By skipping medications for a few days, however, he can bring the feeling back. Unfortunately, however, the torturing voices also return, frightening him even more. His reaction of swallowing several pills at once is a desperate effort to appease these voices. Thus, a cyclical pattern of emotions and behaviors to control them has become the entire focus of his existence, drains his energy, and blocks any attempt at individuation.

In summary, Figure 14.1a shows that Tim's systemic process lacks growth and is extremely labile. Nevertheless, there are remainders of strengths dating back to his academic success in school and college. They are overshadowed by tremendous anxiety but could be mobilized carefully within a supportive environment. The question now arises whether the family is able to provide such an environment. The nurse arranges for a visit with the family with all members present.

Assessment of the Family

System Maintenance. Tim's family is composed of his parents and himself. This is an isolated nuclear system, because both parents have broken off relationships with the extended family. In the father's working-class family, alcohol was a serious problem, and Tim's mother was disinherited by her wealthy parents because she insisted on marrying against their advice. Tim's father has educated himself and is now employed as an engineer. His wife has never worked outside the house. Raising Tim was her calling. She is the intellectual leader in the family and makes or at least influences all major decisions.

Tim's problems have been difficult for both. Although Tim's mother has strengthened her bond with Tim as he became more needy, the father feels left out and has distanced himself increasingly. Having been proud of Tim's previous achievements, Tim's father now blames his wife for spoiling Tim and preventing him from becoming a man. Tim's mother suffers because no matter what she does, it never seems right. She is terribly worried about Tim, follows his moves carefully, and tries to avoid conflicts at all costs. She hides her own anger and pain evoked by Tim's ruthless behaviors and insensitivity toward her out of fear of bringing

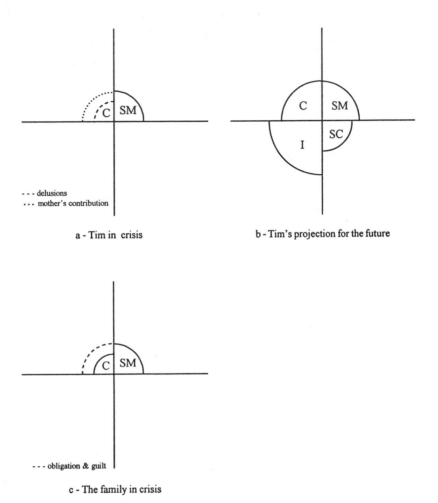

a - Tim in crisis

--- delusions
... mother's contribution

b - Tim's projection for the future

c - The family in crisis

--- obligation & guilt

Figure 14.1. Systemic Processes of Tim and Tim's Family

about another psychosis. Tim, who is striving to regain control, senses that he can do so only by escaping this bondage of love. Therefore, he expresses anger and rejection only to come back to his mother helplessly.

The dynamics of skipping and taking medications are also influenced by this conflict around control. His mother's reminding him about the drugs triggers rebellion. As a result, Tim "forgets" to take the pills and the mother nags him more. This generally produces an angry outbreak with unjust accusations that the mother swallows quietly. This leaves Tim overwhelmed by guilt and worthlessness. His swallowing too many pills at once not only represents a measure to control the increasing intensity of the voices punishing him for being bad but also is a symbolic attempt to end his life. To Tim's mother, such behavior proves that her control is absolutely indispensable. Then, the cycle begins again.

The family members' physical needs are well taken care of, but the family's life process is dominated by intense anxiety about destruction and dissolution of the system. Despite inordinate amounts of energy being spent on system maintenance, the behaviors within the dimension are ineffective. The parents use silencing and distancing, a process that turns them into martyrs with an intense craving for warmth and closeness. Tim's angry outbreaks are an attack on the unbearable silence, tension, and incongruence of the family. The family, involved in stifling repetitive cycles that consume all of its available energy, finds it impossible to change.

Coherence. Tim and his mother's relationship is strong, almost to the point of being fused. Outside of it, there is a lack of understanding for each other's pain. All family members are captives within a destructive family process that ties them together emotionally through a common sense of failure and guilt. As persons, they are not free and need to participate in the dynamic cycles described earlier for the sake of maintaining their own congruence. Bound together in isolation, they lack the ability to individuate.

Individuation and System Change. The family process is frozen in place and individuation in the family system has become impossible. Tim's father goes to work every day but his work has lost meaning, and he has become empty and hopeless about the purpose of his life in general. The other members are equally hopeless.

Assessment of Health

Tim's nurse has jotted down the crisis diagrams of Tim and his family pictured in Figure 14.1 and notices a striking similarity. She envisions the individual diagrams of both mother and father and suspects that they are very similar to Tim's. It seems that there is more than one patient in this family, an observation frequently made by family therapists (Bateson & Jackson, 1964). Meanwhile, the nurse has a conversation with Tim's primary nurse in the hospital unit. Supposedly, Tim communicated well with other patients and seemed quite relaxed during certain activities. None of the family behaviors seemed to be carried over. The nurse noted this as a definite strength.

The nurse realizes that these family interactions could predictably exacerbate another acute episode soon if the family is not helped to loosen its fixed patterns and find congruence. The solution is seen as some kind of individuation of Tim's mother as a beginning, which would permit a necessary emotional distance between Tim and her. The parents' willingness to sacrifice for the sake of the family is considered a strong point. This willingness now needs to be converted into mutual support to build a healthy coherence strong enough to be maintained despite Tim's disturbed behavior.

Nursing Care

After sharing the synthesis with the mental health team and feeling supported by the members who also know Tim, the nurse invites Tim's mother to her office. His father refused to come. She presents her analysis, tentatively making certain not to blame anyone. The mother breaks down crying, excuses herself, and asks the nurse to forgive her. "This is the first time that somebody really understands my problems," she states. She tells of her great pain to live isolated not only from the rest of the world but from her family, too. Talking about her difficulties, she brings her own life process into focus, and the nurse helps her to gain understanding. What does health mean for her? What does she need to be happy? She does not expect that Tim will change much and tells of nightmares she had about his coming home. She also fears that Tim's increasingly violent impulses may lead to a family disaster. She has toiled with the thought of a group home but knows how much Tim needs her. A placement not only would mean to Tim that his family rejects him but would leave her feeling that she had failed him. The nurse helps her to understand Tim's life process with the diagram. She explains that Tim needs a change to grow up and gain self-confidence. She asks Tim's mother to think the group home issue over and not to forget that a home does not mean that their close relationship would have to stop.

In the next days, the nurse calls twice, and each time Tim's mother is grateful to share the difficulties she has had that day. The second time, she mentions that she really would like to become a volunteer in a hospital, because that would be a challenge and she could get to know people. Supposedly, her husband has no strong opinion against this, which has given her the courage to excitedly inquire about the application process. Tim's father seems relieved that she has found new hope and happiness, and he could be talked into being present for a visit by the nurse.

The plan is to let Tim decide for himself what living situation is best for him. Tim has also sensed the easing of family tension and looks more relaxed than before. With the help of the diagram (see Figure 14.1a and b), the nurse shows him where his strengths are: his striving to become independent, his ability to be sociable, his intelligence, and his love of his parents all assist with individuation. Then, they discuss his need to learn how to be independent (system maintenance) and feel good about himself (coherence). The idea of a group home is presented, and the nurse and the parents make sure he understands that the purpose is not to push him out of the parental house but to help him grow. No pressure is exerted and Tim is given as much time as he wants to decide.

At the next joint home visit of the mental health team, the psychologist brings up the subject of a group home and asks Tim what his feelings are about it. Tim is still very anxious about leaving the family but is willing to talk with the social worker about possibilities. A visit to a group home follows, and Tim is delighted about the friendly reception and the rehabilitation program. He is finally ready for a move after his mother assures him that she will take him home for visits every weekend.

This example explains Tim's symptoms from a perspective that differs significantly from the medical understanding. Although the essence of a cure in the medical model is the cessation of Tim's symptoms, a close examination of the life process reveals a chronic core problem of powerlessness, helplessness, and anxiety associated with these feelings. A recent hermeneutic study of power experienced by schizophrenic patients (Cox Dzurec, 1994) seems relevant here. It was found that, generally, a sense of power was derived if individuals viewed themselves as active players in their own life process. In contrast, patients who saw their life as a product ruled by external forces felt powerless. Furthermore, power seemed dependent on integrality. People with schizophrenia seemed to be severely curtailed in that their power was restricted to mundane acts, such as taking medications on time, whereas meaningful acts that promote integrality, such as finding a job or independent living, were generally beyond their reach (Cox Dzurec, 1994).

If integrality expresses active and meaningful interactions with one's environment, it has much resemblance to the construct of spirituality of this framework. Tim, no different from other people, has a strong drive to find congruence through spirituality by connecting to other systems. Being emotionally fused with his mother, however, he lacks the necessary coherence or autonomy to individuate and make a meaningful connection with the environment. Could this be the reason why Tim uses his mundane power and transforms it into an environmental issue, thereby controlling his family members in very subtle ways? If so, the process occurs subconsciously, and the family slides into reactive patterns without being able to control them.

In the same line, Tim's family members tend to view themselves as victims rather than as active agents in the life process. Theirs is the same struggle between autonomy and connectedness, of control versus spirituality. These elements are considered key in the therapy of families with psychotic members (Retzer, Simon, Weber, Stierlin, & Schmidt, 1991), and the recommended approach addresses empowerment and individuation.

It is naive to think that Tim's move to a group home will solve all family problems. Existing studies of families with mental illness view caregiving as a lifelong process (Baker, 1989; Malone, 1990). The burden of these families has been related to stigma, fears, worries, and loss (Cook, 1988; Hatfield, 1978; Lefley, 1987). Grief over lost hopes, adjustment of expectations, redefining relationships, and fear about the future are comparable to the challenges of families with developmentally disabled members described earlier. Likewise, the process of adjustment bears similarities. Howard's grounded theory study of mothers reports a process of searching, learning about the illness and the self, and eventually adjusting by accepting the role of long-term caregiver (Howard, 1994). Families take on the charge of society to monitor and control the behavior of the afflicted member (Caplan, 1982). Even though the odds of families being stigmatized by neighbors and the community may be greater in mental illness, studies report an overall successful adjustment of families. Crotty and Kulys (1986), who interviewed families at a community mental health facility, reported a generally low subjective burden of family members, and the study of Wilk (1988) revealed that families with mentally ill adults living at home were strongly cohesive.

The framework of systemic organization suggests the need for an open systems view. The above studies suggest that some families may be well able to provide the support and encouragement a patient needs, but the conflicts occurring in others will inhibit learning and progress. The ill relative's deficits, such as bizarre behaviors or patterns of relating to people, stand in stark contrast to societal norms (Horwitz, Tessler, Fisher, & Gamache, 1992). Therefore, a healthy integration of such diversity is difficult for many families, and little help is offered by the mental health system (Reinhard, 1994).

Nursing of families, with the aim of enabling them to become the needed environment that provides monitoring, loving control, and support asks for changed models. New models address the collaboration between families and the formal care system (Reinhard, 1994). Family consultation goes in the direction of offering guidance to families who request it to solve caregiving problems (Bernheim, 1989), but a psychoeducational approach combines information sharing with coordination of resources and support in mastering crises (Sloman & Konstantareas, 1990). Nursing with this framework is clearly psychoeducational. Interventions follow a thorough assessment of the family and key individuals and proceed according to the steps indicated in Chapter 2. In the case of Tim's family, the nurse followed the family's lead and reacted cautiously to the mother's indication that she might be willing to make changes. With the help of the diagram, the nurse discussed the needed changes with the mother, later shared them with Tim, and finally discussed them with the father. The nurse refrained from pressuring Tim or the family, even though she recognized that no change would be harmful for Tim's future. The nurse relied on other team members' expertise in assisting the family to move toward individuation when they were ready. The nursing process will have to continue after Tim's move to the group home. A new assessment will show how family roles have shifted and how each member responds to the changes. Attention will be paid to the mother, because she is giving up responsibilities that previously contributed to her sense of competency and coherence. It is to be hoped that her activities as a hospital volunteer will compensate for some feelings of loss.

The relationship between the mother and father also warrants attention. Although the decrease in immediate family conflict may be a relief to both, improvement of intimacy and mutual trust does not necessarily follow. The two will have to work out new roles in a smaller family in which Tim no longer acts to distract from marital conflicts. Tim's well-being and the balance of autonomy versus dependency (control vs. spirituality) will have to be reevaluated frequently, and visits to his home will need to be arranged accordingly. If the intervention proves successful, the nurse will observe a process of growth of each individual but also within their relationships. A process of continuing growth through readjustment within the relationship between the parents, who now act in a distinctly different caregiving role, and Tim will need to take place. A similar process occurring in the most difficult situation of caring for a victim of dementia will be discussed in the following section.

Families Caring
for a Member With Dementia

Families caring for victims of Alzheimer's disease (AD) and related dementias are described as hidden victims (Zarit & Anthony, 1986). These families are helplessly witnessing the cognitive, social, and physical deterioration of their loved one, a process believed to place an inordinate burden on the family (Kuhlman, Wilson, Hutchinson, & Wallhagen, 1991). As explained in the preceding chapter, there is no legal responsibility of spouses or children to give care, but a social and moral obligation is strongly embedded in family life. The tendency for families to accept caregiving responsibilities, even under the most difficult circumstances, is great. This is shown by the fact that only a small percentage of elders in need of care are found in institutions

(Bleathman, 1987; Hall, 1988). The families' expression of this sense of responsibility, however, varies widely and ranges from coercing a member into caregiving to voluntarily giving care to express affection or return a gift of love (Oden, 1986).

The major responsibilities for caregiving are frequently taken on by one person. Thus, an extensive body of literature describes the caregiving process in terms of the experience of a primary caregiver, who is often elderly as well and may have physical, social, and financial problems (Daniels & Irwin, 1989) that intensify the stress associated with the demands of around-the-clock caregiving (Motenko, 1989). Many studies have examined factors likely to influence stress and burden, such as demographics, symptoms of the disease, or the extent of physical and cognitive incapacity of the patient. Evidence provided is contradictory, however (Kuhlman et al., 1991), indicating that the diversity among families and the differing reactions to the caregiving demands may make generalizations difficult.

Giving care to an AD patient is believed to involve a series of choices, all of which are undesirable (Wilson, 1993). On the basis of a grounded theory study, Wilson (1993) describes caregiving to AD patients as a process of "surviving on the brink" (p. 197) and occurring in three stages: taking it on, going through it, and turning it over. Such a negative view may be understandable from a perspective of coping with stress. Nevertheless, it neglects the fact that the drama unfolds on the interpersonal and family levels and that it may involve not only pain and grief but a great deal of personal growth and wisdom.

How such wisdom can grow is not well understood. According to Hirschfeld (1983), caregiving families exhibit the capacity for mutuality. Hirschfeld describes mutuality as a process through which caregivers are rewarded threefold: They find gratification, a positive meaning of caregiving, and reciprocity. These rewards are possible if the caregiver sustains a quality relationship with the afflicted person.

Sustaining the relationship runs counter to the medical model, according to which professionals emphasize biomedical phenomena of the disease and the loss of personhood of the patient. Thinking of the patient as sick and no longer human discourages family members from relating to the patient as they did previously. This mechanism of distancing, however, does not seem to be the choice of the majority of healthy families. In the study of Grafstrom, Norberg, and Hagberg

(1993), even families who had reported abuse in the past were not likely to radically distance themselves emotionally from the patient. The authors suspect that those families who did had long-standing relationship problems and found the distancing necessary as a psychological defense against intolerable pain and grief. According to Chesla, Martinson, and Muwaswes (1994), troubled families fail to be rewarded with gratification and reciprocity, both of which depend on continuing intimate interactions with the patient. The nature of such interactions will be explained in-depth with the example in this chapter.

Grief of AD caregivers is described as having distinguishing characteristics. Rather than anticipatory, grief seems acute and related to the permanent loss of personhood, even though the person is still alive. Over time, many families have increasing difficulties in maintaining reciprocity in the relationship with the patient, and the question arises whether the person who is relatively intact physically but unavailable mentally is still part of the family. The physical presence and intellectual absence lead to a phenomenon called boundary ambiguity in the family system (Jones & Martinson, 1992). Such ambiguity has been found to be related to a low sense of mastery and helplessness (Boss, Caron, Horbal, & Mortimer, 1990).

Although these research findings present a beginning toward a fuller understanding of the complex, long-term adjustment of the patient, primary caregiver, and family, much remains unexplored. The framework of systemic organization has a high potential of being useful for the derivation of interventions that can then be tested. This framework encourages the careful assessment of families in terms of their specific life process and relationships with the patient. Interventions for a family who seeks distancing from the patient may focus on exploring possibilities for institutionalization if it promises relief rather than excessive guilt. In contrast, families who want to continue care and seek reciprocity in the relationship with the patient may benefit from resources that ease their task and consultations about ways to maintain the wholeness of the patient. Such families will find satisfaction through individuation. The following example illustrates the second approach.

Dee is 77 years old and has been widowed for 10 years. Since the death of her husband, she has had little energy, and her life appears without joy. About 5 years ago, she started to forget things and neglect her daily duties. At that point, her son and daughter-in-law, worried about the safety of her living by herself, convinced her to move in with them. Dee's son, Phil, feels very attached to her, and for his wife, Laura, who was orphaned in childhood, Dee has long served in the role of a mother. Four years ago, Dee was taken to a clinic, where she underwent intensive testing and was tentatively diagnosed with Alzheimer's disease. While Dee lived with her son and family, her condition deteriorated rather rapidly. Her behaviors were difficult to tolerate. Dee accused Laura of stealing her money and locking her in to keep her prisoner. She kept calling her friend to come and get her out of the prison. One year later, she did not recognize her family members any more and spent every evening packing her suitcase to go look for her husband. Both Laura and Phil tried hard to talk her out of these ideas but without success. Instead, Dee became more irritated and saw Phil as a policeman who tried to arrest her without justification. She became increasingly stubborn and wandered around the house at night so that the various rooms needed to be locked for safety reasons. Dee's hygiene presented a challenge as well. She refused to change her clothes or take a bath. As a result of all this, Laura became irritable and accused Phil of expecting the impossible of her. The two argued frequently until they finally asked for help from their physician.

As a result, a visiting nurse visit is ordered to set up a care plan with the family and help is arranged with activities of daily living (ADL) and a bath twice a week. After discussing the plan with Phil and Laura, the nurse arranges for the admission of Dee to a day treatment center. This is ideal for Laura, who now has some time for herself again. The visiting nurse is a practitioner in geriatric nursing who also spends some of her time practicing in the day treatment program. The nurse instructs Laura to earn Dee's cooperation by gently leading Dee to believe that they would go on a pleasure trip, something Dee used to do often in the past. Dee would then go to the center without resistance. A few days later, the nurse asks for a lengthy time period for the purpose of an extensive assessment. In addition, she observes Dee on three different occasions in the center, as she interacts with the staff and the other patients. She wants to understand Dee's life process as it unfolds, because she assumes that Dee, plagued by anxiety as she loses more and more of her ability to control her situation, is somehow attempting stability. The nurse, on the basis of the framework of systemic organization, assumes that Dee can be assisted in maintaining her dignity. The strong bonding with the family is a valuable resource that needs to be nurtured at all costs. Dee needs the family to support her system maintenance, and help has to be offered in such a way that her coherence is not threatened. The nurse senses a need for intensive work with the family, because they have little understanding of the true nature of Dee's condition at the present time. Before they can give more of themselves, their own needs have to be attended to. They feel hurt and exhausted as a result of being bombarded with accusations by Dee and faced with her unexpected angry outbreaks. Nevertheless, they are preoccupied with Dee and willing to report all they know in great detail.

Assessment of the Individuum

System Maintenance. Dee's organic problems have led to serious memory deficiencies and loss of orientation to place or time. Dee lives in the past and the present at the same time. Her confusion is not without meaning. It seems that she tries to create a world for herself that grants her some stability and prevents chaos. She calls on the stability she has experienced in the past in compensation for her inability to perceive and absorb what is happening to her at the present. This created world is one in which Dee can sense wholeness and satisfaction that reach beyond her disability and rid herself of anxiety. In her new world, Dee feels some congruence, which explains why her reality is of extreme importance to her and why attempts to talk her out of it are met with vicious counterattacks. If family tension rises because of her reactions, her anxiety becomes uncontrollable and her behavior becomes extreme.

Dee is unable to care for herself. She may start with an activity but forgets what she is doing in the middle of it. Furthermore, she has problems with eye, hand, and motor coordination that render many activities impossible. In better times, Dee liked to work and feel useful. Her fantasies are witness to these values that have been kept intact. Even now, Dee wants to help with tasks, and she accepts assistance willingly. For example, she can brush her teeth after meals if she is reminded of the activity several times and her hand is gently guided back to her mouth. She has always been meticulous about hygiene and appearance, so her latest refusal to take a bath seems unrelated to the actual activity. In day care, she likes to comb other patients' hair or decorate them with necklaces or flowers. Dee can still perform simple household tasks, such as drying a plate or even cutting vegetables under very close supervision. She has never liked crafts, games, or other "useless" activities.

Coherence. Dee needs structure to maintain her stability. A daily routine is important, because her participation in familiar tasks strengthens her sense of worth. Activities need to be considered useful by Dee to deserve her attention. Dee used to be a good dancer. Even now, she loves to listen to dance music and tunes of her youth and hums along. Sometimes, Dee remembers the tunes even after some time has passed. Music seems to engulf her with patterns and rhythms, a structure that provides her with a temporary stability. One can observe Dee relax her tense muscles, tap the rhythm with her feet, and swing with the music. Her facial expression is happy because she seems inwardly directed, absorbed, and concentrated, as if ascending to a world of peace that confirms her humanness. Could it be that music presents a medium for transcendence through which Dee can experience the structure and rhythm of systemic congruence with the universal order?

Individuation. Dee's need for human connectedness is intact. She wants to be with people and be useful. In the group at the day treatment center, she reacts positively to persons who understand her world, and in her fantasies she turns these persons into friends from the past with whom she can find pleasure and joy. In times when she feels threatened and misunderstood, however, Dee searches for what she has lost. For example, she wanders restlessly searching for her husband, her most important source of love, comfort, and consolation.

System Change. If it is true that pain and suffering lead to system change in that they open new ways to reach congruence, one may suspect that this holds true for Dee. A possibility exists that her disability opens up a reality inaccessible to others and that Dee may be one step closer to sensing universal order, for the perception of which full cognition is a hindrance. No nurse will ever know. What is observable, however, is a process of continuous adjustment to ever-increasing losses in the search of new congruence, much of which occurs on a subconscious level. The absence of anxiety and uncontrolled impulsive behaviors, as well as her occasional apparent state of bliss, seems to suggest that Dee is succeeding at least for short periods of time. Therefore, Dee's life process needs to be supported as it unfolds, and, in interacting with Dee, nurses and the family need to exert extreme caution not to interfere with her reality.

Assessment of Individual Health

Dee's life process signifies health in that it enables Dee to find congruence despite physical change. To successfully understand the life process of Dee and others like her, the nurse uses a perception that goes beyond the actual behavioral manifestation. It involves an intense probing for meaning, a search for symbols connected to the patient's life history, and careful attempts to enter the patient's reality to become part of it.

Nursing Care of the Family

It is particularly important that families who cannot intuitively enter the world of their loved one be assisted if they have the willingness and capacity to do so. Nursing of this family involves two goals: (a) The nurse's perception of Dee's life process is shared with the family and possible misunderstandings are corrected, and (b) the family needs to be instructed in creative caregiving based on Dee's life process and the family's own patterns and needs.

The nurse realizes her need to understand the family better, but both Laura and Phil's major concern is Dee. Therefore, the nurse plans to work with them in the day care setting and collect necessary data in the process. She invites Laura and Phil to join her for 2 days for a minipracticum in caring for Dee. Although Laura is excited, Phil has to decline because his work situation does not allow it. In preparation for Laura's practicum, they both receive literature about the care of patients with Alzheimer's disease. On the first day, Laura mainly observes and asks questions. The nurse demonstrates communicating with Dee. The nurse also explains to Laura that Dee's thought process transfers her into a better world, and she shows her how to divert Dee to other thoughts that are also compatible with her reality and usual patterns of thinking. For example, when Dee stubbornly wants to leave to visit her husband, the nurse tells Dee that this trip makes sense, but because the train is not leaving yet, she has much time to eat a snack before going. Besides, she would like to meet Dee's husband also but needs something to eat first. Dee is easily distracted by the smell of fresh coffee and sits down at the table with Laura and the nurse. During the rest of the day, the nurse demonstrates ways to gain cooperation, assistance in task completion, and other interventions. On the second day, Laura is encouraged and supported as she tries to approach Dee in a similar way and is very excited about Dee's positive response. Because Laura wonders why Dee does so well in the day treatment center but is very difficult at home, the nurse invites both Laura and Phil to a meeting to assess the family and discuss the problems.

Assessment of the Family

System Maintenance. Daily routine starts early because Dee wanders around before sunrise. A difficult situation may develop as follows: Laura prepares breakfast for Dee at 6 a.m. so Phil can sleep a little longer. Usually, she encounters difficulties, for example, when Dee waves the spoon in the air after filling it with cereal and milk. Laura tries to take Dee's hand and guide the spoon to her mouth, to which Dee reacts by screeching and cursing and flinging cereal onto the floor. Then Phil enters to complain about the disturbance and leads Dee to the armchair while arguing with his wife. He then feeds Dee, which may work for some time, but he tends to rush her, to which Dee responds by spitting the food out. Phil then stomps out of the kitchen and leaves for work. On weekends, Phil and Laura share responsibilities. Successful are walks with Dee outside, playing Dee's favorite songs, or letting her fold towels, which she does over and over. They used to take Dee shopping but that stopped because she made scenes in public that embarrassed them greatly.

Coherence. Caring for Dee is a difficult test of the marital relationship. Both feel guilty about their failure to control Dee's behaviors. There is a strong sense of responsibility on the side of Phil that Laura can understand well. Laura, however, has to swallow a lot and feels burnt out and without energy. Day care is a great relief, but Phil still has difficulties getting enough sleep, because he is expected to participate in Dee's care in the evenings and on weekends. His work situation has become more stressful as well. He is longing for a vacation, a chance to do as he pleases, and an evening of fun with Laura. They have no extended family in the vicinity. Laura's two brothers are in another state and Phil has no siblings. There used to be friends who came over to play cards or joined them on a weekend trip. They also used to enjoy gardening, but they have not found time lately.

Individuation. The discussion is filled with reports of problems, worries, and unhappiness about the situation. When asked about the possible benefits in relation to the mother's living with them, Laura and Phil hesitantly state that they have matured a great deal and have gained insight into their true nature—something that is less than pleasant. They have thought much about the meaning of suffering, but they have not shared these thoughts with each other. What was important for them earlier—relaxation, sports, fun, travel—they don't miss too much any more. Somehow, their priorities have shifted.

System Change. Dee has significantly changed the family system. Laura and Phil have lost control. Change has occurred quickly, and the family members are anxious about future developments, even within their partnership, that seem to be unpredictable. They have tried to get Dee to adjust to their routines without success and have resigned in desperation. Day treatment has helped, but they know they need to make other changes to prevent being victimized by the situation.

Assessment of Family Health

The nurse realizes that the family is in need of a basic change. In her condition, Dee cannot be expected to adjust to the family's daily routine. Laura and Phil need to learn how to individuate by accepting Dee's reality as a target to exercise spirituality. They need to steer away from controlling symptoms of the disease and instead strive to gain quality in a life that integrates the disease. Such acceptance may lead them to unforeseen insight and experiences that promote a new coherence.

First, the nurse explains to the couple the systemic diagram and uses the terms to explain to them how she understands Dee's life

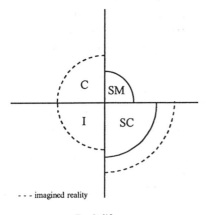

a - Dee's life process

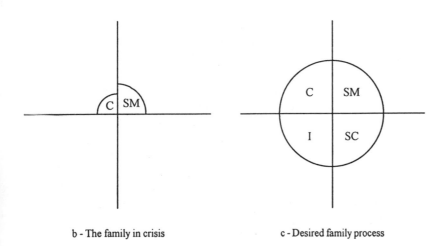

b - The family in crisis   c - Desired family process

Figure 14.2. Systemic Processes of Dee and Dee's Family

process and struggle to counteract the unavoidable physical changes. Using the diagram pictured in Figure 14.2a, she explains that Dee's imagined reality assists in reducing the effect of system change and allows individuation by creating a world in which old relationships are relived and rewards are reearned. In this world, coherence can be nourished and wholeness attained. The nurse stresses Dee's remaining strengths within system maintenance and points out how they can be supported. Furthermore, she stresses that Dee's outbreaks are not personal attacks but reactions to a threat of losing stability or congruence. All along, the nurse expresses her admiration for Laura and Phil's commitment to facing these difficulties.

Next, the family process is discussed. Figure 14.2 points to the needed change process of the family. Diagram b shows the family in crisis. Change is overwhelming and uncontrolled. Instead of adjusting to it, the family adheres to its old patterns and values. The greatest part of the family's energy goes toward system maintenance, but the old strategies are no longer useful. The desperate family members' individuation is blocked as they find themselves in crisis. Diagram c is their desired outcome: new coherence through better understanding of Dee and satisfaction with caregiving, individuation brought about by meaningful experiences in the caregiving process and mastery of the situation, and new system maintenance strategies that ease the fulfillment of everyone's needs. Much additional system change expected in connection with ongoing personality changes of Dee is anticipated, but this time, the family wants to meet it head-on with the ongoing assistance of the nurse.

During the second practicum in the day care center, the nurse guides Laura as she attempts to communicate with Dee. Together, the nurse and Laura engage in hypothesizing the meaning of Dee's confusion and experimenting with strategies that would calm her down or support her memory. Growth occurs slowly and needs to be guided over a longer period of time. The nurse hopes that feelings of guilt and shame in relation to Laura's episodes of lost control will diminish with time and that the family may eventually take Dee outside for walks again and for visits to a store. Furthermore, she explores the couple's willingness to join a support group or accept respite care for Dee so they can take a short vacation together.

The example illustrates the fragile balance of a family struggling to integrate a cognitively impaired mother into the system and seeking renewed congruence. The integration of new members ordinarily occurs through the spirituality process, in which all parties carefully feel each other out and mutually attune themselves to the family's system maintenance and its underlying values. Laura and Phil had expected

Dee to make certain concessions, but Dee's impediment prevented any type of mutuality in the adjustment process. The constant physical and emotional demands altered rhythms and patterns in the family and evoked anxiety and fear of what the future might bring. Without reciprocity, the necessary changes in system maintenance signified a sacrifice of Laura's and Phil's personal rights, time, and space. Such sacrifices ordinarily have limits if they do not concurrently earn some of the anticipated rewards, such as signs of happiness and gratitude by the mother. Because strides toward growth and spirituality had failed, this family sensed the threat of destruction of harmony, coherence, and the personal autonomy of each member. A natural reaction to the loss of congruence is control, which in this case signified the use of methods to control Dee.

The framework of systemic organization explains control as a response to helplessness and an attempt to prevent the breakdown of system maintenance. However, the ensuing pattern effects the opposite. The findings of two relevant research studies illustrate this central issue. These researchers report that, generally, caregivers, unaware of the need for change, perform their daily routine, physical care, and social activities and expect the patient to cooperate. Although this may operate successfully in the initial stages, with increasing dementia, as the patient loses the ability to live up to the expectations, the anxious and threatened patient begins to obstruct routine tasks in defense of personal integrity. Realizing the need for change, some caregivers may turn progressively more rigid in controlling the activities and the patient's behaviors (Phillips & Rempusheski, 1986; Smith, Smith, & Toseland, 1991). It is easy to recognize that in this manner the line between caring and abuse can become a fine one. Even Laura, basically good-natured and committed to help, lost her composure as she recognized the futility of controlling Dee.

The process of individuation is critical to quality caregiving and the prevention of abuse (Phillips & Rempusheski, 1986). In Laura's case, the nurse targeted reciprocity. Laura was helped to find meaning in caregiving not only through efficient physical care but through a new understanding of her role as a protector of Dee's remaining personhood. With much sensitivity and consideration of Laura's own needs, the nurse has introduced her to individuation, the ongoing process of discovering and rediscovering Dee's life patterns. It amounts to

Laura's continuing adjustment of expectations and exploration of new ways of relating. As a result, the nurse hopes that Laura will gain appreciation of Dee's creativity in compensating and compromising and that she will share her insights with Phil. This example shows clearly that the key to health is the sustenance of reciprocity rather than radical distancing from the person.

Using the framework of systemic organization, however, leads nurses to acknowledge significant differences among families. It becomes evident that individuation cannot be taught to all. In fact, evidence exists that relationships with the patients are transformed and sometimes lost and that the resolution of grief over such losses necessitates one's distancing from these painful aspects (Chesla et al., 1994). Although distancing seems necessary to maintain personal coherence, the extent of it and the aspects of the patient from which caregivers seek distance differ greatly. Nursing care varies accordingly. Through the process of nursing described in Chapter 2, nurses need to gain understanding of the potential of families to individuate with the patient. Families who radically distance themselves from the patient and have lost their ability to perceive the patient's personhood may be better advised to seek institutionalization and leave the care to others. In fact, honesty and objectivity of such assessments with a built-in understanding that problems are likely to intensify with time are critical for the prevention of abuse and despair.

15

Research With Families
Who Experience Disease and Illness

Research relative to the topic of this chapter concerns the very core of nursing. It addresses the following questions: How do families function when they have a member with an illness? What is family caregiving? How can nurses best assist families in situations of illness and death? All three questions refer to processes that have remarkable similarity. The first question centers around the most basic process, the systemic process of families and all that is involved in the family's pursuit of renewed health. The second question refers to the families' caring for an ill member. The process relates to attitudes, beliefs, behaviors, interactions, relationships, and exchanges with the environment that are specific to giving care but at the same time are inseparable from the overall life process. The third question addresses the nursing process with families that aims at strengthening and enhancing the family life process. Therefore, the study of family nursing has the task of unfolding processes that form the basis of family life, examining the nurse-family interface, and discovering how the process facilitates or hinders the families' very private struggle to attain the four systemic targets, congruence, and health.

The second aim of research in this area is evaluation or the examination of the process outcome, which is health. It is of vital importance for nurses to understand how their actions and the conditions of the health care setting in which they work contribute to the systemic process of families and what results from it. Although pure experimental designs may be most trustworthy in providing answers about direct effects of nursing interventions on groups of families, they are deficient in explaining variations among families. The same nursing action can result in drastically different outcomes, depending on how new information, suggestions for behavior change, or addition of resources are accepted and integrated into family knowledge and processes. Furthermore, outcomes depend on perception, that is, the families' interpretation of their situation, definition of their needs, and willingness to accept support and assistance. It follows that to be truly informative, evaluations need to focus on the families' own perception of their situation and provide answers about when to do what for which type of family. Consequently, this chapter includes discussions of research design and implementation issues around both the exploration of family and nursing processes and the evaluation of their effectiveness.

Research of the
Family Life Process and Nursing

In preparation for the large California Family Health Project that focused on family functioning in relation to various health outcomes, the researchers reviewed the literature on families and health. They identified several major problems. First, they noted that most research addresses only fragments of the family and health processes, that is, one or two family dimensions, structural characteristics, or behaviors in relation to one or more health measures. Often, constructs are labeled unclearly. Sometimes, constructs labeled differently across studies are actually the same, but other constructs that claimed to be similar consist of different components. Generally, there is no indication about how certain family dimensions are connected with each other. Other problems are the limited range of variables examined that serve as indicators of health, and finally the narrowly defined populations, all of which have specific, identified health problems. Such studies preclude the detection of factors common to families across various populations (Fisher, Ransom, Terry, Lipkin, & Weiss, 1992).

Discussing the concept of social support, Krahn (1993) assessed similar problems, mainly a narrow focus in research, and urged investigators to conceptualize families who have children with developmental disorders as being no different from families in general. Such families had functions and dysfunctions similar to others and were subjected to a series of crises influencing their system like most others. Consequently, research, to provide sufficient insight into the family process and clinical guidance for nurses, needs to take on a broad perspective (i.e., a systemic look at various patterns and rhythms and descriptions of how persons act, feel, and value family life within the context of their environment).

The reader is referred to the previous discussions about systemic research in Chapter 10. Specifically, issues of individual system interface, diversity, and evolution of systems over time are relevant here. Furthermore, what has been said about methods to overcome the shortcomings of quantitative methods, for example, linearity, central tendency, and difficulties assessing change in the life process, can be applied here as well. Likewise, problems with qualitative research, such as reactivity and generalizability, are of great relevance for the study of family process and nursing.

The case examples described in the previous chapters represent nursing process in action. With Ralph's family, the nurse is actively involved in facilitating interpersonal growth through Ralph's and Betty's mutual acceptance of each other's values and beliefs. The next example refers to a process of the nurse finding a brief spiritual union with Harry, the patient, at the time of his death. In the third example, the nurse becomes an actress in an interpersonal system through which individuation and a beginning acceptance of Amanda's death becomes possible for Maureen, Amanda's mother. Edith's case describes nursing at both the individual level in terms of facilitation of system change and at the family level, at which Edith becomes reintegrated into her family system. The example of Tim describes the family's ongoing struggle to find a new level of health and crisis resolution as the nurse introduces new meanings and perceptions that allow a change of course in the family process. Finally, the example of Dee and her family illuminates the need for ongoing mutuality and individuation in the caregiver-patient relationship and the great challenge for continuous spiritual reconnection with Dee as her perception of the world shifts further away from the norm. Questions surrounding such processes involve the nature, meaning, and experience of nursing as it brings about individuation and system change in both client and nurse.

If research is evolving through the direct interaction of the researcher with the subjects, it becomes a clinical process. This means that the changes in perceptions of reality that accompany the qualitative research process and are viewed as a distortion of the subjects' reality (Sandelowski, 1993) may be advantageous. They may constitute the actual evolutionary force that bridges practice and research and, consequently, represent an asset in the research process rather than a limitation (Oiler Boyd, 1993). Newman (1990) describes such evolving research as an expansion of consciousness, and Berg and Smith (1988) stress its ethical value in providing knowledge and insight to both subjects and the researcher. In terms of the framework of systemic organization, this growth-promoting experience is termed *individuation.*

Oiler Boyd (1993) proposes that qualitative clinical research can be done concurrently with nursing practice and that its emphasis is on questions about the families' and family members' experience of their own health, nursing care, and interactions with the health care system and with other societal institutions. Practitioners scramble with the same questions as they explore and assess their clients' life process and perceptions of their situation. Oiler Boyd (1993) suggests that adding a research focus to one's usual practice simply communicates to others what is learned in the process to the benefit of all involved.

Along the same line, the case examples of the preceding chapters could be intensified in detail and rigor to qualify as case studies. Multiple case studies can serve as a means to test theory centering around a common phenomenon. For example, because individuation in the caregiver-client relationship is key to health and congruence, according to the framework of systemic organization, a researcher may want to contrast those families who succeed in maintaining a high level of health with those who are plagued by anxiety, guilt, and resentment. Among a number of case studies of families in different types of caregiving situations, the nurse may identify certain caregivers who feel rewarded by their task, report satisfaction, and tell both humorous and sad stories of discoveries, amazement, or positive responses of the person they care for. Even though these caregivers are likely to talk about periods of severe distress, overall, they will express confidence and courage about the future. Such cases can be contrasted with families in crisis in which individuation is shown to be lacking. The researcher will compare individual and family life processes, specifically values and beliefs, interpretations of the situation, system maintenance behaviors, and readiness to make changes, to detect the remarkable features of families who succeed with their difficult task and the shortcomings in the others. The practical value and comprehensiveness of such research depend on their theoretical foundation. The researcher is guided by the theoretical framework to the phenomena of interest and the observations to be expected and to the characteristics along which the cases should be compared. In all of the previous case examples, the theory leads to the operationalization of individuation as a positive process of evolution connected to caregiving. The research findings provide the specifics with which the process gains texture and color.

This type of research also allows nurses to gain valuable insight into purely experiential phenomena, such as the process of individuation in a spiritual union with a patient (e.g., Harry in the previous example). Nurses' stories about profound experiences could open up the willingness of others to share their own stories. Qualitative research in this area could specify shared philosophical tenets about the meaning of life and death and much-needed open discussion that allows self-examination and leads to maturation of the nurses who care for dying patients and their families. Open sharing would undoubtedly lead to change in certain health care settings, in that the process of individuation through means of spirituality within nursing care would become legitimate.

If research is done for the purpose of testing theory, two issues are of major importance in terms of validity of the findings. The first is self-scrutiny, a matter of importance with regard to ethics. Self-scrutiny refers to the willingness to examine one's own values and the honesty and flexibility to change theory if the results run contrary to one's expectations. Honesty is endangered if the investigator has invested much commitment and energy in a certain theory. For example, temptation may become considerable if all that is needed to support the theory and make the story coherent are a few details of the stories that the respondent has "forgotten to report." The second issue is related. In listening to stories, analyzing them, or examining additional evidence, researchers cannot attend to all details. Investigators bring into the study their own worldview and culture, prior knowledge, and experience, which they use to focus on selected details and create order among them. The cost of ordering along one's own paradigm is a narrow focus due to the loss of alternative perceptions (Sadler & Hulgus, 1991).

The interference of an inflexible mind-set can be prevented to some extent by validation of research conclusions by the subjects. Another mechanism to protect against bias is investigator triangulation. This method is useful, however, only if the investigators have truly divergent mind-sets derived from different backgrounds and schools of thought. Institutions tend to shape individuals who work within them. Therefore, triangulation may be ineffective in providing depth of understanding if research associates are socialized in the same discipline, have worked with similar role models, and have developed a homogeneous thinking process about phenomena.

Interventions with individuals and families can also be studied by action-oriented research approaches. Hospital units, hospice teams, nursing home care teams, or home care agencies may experiment with new approaches. For example, a family assessment of all-new clinic patients with the framework of systemic organization may be a new procedure introduced on a trial basis. New assessment data are compared with data collected in the traditional way to evaluate the merit of the new procedure. For example, qualitative data, such as self-evaluations of client health, which are now part of the new theory-based assessments, are compared with data collected with the old structured assessment tools. Then, two separate focus groups of patients and nurses critique the value and comprehensiveness of both methods and ultimately suggest what they see as the optimal procedure. Emotional responses of staff and clients to the new method are carefully noted when analyzing the audiotaped focus group sessions and staff and patient opinion surveys. These data are taken into consideration by the action team in making decisions to expand, modify, or discontinue the new assessment procedure. Finally, quantitative data derived from instruments evaluating treatment outcomes can be used to provide feedback to the action team to adjust the assessment process accordingly.

Other research methods are equally useful for the study of processes. Ethnography was cited in previous chapters and deserves mentioning again. In exploring the life process of families and the support nurses are able to provide, culture is exceedingly important, first to account for variation among families, and second, to explore culture as the context in which families and nurses function. The area of cultural differences among families remains largely unreported (Krahn, 1993). According to the framework of systemic organization, culture is lived in families. In fact, ethnicity as a unique variable may be of minor importance in predicting health outcomes, compared with the more basic family processes that subsume its effects (Bowen, 1976). Consequently, family variability, or the family type defined in terms of the four process dimensions and the values that provide meaning to the behaviors, promises to be a strong predictor of family health-seeking behaviors. In fact, the California Family Health Project (Ransom, Fisher, & Terry, 1992) yielded such findings. On the basis of a search of the literature, the investigators inductively arrived at a concept they called "family worldview." They then tested the relationship of eight variables pertaining to the concept with family health variables. The variable "life engagement" expressed the "belief that it is reasonable to take calculated risks, try new things, and enjoy change" (p. 255). This variable seems to be similar to system change in terms of the family's readiness to make changes. Another construct, called "family coherence," resembles system maintenance or control. Both variables were significantly related to several health indicators, such as health perceptions, preventive behaviors, self-esteem, low anxiety, and depression. More research in this area is needed.

The framework of systemic organization suggests a structure of family types that varies according to the emphasis families put on behaviors relative to the four process dimensions. Because such a family type constitutes the actual life process, one would expect it to be a strong predictor of certain process outcomes. The development of a useful screening tool for family type, however, presents a challenge still to be undertaken. First, items pertaining to each process dimension should be neutral because the issue is the family's preference for the behaviors rather than the success or effectiveness in using them.

Furthermore, a still greater challenge is presented by the fact that most observed behaviors cannot be objectively grouped into the four dimensions without considering the motivations that drive them. For example, the activity of watching television can pertain to system maintenance, if it is part of the family's activity-rest pattern; to coherence, if members see it as an opportunity for togetherness and sharing of impressions about the programs; or to individuation, if families watch selectively those programs that are educational. The task, therefore, will be to construct a tool for screening families according to their type with items pertaining to activities that clearly express only one dimension and are equally accepted by families of various cultures and educational levels. In addition, the activities need to be scored on a Likert-type scale expressing degrees of intensity or frequency with which these behaviors are used.

A quantitative tool to assess family types along the four process dimensions would be useful in finding answers to diverse questions about nursing interventions. A few include the following: How do needs for information, resources, health education, or emotional support differ among families? How do various families want to be involved in the care of their loved ones at home, in the hospital, or in the nursing home? How do families differ in their ability to interact with the hospital unit staff? How do families differ in their ability to resolve a crisis brought on by mental illness?

Even though the typical research design to address these questions is structural modeling with the limitations cited earlier, studies of this nature would present a large step away from creating one intervention applicable to all and programs that clients are expected to accept, whether or not they are congruent with their life process.

Problems with noncompliance or refusal to accept help in one form or another are far from being solved. There is no concept such as noncompliance in terms of the framework of systemic organization because the nurse does not order the patient of the family to do certain things or follow instructions. Instead, the regime is negotiated and fine-tuned with the family life process. Consequently, nurses need to know how information and available resources should be packaged to be suitable for use with specific types of families. If research findings were available that show how specific family types could be matched with their preferred resources and nursing interventions, a considerable proportion of nursing energy, time, and money could be saved. Such a research program driven by this framework presents a worthwhile goal for the future.

In designing studies to explore family process, a longitudinal focus is desperately needed. The volume of reported research using longitudinal data collections is still small (Campbell, Mutran, & Parker, 1987). Prospective studies are useful in investigating family patterns such as support seeking, caregiving, using resources, and others as they evolve over time and in response to the afflicted person's change of condition (Turner, 1983). In the caregiving process, for example, variables that vary with time are of particular importance because they influence the ultimate decision of institutionalization (Montgomery & Kosloski, 1994).

Within the systemic process, however, such variables change in ways that are difficult to predict. There is little stability in that even the family type variable may change in difficult situations as culture becomes transformed and the life process takes a different course. Although multivariate techniques such as MANOVA or event history analysis allow for the assessment of change in predictor variables, the designs represent comparisons of a situation frozen at various points in time rather than an account of process and movement. The understanding of the process in motion can be enhanced by methods triangulation as it was described in Chapter 6. There is a need to know what happened between time one and two, the ups and downs a caregiver has experienced, the changes of perceptions, and the feelings of burden. Only through their stories can subjects report how their priorities have shifted and how life takes on a different meaning. Such information can be skillfully used by researchers to interpret quantitative findings scientifically. The information precludes educated guessing that often results in "overinterpretation" of quantitative findings. Furthermore, if analysis and interpretation of longitudinal processes are firmly grounded in theory, the likelihood of their validity is greatly enhanced and the methods of analysis can be safely considered tests of the theoretical model.

Up to this point, the discussion has involved the exploration of family and nursing processes with various methods. The second type of research indicated in the introductory part of this chapter is evaluation of nursing modalities and programs.

Evaluation Research

Evaluation studies are undertaken to validate the single or comparative usefulness of interventions or programs. Their designs historically have been atheoretical. Evaluation and survey tools are constructed for the assessment of opinions and satisfaction, records are compared with quality criteria, and the ultimate design for a credible outcome is considered a classical experiment with controls and random sampling (Patton, 1987).

Experiments and quasi-experiments do not conflict with the framework of systemic organization. They are suitable for clearly defined and structured programs that are administered identically time after time. Examples are teaching modalities, demonstration projects, parent training with structured content, or a systematic orientation for families of new patients in a nursing home. The expense of a rigorous experiment is considerable and a statistical validation of benefit to the participants is influenced by many factors. Furthermore, a program that fares best in an experiment is one designed to meet the needs of the average client. Even then, findings that result from an extensive program may be disappointing, unclear, or doubtful. Reasons may be quantitative instruments of questionable quality in terms of assessing the essential and changes over time or methodological flaws, such as high drop-out rates or situational changes over time. Therefore, the use of accompanying descriptive, evaluative, or phenomenological studies to produce data that assist the interpretation of quantitative findings is almost indispensable.

If the interest is in tailoring flexible programs that respond to the needs of diverse client groups, however, other methods of evaluation have to be used. My evaluation of the theory-based Congruence Model (Friedemann, 1992) presents an example that combines both structure and flexibility and therefore uses a quasi-experimental design with multiple measures over time in combination with a method to assess the attainment of individual and family goals set in treatment. The psychoeducational modality used with families of substance abusers in rehabilitation is made up of eight sessions with highly structured objectives, educational content, and experiential exercises. Within this structured format, however, time is provided for clients to set their own goals and define ways to meet them, all of which is highly individualized. For the evaluation, a quasi-experimental design was used that involved comparable controls from the same treatment center. Outcome was defined as family health measured in terms of a subjective assessment of the family's effectiveness of processes pertaining to the four dimensions of system maintenance, system change, coherence, and individuation as well as general satisfaction with the family. Consequently, family health was operationalized by using the scores on the Assessment of Strategies in Families (ASF) instrument (Friedemann, 1991a) and the Family Apgar with five global items expressing satisfaction with the family (Smilkstein, 1978). Data were collected at the beginning and end of treatment and 1 month after treatment, with equal intervals for repeated measures in the control group.

The individualized approach and flexibility in the program were evaluated differently. Progress with personal and family goals during and after treatment was measured with the goal attainment scaling method developed by Kiresuk and Sherman (1975). This method allows for individualized descriptions of steps of partial goal attainment that lead to optimal goal attainment and assigns numerical values to the steps that can then be statistically evaluated. Consequently, the method is longitudinal, allows for the consideration of individual differences, and allows for quantitative statistical methods, in this case multiple measure analysis of variance. The findings of this study are described elsewhere (Friedemann, 1994).

In the above evaluation, no rigorous qualitative component was added; however, the findings suggested a definite need. For example, after eight sessions, the scores of family effectiveness in the treatment group were somewhat lower than before treatment. In comparison, change in the control group was minimal. This was unexpected but could be explained by an increased awareness of the treatment group subjects. This could have happened through a process of individuation and a subsequent change in their self-evaluation. Thus, an apparently unfavorable statistic might have been a desired effect of treatment, but there was no scientific evidence to support this. Additional interviews with the subjects with the purpose of clarifying the phenomenon of individuation would have lent the study more depth and value.

In evaluations of this nature, controls need to be rigorous. This then may raise the question of beneficence and ethics of experiments. For example, certain families may suffer a delay in treatment due to their assignment to a control group or receive a less desirable intervention if they constitute part of a comparison group. Consequently, there may be a need for other designs. Much of what was previously said about the study of process can be applied here, too, to gain depth without rigor that exceeds usefulness. Patton (1987) suggests the use of qualitative methods in evaluation to assess perceptions of the clients and staff and explore the diversity among those perceptions for the purpose of gaining depth and insight. Furthermore, qualitative data can ensure quality of treatment by providing evidence that standards are met and promises are kept.

An evaluation approach with methods triangulation is in keeping with this framework. Although the experiment measures the outcome of the final product, there is a need for additional study to assess the process leading to the product. The program or intervention itself is a process. Once instituted, it unfolds and the researcher is encouraged to promote a formative or process evaluation with techniques much like the ones described earlier. This is absolutely necessary if the program is not entirely living up to its promises, and, in reality, this rarely happens. With additional surveys, interviews, case studies, and more, researchers can point to possible problems and guide the way to make improvements. Of particular interest is the diversification of interventions for the sake of accommodating various types of individuals and families.

The methods used in evaluation are driven by the questions, and the purpose of the project within its context will determine the questions to be asked (Asen et al., 1991). Therefore, many creative possibilities exist, but necessary standards and controls have to be strictly enforced. For example, Aaronson and Burman (1994) urge researchers who use client records, a highly popular data source in evaluation studies, to assess the quality and validity of the data in the records before using them and possibly supplement them with alternative information.

In summary, the framework of systemic organization leads the researcher to examine multiple methods and combine them to yield the broadest possible and most complete information about the unfolding of the processes under study. Asen and his associates (1991) indicate that the planning of an evaluation design is no simple matter. They describe a complex process of planning an evaluation of their family therapy interventions. This planning process turned out to constitute a series of preliminary research studies to determine what kind of evaluation components would be most suitable to use systematically over time. Much thought and preparation go into a complex evaluation design, including the development of necessary assessment scales and opinion surveys. Researchers are advised to provide ample time for these preliminary activities and carefully examine all issues related to complex methodologies. Questions asked are whether data to be explored need to be factual or subjective, emic or etic, and from whose perspective they should be derived (Asen et al., 1991). Furthermore, issues discussed earlier about multiple respondents of the same family and the analysis of their data as well as the unit of analysis are also relevant for this area of research.

Ultimately, validation of theories and nursing interventions calls us to define a sense of coherence, correspondence, and pragmatism. If the theory has meaning and truth, it must be logically consistent within itself and finally help families solve problems (Silva & Sorrel, 1992). The framework of systemic organization has the potential to help researchers accomplish these tasks.

PART
5

Families in Crisis:
Crises From the Environment

Introduction

Crises from the environment are evoked by detrimental influences on individuals and the family system. Common to all such crises is the victimization of the people involved and, in terms of the framework of systemic organization, a forced system change. Victims often change their view of the world radically in that their self-confidence or sense of power and control gives way to helplessness and a new realization that justice is nonexistent. Such changes have serious repercussions on the individual's role perceptions and the entire family process. Specific environmental crises differ in various aspects: They may be sudden, as in a natural disaster, a traffic accident, a crime, or an arrest of a family member, or they may develop insidiously as the victims' life process attempts to remain stable and becomes incapable of reaching a satisfactory level of congruence. Examples of the latter are intolerable work conditions or forced retirement. Both types of crises eventually force the victims to radically change their systems, get out of the situation, or suffer the consequences. A similar variant is presented by sudden events that result in a delayed crisis, as in a job loss situation that becomes hopeless after insurance money runs out and no new employment can be obtained.

Crises with severe economic repercussions that cannot be resolved drive people into a marginal lifestyle in which family systems change their priorities to day-to-day survival and most mainstream values become irrelevant. The framework of systemic organization purports that in those situations, the development of a lifestyle centered around adaptation to deprivation occurs through culture transformation and results in a pervasive, self-defeating culture of poverty. The prevention of such culture transformation should be a priority in public policy in that families need the resources to avoid economic crises or reverse them, if they occur (Bane, 1986).

This part will illustrate the nursing process with relevant case examples. Chapter 16 describes the impact of a crime. Chapter 17 discusses the role of employment and work conditions in the life process of women, men, and the family system, and Chapter 18 highlights responses to loss of work, unemployment, and economic hardship. Chapter 19 discusses the family life process with chronic poverty and homelessness.

16

Affront From a Hostile Environment

Violent crimes hit individuals and families like a bolt from the blue (Pittman, 1987). The event signifies a serious loss, possibly of property and physical health, but most of all of such intangible properties as dignity, self-respect, security, and sense of control. Furthermore, the event destroys the belief in the predictability of the future and one's power to influence events. A family's expectation of its course in time is rooted in the values underlying system maintenance and coherence. Expectations represent family norms grown out of historical events, cultural beliefs, and personal and societal ideals. The extent of disruption after a bolt from the blue seems to be related to how much deviation it represents from the expected course of events (Neugarten, 1979). The following example involves a family living in a safe community who had never envisioned an assault on one of its members as a possibility.

Alice is the eldest daughter of the family and a psychology student at a major university. Her father, Harry V., has been working for a building contractor for over 20 years. The family lives in a semirural community where Alice's mother, Ruth, takes care of the house and garden. Alice's younger brother and sister are high school students. Alice is the pride of the family and the model for her younger siblings. She is the recipient of a competitive scholarship that enables her to study full-time. No other family member has ever succeeded in an academic career. Ruth has encouraged and supported her daughter throughout her school years, often against her husband's wish to keep Alice in line with the family's tradition of hard and honest work. Harry does not understand why Alice has such high aspirations, and besides, if Alice earned some money, it would serve the family better.

Two weeks ago, something incredible happened. Alice lived in the city, near the university in a small apartment with a classmate. Both women were studying in their own rooms late at night when they noticed two men prying open the kitchen window and about to climb in. In panic, Alice's friend screamed as loud as she could. One of the men pulled a gun and fired into the two bedrooms. Both girls were shot and fell on the floor while the two men took off as fast as they could. When Alice felt safe enough, she crept over to her friend's room. Coming closer, she noticed that blood was flowing from her friend's nose and there were no signs of life. Alice does not remember what happened next. She woke up in a hospital bed after surgery because her arm had been injured by a bullet. Alice had not even noticed the injury or any pain connected with it.

A nurse practitioner meets Alice with her parents at her first clinic visit. The wound is healing and there is no sign of infection. Alice looks perturbed, however, and the nurse who had read Alice's story in the record feels concerned. Alone with Alice in the treatment room, she asks Alice how she is doing and if she had gone back to her classes yet. Alice mumbles a few words and stares at the floor, then looks at the nurse with wide-open eyes and an expression of desperation. The nurse practitioner pulls up a chair and sits next to Alice, gently putting her arm around Alice's shoulders. "What's the matter? Tell me," she says. Alice looks disturbed and answers, "I don't know." "But I can't let you go home so upset—tell me how I can help you," the nurse replies. At this point, Alice loses her composure. Like a child, she clings to the nurse's arm and sobs. In between sobs, the nurse hears her exclaim, "They have killed my friend! They took off! I'm so scared! Will they come back? I can't sleep—they come back in my dreams. If I had done something, my friend would not be dead!" The nurse grows increasingly anxious and feels her heart pounding. Instinctively, she strokes Alice's hair and wonders what to do next. Then she just makes herself sit quietly.

Alice's sobs are subsiding slowly and she seems calmer. "Do your parents know how hard this is for you?" the nurse asks. Startled, Alice responds, "No, they make my life even harder. My father doesn't understand. He says it is my fault, because I did not follow his advice to stay home and find a job. My mom tries to defend me. Then, they fight with each other and I lock myself in my room." Then, the nurse asks about Alice's future plans. Alice would like to finish her studies, but she does not have the courage to live alone and neither does she have the money to pay the whole monthly rent. Living at home is painful, but she does not dare go to the city. After some questioning, Alice reveals that she knows a young woman, a relative on her father's side, with whom she has a good relationship. She could possibly live with her, but her father would resent this tremendously.

The nurse decides to have a conference with Alice's parents and invites them into the treatment room. After a brief introduction, she informs them that Alice's arm is healing well. She then explains that it is hard to get over a crime like that and that such events change many things in a person's life. Then she asks how the parents have dealt with the crisis. Ruth responds first, stating that it was time to realize that such crimes can happen and that there was nothing one could do about it. "But it didn't have to happen if Alice had listened to me!" Harry interrupted. The nurse states that she can well understand that he was concerned about Alice and tried to prevent her from living in the city. After a short silence, Harry remarks that he also understands how important education is for Alice. Even though he has never really thought it was necessary, he is still proud of his smart daughter. This thing has really messed him up, he admits. The nurse states that she knows from working with many families how easy it is to lose one's temper over such terrible things. She advises them to stick together now, because Alice, who has suffered the most, needs their support.

The nurse then asks Alice whether she can tell her parents what they had talked about. Alice nods and the nurse describes Alice's fear of going back to the city. Harry thinks it is a bad idea to break off the studies and asks Alice whether she has thought of his relative in the city. At this point, Ruth interrupts and asks very angrily why he now, all of a sudden, acts so understanding, after causing all this uproar in the family with his stubbornness. "He just pretends, because he wants to look good," Ruth said. The nurse intervenes by putting herself in the middle. She explains that in a crisis people first try to blame something or someone, because they are upset and powerless and don't want to admit that terrible things just happen to people. Harry has pushed the blame on his family, and Alice has blamed herself for the death of her friend. But the whole thing is over, and she now wonders if anything can be done to prevent something similar from happening.

After reflecting briefly, Harry declares that he will call his relative. Her apartment is safer, in a good district, and on the fourth floor. Ruth thinks Alice should take a class in self-defense. Alice laughs and says that nobody has the funds to pay for this, but Harry jumps in and offers to take the money from his savings. He will also urge his relative to install a burglar alarm at his expense. He wants to sleep without worrying about Alice. The nurse praises the three of them in their ability to find solutions. She suggests that they should continue to talk openly and try to understand each other's way of thinking. Preventing misunderstandings is especially important in trying times like these, when they need to hold together and support each other.

In this case example, the framework of systemic organization has given the nurse the most important insight. She remembered the crisis diagram (see Figure 16.1) and the two principles discussed in previous chapters: (a) In a crisis, existing conflicts are magnified and inhibit a productive cooperation and mutual problem solving necessary to resolve the crisis. (b) Nursing in a crisis situation involves the support of the family's unique processes that lead to new individuation and system change. Both principles let the nurse recover from her initial shock by realizing that no magic solutions were needed. Instead, she expected Alice to calm down by feeling supported. Alice's parents were involved in a long conflict centering on the issue of power to make decisions. Harry had lost his case when the rest of the family decided to support Alice in becoming a university student. The family's action was against his understanding of the father role and his wounded pride was intensified by the tragic event. Feeling supported by the nurse, he could let go of his self-defense and admit that he had felt pain for his daughter. A process leading to spirituality among the three family members took place in the treatment room in that they

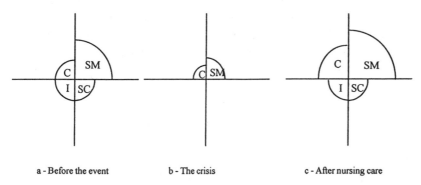

a - Before the event b - The crisis c - After nursing care

Figure 16.1. Systemic Process of Alice's Family

all moved closer to each other to fortify their coherence. As their worldview and expectation of their course of life changed radically, they needed each other more than ever to effect the system change. The situation is typical, because it shows how little is often needed to push desperate family members into action. The solution was simple, but they were not able to see it previously. However, no change was more painful than a move toward system change. Thus, the crisis enhanced family health in that it led to a reorganization of priorities and a new perspective that provided new meaning to the family system. The event, terrible as it was, served as an agent for growth so that the previous autonomy conflict lost its significance, and coherence in the family took on a new meaning—the healing of old wounds.

The diagrams in Figure 16.1 summarize the sequence of events and their effect on the family life process: Family coherence, initially impaired by the father's hurt pride and the ensuing family squabbles, had also affected the family's ability to individuate, grow, and adapt as a system (see Figure 16.1a). As the crisis occurred, everyone froze in a rigid pursuit of disconnected activities in an attempt to meet individual needs. Family coherence became temporarily destroyed, and tempers flared every time members approached each other. The members felt emotionally deprived and unable to meet their developmental needs or grow and individuate. Therefore, individuation and system change were lacking (see Figure 16.1b). After the session with the nurse in the treatment room, the family began to resolve the problem in that members sensed the need for each other and came together through joint problem solving. Consequently, coherence grew. The members felt supported by the nurse, stated their positions, and learned to look at the situation from each other's perspectives. This allowed for individuation and gradual system change (see Figure 16.1c). It would be naive to think, however, that this family's process was totally and permanently corrected. A perceptive nurse recognizes the need for follow-up and ongoing encouragement. Whether this can be provided by the nurse, the extended family, or a therapist depends on the situation.

The resolution of crises caused by disasters is no different from the resolution of all other crises. Disasters hit quickly and unexpectedly. Therefore, it is a rare type of family that does not experience a crisis reaction. After some time, however, it becomes evident whether or not the family is able to pull together and mobilize its resources for the sake of crisis resolution.

In examining the process, researchers have pointed out the relevance of demographic variables, scope, duration of the crisis and perception of the event (Pilisuk & Acredolo, 1988), stress appraisal, and coping methods (Boatright, 1985; Lazarus & Folkman, 1984b) in influencing crisis resolution. Furthermore, in all types of crises brought on by the environment, the role of the victim in their development or prevention seems of paramount importance. In the previous example, Alice's guilt about not having done anything to protect her friend, whether it was reasonable or not, has increased her distress and tortured her by eliciting severe preoccupation with measures she should have undertaken to prevent the crime. Alice's guilt was further intensified by her father's seemingly heartless comments about her being the cause of her own problem. Generally, hostile messages from bystanders, such as, "If you had worked harder, you would still have your job; you asked for trouble when you built the house next to the river; if you had accompanied your child, nothing would have happened," can be devastating because they magnify the victim's already existing guilt, lead to despair, and affect mental health (Murphy, 1991).

Because unforeseen events present a threat to the perception of an expected way of life or the normative unfolding of events (Neugarten, 1979), they are disconcerting to individuals who maintain a view of their world as being controlled, regulated, and predictable. In fact, most people have a strong need to hang on to such a worldview of control to ward off basic anxiety. Despite daily contrary evidence, they somehow seem to rationalize that disasters happen only to others. Consequently, when they become victims, they search for an explanation. Blaming something or someone who may be responsible for the event provides a feeling of control and a sense that it can be prevented in the future (Pittman, 1987). Alice's nurse, familiar with the strong emphasis on the target of control of ordinary people in this society, cautiously introduced the topic of prevention of future crimes in the hope that finding a solution would be easily accepted as a means to reduce anxiety and tension.

Research related to catastrophes is almost entirely based on theories of stress and coping and focuses on the victims' responses. Outcome measures are physical and mental health and, recently, the occurrence of posttraumatic stress disorder (PTSD) (Murphy, 1991). In the third edition of the *Diagnostic and Statistical Manual of Psychiatric Disorders (DSM-III)*, victims are described as reexperiencing the event in thoughts and dreams, attempting to disassociate their feelings from the event, and experiencing symptoms described in Alice's example, such as guilt, sleep disturbance, anxiety, and others (American Psychiatric Association, 1980).

Studies exploring direct relationships between an event and its effect on the individual lack agreement (Melick, 1985) and are generally inconclusive (Murphy, 1991). This is understandable, considering the complexity of systemic reactions and the interaction with other factors intimately involved in the life process. Responses of family systems to traumatic events are even less well understood and remain largely unexplored. No different from family reactions to illness discussed earlier, responses to incongruence due to environmental factors exhibit vast variations. Alice's example shows clearly that the externally induced crisis, if not resolved quickly, becomes a crisis from within and, consequently, a developmental crisis as described in Chapter 7. Generally, sudden events such as fires, earthquakes, and the like are a true test of family resilience. It is difficult for family members to attend to the posttraumatic stress symptoms of others (Verbosky & Ryan, 1988), especially if they have to overcome their own anxiety concurrently. Furthermore, if the disaster involves deaths and loss of property essential for survival, the crisis becomes astronomical. Material and emotional support through extended family, friends, a church, or social agencies are essential for relationships to survive and family systems to readjust and make the necessary changes.

Again, the framework of systemic organization serves as a tool and basis for discussion for the nurse who places actual losses and subjective meanings of the event into the family's total life process and thus moves a step closer to understanding necessary change and offering true help in the family's struggle to regain congruence.

17

Roles in the Workplace and Family Crisis

There is general agreement that employment and work play a major role in the family process. Work outside the home is a necessity for the great majority of families. The importance of work can be estimated by the hours spent by male and female family members who take on roles of workers, employees, managers, or directors in various types of organizations. Today, the dual-earner family has become the predominant arrangement (Hayghe, 1986), with nearly two thirds of mothers with dependent children being employed outside the home (MacEwen & Barling, 1991). As the family interfaces with two workplaces and various child care arrangements, as its living space expands and its family time shrinks, the family's life process becomes increasingly complex (Hoffman, 1988). The shifts in both husbands' and wives' roles and their impact on relationships and activities of the family are far from being understood (Crouter & McHale, 1993).

Historically, work has provided meaning to a person's life and workers today still think that employment should be a means to attain fulfillment and self-worth (Howard & Bray, 1988). Being employed seems to have distinct benefits for a person. In addition to securing the financial survival of the family, the workplace provides essentials such as a time structure, coworkers with whom to socialize, and the opportunity to develop competency and knowledge (Joelson & Wahlquist, 1987). Men and women are experiencing these rewards but the outside responsibilities also have a potential to create conflicts in the family.

Work conditions are seldom ideal. Conditions at the workplace easily become a threat to personal and family stability (Voydanoff, 1990). Crouter and Manke (1994) list the three major workplace changes occurring in the United States, namely, downsizing of businesses that sometimes result in severe budget cuts, closing of plants, or relocation; computer and telecommunication technology that increases the demand for intellectual skills rather than action-centered jobs; and competitive pressure that calls for internal restructuring of the organization, team building, and worker participation.

The implications of these changes are twofold: work overload and job insecurity. Job insecurity has not been sufficiently researched (Voydanoff, 1990; Wilson, Larson, & Stone, 1993). Nevertheless, there are indications that families suffer as they anticipate growing difficulties. A threat of job loss, salary and benefit freezes, loss of potential promotions, or forced relocations erode their sense of security (Larson, Wilson, & Beley, 1988) because they are preoccupied with the current situation and the future (Wilson et al., 1993). Job insecurity has been found to be related to self-reported symptoms of ill health (Kuhnert, Sims, & Lahey, 1989). In fact, in their classic study of reactions to plant closure, Cobb and Kasl (1977) found that the anticipation had a greater impact on mental and physical health than the actual job loss. Furthermore, findings of a study by Voydanoff and Donnelly (1988) suggested effects on spouses, in that wives who reported job insecurity, either in their own job or in their husband's, were less satisfied with their marital relationship.

Similar effects are expected with work overload as companies downsize and dislocate and those left behind encounter greater responsibilities (Price, 1990). High work demand coupled with a low level of control seems to be a most harmful combination of job factors with respect to the workers' physical and mental health (Ironson, 1992). Problems are not eliminated, however, when employers ask for more involvement and participation in decision making (Lawler, 1990). Employees spend more energy at the workplace, and because it is difficult to put limits on work if one is committed to progress

(Ronco & Peattie, 1988), energy for family responsibilities may be compromised (Bolger, DeLongis, Kessler, & Wethington, 1989; Small & Riley, 1990). Spillover theory maintains that overload experienced at work carries over into the family system, thereby affecting the quality of marriage and family life (Rousseau, 1978; Staines & O'Connor, 1980). Especially in dual-earner families, it becomes increasingly difficult to balance high work demands when both partners experience similar trends.

Spillover theory has become the basis of many studies, specifically on the interface of work and family management. Much has been written about role conflicts between spouses. Work-family conflict is viewed differently by various groups of professionals. Some researchers claim a direct relationship between the amount of outside work and the extent of interference with family tasks (Greenhaus & Beutell, 1985; Gutek, Searle, & Kelpa, 1991). Many studies show that women spend disproportionate amounts of time in the household whether or not they are gainfully employed (e.g., Hochschild, 1989; Voydanoff, 1988), and men spend more time than women in paid jobs (Duxbury, Lee, Higgins, & Mills, 1992; Voydanoff, 1988). This inequality has led many researchers to focus on gender roles.

Traditionally, men have fulfilled family expectations by being good providers, but women see the family operation as their major obligation (Barnett & Baruch, 1987). These ideologies have become increasingly liberal. But many women, even today, work for pay not because of liberal views about female roles but for economic reasons, and their ideology conflicts with the actual role. Likewise, men may be forced into sharing household work against their traditional understanding of their role (Zvonkovic, Schmiege, & Hall, 1994). This suggests that spillover is a complex process that reaches beyond simple task overload and involves values and attitudes (Perry-Jenkins & Crouter, 1990) as well as interactional and family system factors.

Ferree (1988), for example, discusses the breadwinner role in the family and maintains that women could gain status if the role was shared. The social construction of the role, however, involves strict boundaries and a process of assigning different behaviors and meanings to the construct for men and women (Potuchek, 1992). Hood (1983) claims that change toward equality of women who participate in the labor force is not a given but entails a process of continuous renegotiation necessary to maintain coherence within the family. Thus, change is slow and depends on the success of contesting gender boundaries (Gerson & Peiss, 1985).

The idea of boundary competition has changed the view of the family process from sharing goals to competing for interests (Ferree, 1990). Women seem less eager to participate in such competition than anticipated by social scientists. Potuchek (1992), on the basis of her study of 153 working wives, observed that the great majority of the subjects maintained the belief that the breadwinner role was a male role, even though most reported that their job was financially important for the family.

A related theme in recent research is the conflict of the partners' role expectations as a threat to family coherence. McHale and Crouter (1992), measuring attitudes of spouses and behaviors in getting household tasks done, found that marital dissatisfaction was more likely to arise because the partner did not live up to the role expected by the other than because of work overload. This theme of conflict supports the systemic process explicated by the framework of systemic organization.

On the basis of this framework, one would assume that spouses who have differing ideas about essential family roles would have difficulties establishing coherence and mutually valid system maintenance strategies. Likewise, if spouses are forced by their partner into behaviors incongruent with their own values, systemic tension and anxiety are likely to occur. For example, one predicts that women who work for economic reasons but believe in the need to stay at home with their children are likely to feel guilty and suffer anxiety and mental health consequences.

Research has shown that, like the breadwinner role of husbands, the traditional female role of household manager and emotional caretaker of the family members has maintained itself rather strongly. Several studies have shown that women view housework as something more than mere physical tasks. Wives and mothers think of their housework as taking care of or managing the family (Hochschild, 1989), which gives them a sense of power and is embedded in their self-concept (Mederer, 1993). In addition, Thompson (1991) found that they value interactional outcomes of their family work. Nevertheless, interpersonal work is "emotion work" and may, without sufficient support from others, lead to exhaustion (Kessler, McLeod, & Wethington,

1985). The findings of a study by Erickson (1993) suggest that today's work trends encourage a loosening of gender boundaries in this area. Emotion work performed by husbands with the children seems to compensate for an unequal share of household labor and is the best predictor of the wives' marital well-being.

In terms of the framework of systemic organization, emotion work falls within the coherence dimension. Although it seems logical that a mutually supportive couple or family has the necessary energy to accomplish needed tasks, a system in disarray finds even simple tasks extremely burdensome. This leads back to the mediating effect of a sound marital relationship discussed in previous chapters. In the area of work-related stress, strong marital coherence has been found to prevent psychological distress with job insecurity (Rook, Dooley, & Catalano, 1991).

The above discussion of the literature illustrates the complexity of work conflict spillover into the family process. Each individual participating in the family process brings along gender-based attitudes and behaviors that enter into cooperative or competitive interactions that promote or prohibit coherence of the family. A severe threat to personal coherence through role overload at work and in the family, or a threat to system maintenance due to job insecurity, can create a crisis situation as individuals defend their own needs and are no longer able to understand each other's reactions. When chronic interpersonal conflicts exist, a marital relationship will present an additional source of distress in the difficult situation, but a new balance may be found with relative ease if the family members are connected by strong emotional bonds.

As was the case with changes brought on by illness, external influences from the work world are further modified and dependent on cultural patterns and attitudes, the member's developmental needs (Karasek, 1979), and the availability of resources, such as education, socioeconomic status (Symons & McLeod, 1993), operational support (Atkinson, 1992), and, most of all, the family's total life pattern. By means of the assessment of the family life patterns, nurses can estimate the extent by which the work situation in interaction with other factors exerts an influence on the individual's and family's ability to remain stable and learn, grow, and change as the situation demands it. What follows is an example of a work-related crisis situation.

Allison, age 17 and 5 months pregnant, starts to cry as she tells the nurse who interviews her in a prenatal clinic of her family situation. Allison had kept the pregnancy a secret until recently. Her father, Herb, when he heard the news, announced that he wanted no part of it. It was Allison's problem, and she had to live with it. The family was in no position to help her care for this baby. Her mother, Margaret, listened to Herb's raving and kept silent. Then she went to the bedroom to cry. Allison reports that neither of them cares about her. She has to be good to please them, but her achievements are never recognized. Now she does not know what will happen; nobody talks to her anymore. When the nurse asks Allison to tell her more about her father, she describes him as a hard-working businessman. After losing his managerial position in a major industrial company, he attempted an export business of his own. Even though the business is now in its third year, he still cannot pay himself a salary. Allison is constantly told that there is no money and if she wants luxuries, she has to work for them. Margaret is the breadwinner even though Herb has maintained the role of deciding how the money is spent. Margaret is an administrator in an academic setting and earns a relatively high salary. She has long workdays, presumably very stressful, and often returns home as late as nine or ten o'clock. On weekends, she usually takes home a stack of papers to take care of. Margaret looks and acts exhausted. She gets angry if family members demand her time, argue, leave messes, or refuse to be helpful. She complains about lack of support, having to be in charge of everything, and having to provide money for everyone without being able to spend any for herself. The remaining family members are Kelly and Steven. Both are college students, commuting to class and working part-time.

The nurse invites Allison's parents to a conference. Both find it impossible to miss work but consent to a visit of the nurse to their home. They own a lovely house in the suburbs. The nurse collects the following family data.

Assessment of the Family

System Maintenance. The household is structured reasonably well and organized. The three kids do their own laundry, Kelly cleans the house for money, and Herb is in charge of the parents' laundry and shopping for groceries. All three kids have their own schedules, eat out, or prepare food to their liking. A family meal used to be the tradition but rarely happens anymore. Margaret cooks for Herb and herself and gets assistance from Kelly once or twice a week. Herb works until late, because there is nothing to do at home anyway. If he comes home early, it is because one of the kids needs the car. Allison, until recently, took part in numerous after-school functions and needed transportation frequently. Herb was in charge of assuring, arranging, or giving Allison the necessary rides. The family has no time to entertain guests. Friends of the kids go in and out but seldom stay in the house for long periods of time. Each member, with the exception of Margaret, has private space—the kids have rooms and Herb has an office. Margaret does her work using the living room table, which keeps the rest of the family out of the shared living area. Conflicts arise around watching TV, because the TV room has no door and Margaret feels disturbed by the noise.

Coherence. This family consists of a group of headstrong individuals who are more committed to self-development than a joint family operation. Nevertheless, there is a feeling of togetherness in that members feel different from ordinary people and are therefore united "as they are all crazy." There is tolerance for opposing attitudes within limits. Kelly and Steven have taken great strides in finding a life course of their own, and the parents have lived through emotional upheavals and "rocky" times during their children's adolescence. Allison, being the youngest, has felt more pressure to comply with the parents' wishes than the other two. She has always been "the good kid" and her father's favorite. For the past 3 years, however, she has been in a state of rebellion. Her mood swings and increasingly belligerent demeanor have turned the household into a battlefield. Margaret reacts by vacillating between anger, uncontrolled accusations, and attacks of guilt that are followed by attempts to make up for what was said. Herb removes himself from these scenes but attacks Margaret after the altercations, accusing her of improper responses. If Margaret is not present, however, he reacts to Allison's behaviors equally direct and angry. Conflicts between the two have always revolved around the kids in that Margaret wants Herb to be more assertive with discipline. Herb, however, has shied away from the role of disciplinarian. He has a strong urge of being liked and accepted and consequently has been very lenient and accommodating with the children. Despite tension, the marital relationship has considerable strengths. Herb and Margaret talk things out and share concerns. In fact, they have been a mutual source of comfort in adjusting to their difficult work situations.

Individuation. Both Herb and Margaret have strong work values. Work is considered their purpose and mission in life. Individuation and growth have occurred through work, contribution to the workplace, leadership, and competency. There is an honest pride in accomplishment, diligence, and trustworthiness. Herb looked at his loss of employment as a challenge, because it gave him the opportunity to build a business of his own, something he could really be proud of. Since then, he has worked incessantly. Progress has been much more difficult than anticipated, and had it not been for Margaret's career success and promotions, the family would have had serious economic difficulties. Herb has moments of discouragement and anxiety about the future. The value of being the breadwinner is deeply ingrained in him, and he suffers when he sees Margaret struggle with an excessive work load and responsibilities for the sake of the family. His self-esteem is especially wounded when Allison tells him outright that he has no right to tell her what to do because he brings no money home. Margaret tries to protect his status and autonomy by not claiming financial authority in the household. She sends the kids to him if they ask for money. Sometimes, however, when she feels overwhelmed and pities herself, she makes him responsible for having no time to herself, no money to spare, no opportunity to send the kids to a topnotch college, or no time to take a good, long vacation.

System Change. All things considered, this family is a flexible system. It has experienced a reversal of roles and responsibilities. The members have not accepted this as a permanent feature, but they are willing to live with it as long as necessary. Margaret vacillates between a sense of pride about abilities she never knew she had and anxiety about the future. Herb has accepted household responsibilities grudgingly, but a shift of commitment from work to family seems unthinkable for him. The family seems deadlocked in patterns that control the economic situation and maintain stability. Allison's recent acting out seemed to arise from a need for system change away from excessive control to emotional confrontation. This latest crisis, however, has locked the parents even firmer in their controlling positions, and Allison seems in danger of being ousted from the system without concerns for her emotional well-being.

Assessment of Family Health

A mutual assessment with the help of the system diagram shows the picture of the family in crisis (Figure 17.1c), in which family incongruence has become a barrier to individuation of the members and growth of the system. In fact, members are so excessively concerned about maintaining personal control in the situation that family coherence has become minimal. Members report that it feels better to stay away. If we look at each member at the personal system level, evidence shows that all respond to the emotional paucity by disconnecting from the family, overinvolving themselves with work and school, and shielding themselves from hostility by keeping family matters to the basics of providing and channeling resources. There is some strength in the parental relationship. Herb and Margaret have frequent discussions about their situation, and even after an argument, they try to talk and make peace with each other. After this latest crisis, however, interaction has become difficult, the atmosphere is tense, and Allison's pregnancy has not been addressed to avoid serious emotional outbursts.

In contrast, the basic family pattern before Herb's problems (see Figure 17.1 a) shows strong system maintenance on the family and individual levels. With its focus on individuation, the family encouraged self-development of the members and an orientation external to the family. Their coherence was satisfactory for their system built on success and pride in independent problem solving. It is easy to recognize the important role that work and education played in the life processes of the family members, because work served as the target of spirituality and represented that part of personal coherence related to connectedness within and with the environment. When Herb's problems came into play (see Figure 17.1b), his external rewards disappeared and Margaret's lost their attractiveness as family coher-

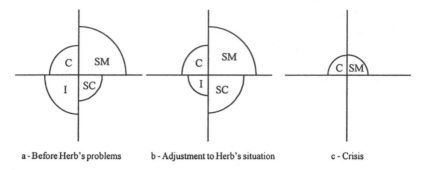

a - Before Herb's problems   b - Adjustment to Herb's situation   c - Crisis

Figure 17.1. Systemic Process of Herb's Family

ence became seriously disturbed. Being immersed in controlling the family business, members failed to provide or receive necessary emotional support. Although they managed to provide financial security through efficient system maintenance and well-controlled operational changes, efforts depleted their energy and impaired their personal growth. Because these processes occurred in a cyclical, self-reinforcing fashion, a crisis was inevitable.

Allison's crisis has the potential to act as a motivating force to effect system change by bringing the members back together and setting new priorities. The nurse's approach is no different from the interventions described earlier in crisis situations. In fact, the members may be very receptive to restructuring their relationships, because the situation has made them painfully aware of inadequate family processes.

The central focus of work in the life process is typical for many families. Many will go through life without ever noticing a problem. Herb's family experienced difficulties with unemployment and the subsequent struggle to regain economic footing. Herb's problem could be described as a role conflict in that he executed a role in the family that was incongruent with his values or the understanding of what his role should be. The same can be said of Margaret, whose feelings reflected the working woman's dilemma described in the literature. Although Margaret basically enjoyed her work, she also resented losing control within the family and had little energy to catalyze emotion work. Because Herb was not willing or able to take on the emotional support role in the family, the loss was sensed by the children. As Margaret's work load increased and the family felt emotionally depleted, Allison may have reacted to the void with problem behaviors that at last brought her to the center of attention.

The reconciliation of work demands with the family process is not easy. If it involves change of traditional attitudes, values, and roles, the outcome is system change. In Herb's family, demands changed rapidly with his unemployment and continued to change gradually over time. When work is intertwined with the family process, its interface with the marital relationship can also be visualized. Herb and Margaret, through their discussions, were able to jointly control the impact of economic scarcity and support each other in strategies of financial stabilization, such as Margaret's job and Herb's helping out in the family. Pride about the mastery of such difficulties maintained their coherence. Due to their strong relationship, an emotional deficit in the family became apparent with a delay and was noted only by the members who were not included in the parental subsystem. The example, therefore, clarifies the importance of family coherence that encompasses the whole family, including the children. Such emotional bonding is needed for individuation or personal growth for the prevention of crisis and in Herb's family for the resolution of the crisis. The following chapter on unemployment illustrates this point further.

18

Families and Unemployment

Most of the research on unemployment explores its effects on the unemployed person, usually males. Researchers using available aggregate figures report that high unemployment rates are correlated with higher rates for homicide and suicide (Kasl & Cobb, 1967; Kirby & Luker, 1986; Wasserman, 1984), child abuse (Howze & Kotch, 1984; Steinberg, Catalano, & Dooley, 1981), mental illness (Dooley & Catalano, 1980), and health problems (Clark, 1985; Johnson-Saylor, 1984; Kirby & Luker, 1986; Wright, 1986). The most common correlational studies are cross-sectional and examine psychiatric and somatic symptoms of unemployed men (Hepworth, 1980; Hobbs, Ballinger, McClure, Martin, & Greenwood, 1985; Margolis & Farran, 1984). Evidence of detrimental effects of unemployment on these men recruited for the studies in unemployment offices and registries is strong. Furthermore, there is reason to believe that factors such as age, length of unemployment (Jackson & Warr, 1984), social support (Payne & Hartley, 1987), and the level of job commitment (Rowley & Feather, 1987) play a significant role as modifiers.

These studies give some indication of the complexity of the phenomenon and a need to look at all essential processes in a person's life. A focus on wider ramifications of unemployment, namely, responses of significant others and families, however, has been sorely neglected (Jahoda, 1988; Voydanoff, 1984). A few descriptive studies dating back to the Great Depression are notable exceptions and have become classics. An example is Mirra Komarovsky's (1940) study of 59 families outside New York City. His basic hypothesis that unemployment lowers the status of the husband and makes him less of a role model to the children was supported in 13 of the families. What was different in the others was not made clear, however. The theme of adaptation is wonderfully illustrated in another classic project, the Marienthal study, done after World War I in Austria after the closure of a large textile factory that had served as the source of income for most villagers. The researcher found that the majority of families adapted surprisingly well to extreme hardship by narrowing their wants and desires and focusing on day-to-day survival. Families who had reached the breaking point lacked cultural and spiritual resources (Jahoda, Lazarsfeld, & Zeisel, 1971). The theme of status loss was picked up again in the Oakland Growth Study that was started during the Great Depression and continued over several generations (Elder, 1974). Similar to the Marienthal study, Elder's study described family adaptation as the process of using material, cognitive, and emotional resources to solve problems and gain control over the difficult life situation. Families were observed to generally cope well with hardship. Problems occurred, however, when long-term deprivation had eroded the belief in a predictable future and the self-esteem of family members. Because tensions were played out mainly in the marital relationship, Elder deduced that the reason for the breakdown was the loss of the couple's ability to maintain their desired role in the family, thereby supporting the hypothesis of Komarovsky (1940).

In the late 1970s and in the 1980s, a new enthusiasm for the topic of unemployment had developed, and, more recently, an impetus toward model building has become apparent. Theories of stress and resource management have been used to explain family coping (Weigel, 1988). Researchers have called attention to the complexity of interacting variables (Voydanoff, 1984) and the cumulative impact of life events (Dohrenwend, 1973; Myers, Lindenthal, & Pepper, 1974; Pearlin, 1983). The body of literature focusing on relationship patterns and responses of family members to the unemployment situation is slowly growing in size (Liem & Liem, 1990).

The findings of recent studies generally support explanations of family process explicated with the framework of systemic organization. Therefore, in the following paragraphs, family processes will be theoretically deduced and supported by recent literature as well as by my own work in the area.

The impact of unemployment is first felt by the individual directly affected. The effect depends on the person's life process and therefore varies greatly. Responses reported by unemployed fathers range from happiness about finally having time to spend with the children to despair about the inability to provide for the family or feeling that unemployment was just one more thing in a chain of disasters (Friedemann, 1986). Paying attention to interpretive processes is therefore of paramount importance. For example, the individual's perception of financial strain may be poorly related to the actual economic situation (Locke, 1969), and financial worries rather than bank statements are associated with psychological and physical symptoms (Kessler, Turner, & House, 1987). According to the framework of systemic organization, negative reactions are responses to a threat to personal coherence. Furthermore, individuals who consider the breadwinner role the most important source of satisfaction and sense of worth are most likely to feel a threat to their coherence when losing their job. Thus, men with traditional role perceptions have been shown to have more psychological symptoms after losing their job (Dew, Penkower, & Bromet, 1991; McLoyd, 1989). One can also assume that a particular job that has served as a means for individuation is difficult to replace with another. Reactions are influenced by the macrosystem because the economic context determines the difficulty to find another job and the extent of financial deprivation (Mirowsky & Ross, 1989; Pearlin, 1990).

If system incongruence occurs, unemployed individuals respond to tension in many ways, for example, with anger and hostility, withdrawal, or depression. These responses are acutely felt by others who are in close contact. It seems that wives of unemployed husbands are the foremost targets of their husbands' reactions. Empirical findings from longitudinal studies suggest that wives do not react directly to their husband's unemployment but instead react to their symptoms and consequent marital tension (Friedemann, 1987; Friedemann & Webb, 1995) with psychological symptoms (Dew, Bromet, &

Schulberg, 1987; Friedemann, 1987). Due to the indirect response to unemployment, the wives' symptoms do not appear immediately or concurrently with the husbands' but are delayed several weeks (Dew et al., 1987; Grayson, 1985; Liem & Liem, 1988). Wives in crisis have reported somatic complaints, depression, alcohol use, and low self-esteem (Buss & Redburn, 1983; Larson, 1984).

The role of the marital relationship in the process of adaptation to unemployment has been a research focus since the studies cited earlier. Findings of a number of studies show measurable strain on the marital relationship in the face of the husband's unemployment (Atkinson, Liem, & Liem, 1986; Larson, 1984; Liem & Liem, 1988). This effect is not uniform, however. Although communication often deteriorates initially, many relationships find renewed congruence after some time despite ongoing unemployment (Thomas, McCabe, & Berry, 1980). Recent studies are in agreement with the view of the marriage serving as a stabilizing force if the relationship is strong but being a destructive force if problems existed prior to unemployment. In the latter families, responses to unemployment are severe and marital problems become intensified by the difficult situation (Friedemann, 1987; Moen, Kain, & Elder, 1983; Ray & McLoyd, 1986).

A key to family survival, therefore, seems to be coherence. Of equal importance, however, seems to be a satisfactory stabilization of family system maintenance (Whelan, 1992). As this framework proposes, the first attempt of stabilization is the reinforcement of already existing system maintenance patterns. Thus, several researchers have observed that both husbands and wives tend to keep to their traditional roles instead of finding new ways to divide labor (Marsden, 1982; Shamir, 1986), irrespective of social class. Hartley (1987) reports that wives tend to protect their husbands by not asking for help, and wives in the study of Liem and Liem (1988) left decision making to their husbands.

However, certain changes to maintain the family system need to be made to compensate for income loss. Statistics show that in 1985, wives contributed by finding work or increasing work hours. Thanks to the wives, the rate of families who would have reached poverty levels due to the husband's unemployment was reduced from 24% to 14%. In today's families, such flexibility is becoming more restricted than in the past, because many wives are already working when their husbands are laid off and the opportunity to increase work hours may be limited during an economic recession (Jones, 1991).

Whether or not families succeed in their adjustment depends on available resources and the dimension of individuation. The lability of the economic situation brings challenges to family systems because individuals must redirect their way in an ever-changing job market and develop skills to become or remain "marketable." There is an increasing need for families to support individuation of their members. One third of the men interviewed 6 years after an economic crisis had engaged in additional education, either to change their field of work or as a precautionary measure in case of a permanent layoff from their union job (Friedemann & Webb, 1995). The socioeconomic situation has been found to act as an important mediator in that lack of financial and educational resources may become decisive factors when families are unemployed (Pearlin, Lieberman, Menaghan, & Mullan, 1981). Without essential resources in an unfavorable situation, unemployment becomes a major factor driving families into a marginal existence and chronic poverty (Whelan, 1992), a topic to be discussed later.

In today's society, the proposition of a general trajectory of adjustment to unemployment is practically impossible. External factors, such as interactions with several workplaces, commuting needs, child care facilities, recreational interests, and leisure activities, play an increasing role in people's lives and influence family dynamics.

It is equally difficult to foresee effects of the unemployment of one person in dual-earner and dual-career families, because such effects are substantially more complex. Unemployment of women has traditionally been considered less important (Dew et al., 1991). In the past, only a minority carried the responsibility of primary breadwinners in the family. Single parents, especially vulnerable in today's economic instability, have become an increasingly important group to research, but as of yet, they constitute a neglected population. The few existing studies have shown that unemployed women seem to experience similar psychological reactions as men; however, systematic comparisons with male samples or longitudinal studies are missing (Dew et al., 1991).

Outcomes of unemployment are minimally researched. Most studies done are cross-sectional in nature and cannot begin to address the complexity of an adjustment process. Liem and Liem (1990), evaluating the results of their longitudinal study, concluded that the impact of unemployment was conditioned by vulnerabilities arising from the family's ongoing exchange with its environment. Economic hardship has the potential of damaging the family and its individuals. Long-term effects can be seen even in relatively well-functioning families in which husbands are reemployed and the financial situation is stabilized. The initial crisis, interacting with the quality of the marital relationship and the perception of stress during the 6 years following the crisis, predicted 30% of the variance of the couple's anxiety at the time of the follow-up (Friedemann & Webb, 1995).

Research about the effect of unemployment on children is scarce and largely inconclusive (Barling, 1990). Because the association between the father's unemployment and child abuse is rather strong (Gil, 1970; Taitz, King, Nicholson, & Kessel, 1987), much speculation has ensued with regard to responsible factors, such as the use of alcohol (Gil, 1970) or the sudden, increased contact time with the children (McLoyd, 1989). None have yielded strong associations. In fact, increased time of the father with the child also could present an opportunity to build lasting relationships and compensate for losses (McLoyd, 1989; Shamir, 1986). Relationships between role changes of mothers and the children have remained unexplored (Barling, 1990). Nevertheless, the finding of a moderate relationship between economic stress and anxiety and peer rejection in girls 6 years later (Webb & Friedemann, 1991) suggests the need to focus on mothers who are more intimately involved with the family and tend to be more depressed than the husbands (Friedemann, 1987).

Generally, most research data suggest that the family situation as a whole is responsible for the child's well-being and not necessarily in a negative way. Starting with Elder (1974), there are reports of children growing up to be more responsible and maturing earlier in unemployed families. Recent studies suggest that children exposed to unemployment are more concerned about economic issues in the family and put a lesser emphasis on values of academic achievement (Barling, 1990).

Nurses usually meet unemployed clients in the health care system. Such clients may never reveal their situation, unless an ingenious nurse addresses subtle signs of depression or other problems observed in the client. Once the problem is evident, nurses must assess the uniqueness of each family by asking questions about its life process before and after the job loss. How the family's struggle with the difficult situation occurs over time is the most relevant answer to find (Liem & Liem, 1990). Nurses need to gain clarity by understanding the family members' perceptions about their successes and failures within the context of their situation and supporting the most vulnerable members in the system, the women, and even more so, the children. The following examples illustrate two vastly different situations in which the phenomenon of unemployment is played out.

Example 1

One year ago, James's electronics company was closed due to financial difficulties. Including James, 12 engineers suddenly found themselves without employment. Announcements were made of the closure some time ago, but because these people were highly specialized, the marketability of their skills was low. Consequently, the entire group had difficulty locating new jobs. James was the oldest and had children in high school. The group of engineers met regularly in the bar, where they used to celebrate special events during times of their employment. At first, they met weekly, then monthly, updating each other about disappointments, hopes, and successes in their job search. James found the meetings helpful. The fact that all had similar difficulties helped him to get over the pain of his loss. Soon, however, it showed that his colleagues had better chances for reemployment. A few took courses to learn new skills, while others found an employer who trained them for different work. Most had to move to different cities, even to different states. Being 7 years away from retirement, James did not want to move, especially because his adolescent children would have a very difficult time adjusting to a new school, and intensive retraining was out of the question.

Presently, the group of colleagues no longer meets. James feels useless and depressed, and for a month he has been plagued by the symptoms of a peptic ulcer. His unemployment insurance has run out and his retirement will not kick in until age 65 and will be substantially lower than he had expected. Meanwhile, his wife, Sylvia, who has not worked since age 30, has found a secretarial job and enjoys her new responsibilities. James has never liked the idea of Sylvia working. Because he considers it his duty to support her, he has strongly discouraged her from taking on a job. Now, he can no longer deliver viable arguments against it. He feels like a loser, left out, and ignored. He strongly resents his wife's occupation, especially because she now seems to have the power to make financial decisions.

Actually, Sylvia has always looked after the bills and carefully invested whatever money was left. As a result of James's unemployment, she has set up a reasonable plan to bridge them over the 7 years to his retirement. It means staying away from luxuries such as eating out and common vacations. A major reason for James's anger is the small monthly allowance he receives for personal expenses. Sylvia has shown him the budget and James understands the need to be prudent, but the fact that he can no longer write checks as he pleases or go to the bar for drinks when he wishes has robbed him of his autonomy. On the one hand, he feels that the "punishment" is deserved and he knows that the plan is reasonable, especially because Sylvia has sought his consent and he has reluctantly agreed to it; on the other hand, it evokes anger and resentment as every unattainable desire reminds him of his lowly status. Therefore, James refuses to take part in household work.

James sleeps during the day or lies on the couch listlessly watching TV. He has gained 30 pounds and makes no effort to shed the weight. Often, he leaves the house before his wife comes home from work and sits in the bar for several hours with the one drink he can afford. Sylvia is irate about his behavior. Recently, she yelled at him and called him a worthless bum after she discovered the house in disarray. James had ordered her to clean up his dishes and clothes because she is the "woman of the house." The two argue on weekends and James has hit Sylvia twice. The children side with their mother. Because she has put her whole energy in organizing the household so efficiently to compensate for the loss of income, they feel that James owes her thanks. They do not understand why Sylvia puts up with so much and does not order James out of the house. The daughter suffers from frequent insomnia, is tired in school, and her grades have dropped. The eldest son disappears from the scene whenever possible. Often, he does not come home on weekends and Sylvia lacks the energy to enforce rules or question him. The younger son is extremely worried about his mother, helps her, and stays with her in his free time. He has difficulties finding friends in school.

Norman, a clinical nurse specialist, meets James when he is admitted to the hospital with severe bleeding from his ulcer. After detecting in the medical history the previous diagnosis of a peptic ulcer, he asks James in a matter of fact way what is bothering him. James stutters a few disjointed words about unemployment and feeling displaced. Norman suspects serious ramifications and sits down for a talk. After a few well-targeted questions, James gives him an account of his situation and the nurse shares a summary of his impression with James, namely, that James is hopeless about the situation and very anxious about losing his wife and family.

When he finds an extra few minutes, Norman shows James the system diagram. He explains that from what he knows about James's family, control plays an important role and that his authority in the family used to give him a sense of manliness. Norman suspects that James, by losing his breadwinner role, has also lost control over his own life and his family, especially because his wife is taking over so aptly. Having lost his equilibrium or congruence, his pride, and dignity, he fights back with anger that is hard to take for the family. The nurse sees the crisis as a struggle for control that stifles self-growth and ruins family togetherness. When James agrees with this and adds his own confirming comments, Norman presents the solution in the form of a shift toward spirituality or mutual understanding of each other's needs. He asks James how far back it was that he felt important for the family and well accepted. "Certainly not since I lost my job and probably not for a good many years before that." James feels that he never played a very significant role as a father and that his wife always was the organizer and told him what to do in the house. His income was his leverage and the power base through which he managed to keep Sylvia from working outside the house for all these years.

It is obvious that the family has had problems for a long time and is in need of professional help. The nurse's objective is therefore to warm James to the idea of family therapy and then introduce the plan to Sylvia and the kids.

Example 2

The family consists of Roberta and her common-law husband, Roy; Gilda, age 27; Lamar, age 25; and Sasha, age 19, who has two children. Gilda has moved out of the home. The others live in a house in an inner-city ghetto neighborhood. The family is lucky to own the house. Roy had inherited it from his father, a union autoworker. Roy, following in his father's footsteps, joined the autoworkers' union and worked for 15 years in an assembly plant. Twenty years ago, after his father died, Roy invited Roberta, Gilda, and Lamar to live with him. Roy never legally married Roberta, because she did not want to lose her independence. They then had a child, Sasha. Twelve years ago, Roy was laid off, never to be rehired. Because his house was his most valued possession, he did not want to move from the city. He had some hope of being rehired first, but then he witnessed factories closing all around him. He was able to locate occasional temporary jobs but never worked longer than a month and received no fringe benefits. Today, Roy regularly scavenges resalable materials in abandoned houses. He used to make fairly good money with aluminum siding until its retail price became miserably low. He now goes for scrap metal, oak doors, and whatever else he can find. Roy expresses pride about being an honest man and trying hard to earn money for the family. Even though he has had a lot of time on his hands over the years and has socialized with other men at the street corner and tried street drugs on and off, he has never got heavily involved in drinking or drug selling. He has never left the family and Roberta respects him, because he takes his father role seriously and serves as a role model. She also knows that without him, she may not have a home.

Roberta has done her own share of holding the family together. She works as a clerk in a department store. To get to work, she had to learn how to drive a car. This was a major accomplishment for her, because she was frightened of freeways and had no self-confidence. The first few days before driving to work, she found herself in tears and praying to God before she found the courage to turn the ignition key. Roberta used to be hopeful about the future of her children, but now she looks exhausted and seems depressed. She goes to church regularly. That is where she finds strength and knows that she can ask for some money or food to help her out between paychecks.

Gilda, the eldest daughter of Roberta, is married to a young man with ambition. An X-ray technician with a good job in a local hospital, she is the family's big hope. She supports her husband, who goes to college to earn a degree in business administration.

The two manage to make ends meet but do not have extra funds to support the family. Roy thinks that they are selfish, but Roberta tells Roy that they need to think about their own future and need all the support they can get to make it. Besides, who knows, in the future, they may be able to help the family much better than now. Lamar dropped out of school at age 15. At that time, he thought he did not need school. He had learning difficulties and his parents were in no position to assist him with reading or homework, because they are minimally literate themselves. Seeking help from teachers was painful and his friends teased him about it. As he watched his father struggle with everyday reality, he became convinced that this was not the kind of life he wanted for himself. The poverty of their family led him to value the things that were out of his reach. Lamar wanted to be rich and own what he needs to be admired, starting with the right kind of clothes, then a sporty car, a house, and a beautiful woman. Lamar is selling street drugs. His family does not know where he lives. When he visits, he refuses to talk about his life. For 2 years, Roberta had thought she had lost him, but when he appeared again, everyone figured he must have been in jail. When Lamar visits, he brings presents for the family. He is respected as the rich uncle, especially by Sasha's two children. Sasha, the only child fathered by Roy, lives at home and goes to evening classes to earn a high school equivalency diploma. She too had fallen for the drug scene and became a prostitute to buy drugs. She has had two children, and when the second one was born, Roy gave her a violent beating "to cast the devil out of her." Sasha was so shocked that she turned her life around. After a long talk with the minister, she agreed to follow her parents' command to live with them, stay home at night, take care of the kids, and become something. Sasha now goes to church with Roberta, and the minister encourages her regularly. She has tremendous respect for her parents and feels supported enough to work for a better life, one similar to her sister's.

Both examples show the chronicity of the problem of unemployment. Both families have mobilized in an effort to prevent a family breakdown. Their resources are vastly different, because they are drawn from equally different environments. By continuously modifying system maintenance strategies, they attempt to also maintain

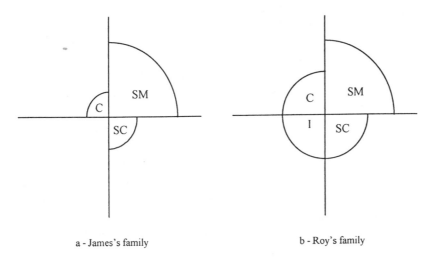

a - James's family   b - Roy's family

Figure 18.1. Comparison of Two Family Systems

coherence of the family system. In James's family, the attempt back-fires as James becomes demoralized due to status loss, and family dynamics ensue as described earlier (Komarovsky, 1940). Strong emphasis on control puts James's wife in a one-up position and results in an internal struggle for power that achieves the opposite of its intended aim: It destroys the family's coherence. Against all odds, despite their incredible financial hardship, Roy's family fares better over time. Their system maintenance includes the needs of all and their emphasis rests on both control and spirituality. Roy's pride is maintained and reinforced by respect from his wife. The children are faced with the difficult choice of honest toiling versus taking enormous risks to get quick wealth. James's family has managed to prevent a slide into marginal existence but has sacrificed mutuality, warmth, and belonging. In contrast, Roy's family, considered an economic failure by the outer world, lives in poverty but has gained strength and resilience unheard of in most systems.

Figure 18.1 illustrates the difference between the families. In addition to the varying degrees of coherence, the two families differ in the way the family members individuate. James's family is in crisis and is depleted of energy for growth and learning. The children's development is equally impaired. Sylvia has always been controlling and to be more so seems necessary and natural for her. Her actions dismiss James's need for system change. The family has become rigid. Both James and Sylvia are deadlocked in their positions, and each argument is a scenario with a stepwise progression that is entirely predictable and always the same. Nobody learns from the situation, nobody wins, and nobody sees a way out.

In contrast, Figure 18.1 shows Roy's family with sound individuation in that members are encouraged to find their own way and are supported in meeting their goals. Individuals learn from experience and interchange with their environment, adjust to changing situations, and attempt to mobilize available resources for a better future. Lamar is a problem in that his double life affects family coherence. The family copes by accepting only one of his lives into the system, thereby denying the other. Lamar knows this and keeps the second life a secret from the family. Nevertheless, tension arises from fear of the unknown future.

Roy's family may never come to a nurse's attention. Seldom are the right questions asked in well-baby clinics, doctor's offices, or agencies in which such families may appear. If they do, family members do not need to be told by professionals what to do better. Instead, they deserve respect and admiration, something that is provided rarely by professionals in such situations. Over and over, nurses in the field cast quick and derogatory judgments about behaviors they do not see in the larger context: stealing contents of abandoned houses is illegal and therefore bad; beating Sasha about having a child is insensitive and abusive; accepting gifts from Lamar is immoral; and Roberta's self-sacrifice shows that the family is enmeshed, unable to launch the kids, and therefore ineffective. Such judgments, verbalized or not, occur much more frequently than anyone dares to admit. Families like Roy's feel misunderstood in the health care system and treated as sick people who have caused their own misery or as poor victims. Neither position is functional and both prevent professionals from treating human beings with the heartfelt respect they deserve.

The use of the framework of systemic organization has the potential to open nurses' eyes to the pain and tribulations of families like Roy's and let them grow and individuate through intimate participation in the family life process. A theory-based, in-depth assessment provides understanding of the dynamics described earlier and seems to be the best guard against value judgments. In this respect, working with the deprived is no different from other populations. However, nurses need to understand that poverty engulfs these people with a culture different from society as a whole in which well-accepted norms easily lose validity. Irrespective of skin color, culture consists of ethnic values and beliefs lived in the family process, and behaviors arise from the backdrop of poverty and their meaning needs to be understood accordingly.

The framework of systemic organization leads professionals to examine each unique situation. Included in system maintenance are strategies of parenting, and within coherence one finds the nurturing behaviors among adults and responses of parents when the child seeks contact and closeness. Because research suggests a connection between depression and emotional instability and punitive and nonnurturative parenting (Jones, 1990), nurses need to carefully observe interactional dynamics and explore the possibility of violence in volatile situations. Nevertheless, this has to be done in the context of the total life pattern. Consequently, extreme caution should be taken when casting judgments without consideration for culturally based behaviors, such as Roy's casting out the devil in Sasha, or punitive disciplinary measures with children that signify the cultural norm and health rather than family tension.

19

Families and Chronic Poverty

Statistics show that poverty is a problem of marginal populations such as women, minorities, or immigrants. Poor families have a low participation in the labor force or a small share of earnings for reasons such as limited access to the labor force, high unemployment rates, and inequity of wages. Public discussion of the problem is dominated by three broad positions: absence of motivation to work, personal circumstances, and unavailability of quality jobs (Osterman, 1993). Researchers have used various methods to weigh the contribution of these positions and have concluded that employment trends are far more significant than family circumstances and that much could be improved by directing public support toward creating jobs and effective retraining programs (Bane & Ellwood, 1986; Sawhill, 1988).

Listening to stories of the poor often shows a chain of events that finally disconnect the individual or family from the working world or society. Mental illness triggers the downturn for some. Homelessness and poverty used to be blamed on the deinstitutionalization movement in the 1960s and 1970s and the inadequate care of chronically mentally ill patients in the community (Mechanic, 1987). The blame is no longer valid today, because the extremely poor and homeless population includes a large proportion of young people as well as women, children, and families who are failed by society and do not have the resources to reverse their economic plight.

Recent years have been marked with an erosion of income in all population segments, most seriously among minorities. The gap between wealthy and poor families has been widening since 1970. This is related to a serious loss of jobs, mainly low-skill labor jobs likely to be occupied by the previously mentioned marginal groups (Malveaux, 1989). The people who lose these jobs first are also the ones likely to suffer unemployment longest due to their low educational level and few reserves and resources (Bullough & Bullough, 1981).

Despite a general awareness of serious repercussions of unemployment on vulnerable families, it is astonishing that unemployment literature pays minimal attention to outcomes of economic hardship (Kelvin & Jarret, 1985). For example, in 1984, only 34% of the 8.5 million unemployed received benefits, and almost two thirds of the benefits fell through the cracks (U.S. Congress, p. 98). Literature further shows that once families slide into a marginal existence, their health status deteriorates and medical care becomes out of reach (Brenner, 1987). Many families are plagued by alcoholism, mental and emotional problems, violence, and abuse (Zlotnick & Cassanego, 1992). Pearlin, Lieberman, Menaghan, and Mullan (1981) describe their circumstances as "economic brinkmanship," whereby psychological health is severely affected by the fusion of acute and chronic stress (Whelan, 1992).

In terms of this framework, a situation so severe that it presents a threat to the most basic needs for survival seems to be the ultimate challenge for system maintenance and often carries severe repercussions in terms of the entire family life process. Poverty changes values in that it rearranges priorities. Individuation occurs by learning to use resources in the environment to one's advantage. Through individuation, individuals and families who are disconnected from the mainstream culture and access to material reward systems seek to reconnect with another culture and find a new purpose in life. The adaptation of individuals to adverse conditions signifies system change and culture transformation. This adaptation process has encouraged the development or strengthening of community organizations and subcultures, some respectable in the eyes of outsiders, such as neighborhood networks or religious organizations, while others are a sore thumb for society (e.g., the drug culture or youth gangs).

The example of Lamar in the previous family case example is typical for many youths in deprived situations. Lamar's life process distinguishes itself from biculturalism as described in Chapter 18. Lamar does not live one culture while aspiring to another. Instead, Lamar lives two cultures simultaneously. As is the case with a split personality, he lives by two sets of conflicting values. When he is with his family, he activates one set; when he is immersed in the drug culture, he lives by the other. For the sake of material rewards, he tolerates a severe lack of coherence and confusion about the meaning of his life.

The literature falls short of describing changes and influences experienced by families with chronic poverty. Some families remain resilient despite all odds, but in vulnerable families members such as Lamar, who ascribe to competing ideologies, destroy their own coherence and chip away their family's. It seems that such families represent a composite of crises outlined in all previous chapters combined into one system, in which economic bleakness forms the backdrop of physical and mental illness, addictions, and structural and developmental family crises.

Upon interviewing a group of rehabilitating drug abusers from poor multiproblem families, almost all of whom had more than one member addicted to drugs or alcohol, I discovered one common trend: The families were in an ongoing severe crisis. They were not connected within; they also did not enjoy the benefit of a wider kin network and did not go to church or make use of the very few resources in the community. This was due to access or availability problems and lack of knowledge and a rigid concentration of the entire family energy on the enforcement of defensive system maintenance. The greatest deficiency in these multiproblem families, however, was the lack of individuation. They had experienced disasters, such as the murder of a father, the arrest of a child, wife abuse, or a death due to AIDS, but these events did not seem to effect any change. There was no culmination of crises through which growth could occur nor was there a notable difference in their chronic level of despair and resignation. These families, numbed by their pain, made great strides to kill flair-ups with drugs, sex, and alcohol, or sought thrills and adventure. Instead of healing wounds, each member continued his or her rigid pattern of suppressing and releasing tensions in an unchanged manner. Although these family members believed in and talked about the soundness of Christian values, different principles ruled their lives. They found stability in recurring chaos and strayed apart, but the illusion of a united family was kept alive and the children became victims (Friedemann & Musgrove, 1994).

This suggests that families, to stay healthy, have to live by a common set of values and use mutually valid strategies for survival to maintain congruence. The traditional African American family system, historically equipped to function amid poverty and in a hostile environment, is described as such a system. As explained in Chapter 9, such families represent a mixture of cultural patterns and values transmitted from the past (Boyd-Franklin, 1989) and experiences made in their ongoing struggle for economic survival (Staples, 1986). The family process interacts with a welfare system that has managed to maintain families at the subsistence level rather than encouraging self-reliance (Zimmerman, 1988). However, struggle for survival has forced females who head families to become strong family managers who are connected to a female neighborhood network that provides mutual functional and emotional support.

Such amazingly resilient systems, however, are increasingly threatened as neighborhoods change, individuals and families become disconnected, and pride is lost. The previous example of Roy and Roberta's family is typical of a system built on a firm foundation of Christian values and connections to the neighborhood and church community. Nevertheless, eroding tensions have to be counteracted continuously. Presently, Lamar leads a dangerous life and Sasha has only recently stabilized hers after having been in the midst of prostitution and drug abuse. Roberta is willing to support Sasha but cannot win Lamar back to the family. In fact, in the face of their poverty, she is rather ambivalent and her integrity is weakened. She does not defy Lamar's image of the rich uncle as a role model for her grandchildren and accepts presents from him for the family. She appreciates Lamar's emotional attachment to his family and the goodness of his heart, but she suppresses the reality of his other life. The example shows further how hard it is for deprived families to make a case for honest toiling if children are exposed to competing ideologies that promise instant gratification. Newspapers report daily about families who neglect or abuse children or whose members commit crimes. Many such family members are already products of families who have lost emotional connectedness and a sense of direction.

In summary, the economic bleakness and high unemployment rates, low wages, and inaccessibility of jobs in the inner cities make the achievement of basic self-respect by earning an honest and comfortable living a formidable task. Added to these problems are psychological effects of chronic deprivation that create resentment, erode the motivation to do menial work (Wilson, 1987), and entice people to break away from families and support systems. Many families' struggle to maintain congruence becomes a losing battle and children raised in such systems never learn the meaning of closeness, caring, and sharing.

Today, poverty reaches beyond the boundaries of the inner city. It is a well-known fact that the poor in homeless shelters are not just alcoholics and mentally deranged individuals. Many are working minimal wage jobs that do not allow them to pay the rent of a suburban dwelling. Osterman (1993), studying the poor in Boston, found almost three quarters to be women, divorced, or never married with children. The poor were less well educated and comprised a high number of high school dropouts. Osterman found that many men accepted work as the opportunity arose, but most women could not because they had to deal with complex situations, family obligations, and the lack of available child care facilities.

This shows that the poor comprise a heterogeneous population of all ages in many different situations. They all have been victimized by society. Some have known a better life and through adverse circumstances have slid into marginality. Others have been born into a situation of material and possibly emotional deprivation. According to the theory of systemic organization, all humans need connectedness. Marginal groups develop their own subcultures through which members regain a sense of belonging after being cut off from mainstream culture. This theory, by way of the culture transformation process, leads to the hypothesis that the longer a subculture exists, the more it will separate its values from the mainstream. With values, patterns, and behaviors functional in a deprived environment but less appreciated in the larger society, the rehabilitation of individuals to become fit for work requires extensive system change and becomes increasingly difficult. Retraining programs that do not consider such cultural factors are likely to be doomed for failure.

In cases of new poverty through unemployment or divorce, it should be of interest to society to reverse the poverty situation as quickly as possible to prevent these individuals, predominantly women and children, from joining marginal groups. Professionals understand such family systems insufficiently. Routinely, nurses assess mothers and children but fail to determine who else may be part of the functional family. Experience in a homeless shelter has shown repeatedly that women who are moved into an apartment disappear from one day to the next, only to come back to the shelter a few months later. For example, one of my clients lived in her new place provided by the shelter for 1 week, until her boyfriend found her again. Three days later, the place was raided by the police because of severe drug trafficking.

The situations of poor women are complex. As single parents, they need to be connected and supported. Some are lucky to be part of a caring extended family; others are vulnerable, because they try to meet their needs for love and belonging, scanning the community for targets. They are in danger of falling prey to abuse and violence. Such situations are described in Part 2 of this book.

The urgency is great to reduce poverty by developing highly effective retraining programs and creating well-paying jobs to serve as a basis for a worthy existence (Whelan, 1992). The situation for women is more complex, however, because they need more help to create the basis for work or education. If women have enough personal congruence to endure their hardship and live an autonomous life, enough strength to run the family business without damaging the children's emotional well-being, they need the resources to maintain their good work. If no extended family is available, women need to be supported by a network of social programs that provides the necessary stability to concentrate on work and education and allows them to reach the goal of a better life in the future.

Nurses can build relationships with poor families and gain their trust. They can serve as their advocate within the health care system if they understand their life process and can interpret their strengths for other professionals. Using the framework of systemic organization in assisting families in poverty, nurses must draw material from all chapters in this book to interpret the complexity of their problems. They must work in conjunction with community supports and agencies, substance abuse treatment centers, child care facilities, head start programs, and the like in helping families to be firmly anchored in the community, meet their needs without resorting to dangerous subcultures, and regain hope for a better future.

Summary

In summary, this chapter presents still more evidence of the multifaceted nature of family problems. This time, they are induced by the environment, and the crisis arises when the change seriously impairs the systemic process of the family and its members. One might assume that radical changes happening abruptly would present the most serious problems. Consequently, unemployment would be more serious than day-to-day work stress, and a disaster, such as a murder or a housefire, may be the worst of all. This may be true in some cases, but not all. The examples and research cited have shown the deleterious results of chronic incongruence that slowly gnaws coherence, instills resentment and hostility, and erodes the quality of relationships. Some families' equilibrium is very fragile and little is needed to embark the family process on a destructive path; others have tremendous resilience. Nurses are presented with the challenge of discovering these differences by exploring each family as it interacts with its very own context. They are offered the unique opportunity to join the inner world of families, discover the secrets, and expand their wisdom.

20

Research on Environmental/Economic Conditions and Families

The preceding chapters focused predominantly on processes of families, the individuals within them, and the nurse interacting with them. The topics of this chapter pose a still greater challenge to the researcher, namely, an expansion of the phenomenon to the environmental systems level. Basic questions to be addressed here include the following: What is the nature of the community life process? How does the community life process interface with individuals? How does the community life process interface with families by way of their members?

Research that attempts to clarify certain aspects pertaining to these questions constitutes an exploration of multiple complex processes in constant movement and ongoing change. Murphy (1991) points out that research about catastrophes affecting individuals and families should investigate community and family processes, but what little research has been done has been atheoretical and lacks control. As a solution for the future, she suggests quasi-experiments with longitudinal designs to allow statistical analyses that reach beyond descriptives. The view of the environment as systemic process—that is, simultaneous, dynamic patterns and rhythms of interacting individuals, groups, organizations, and communities—points to the need for a more significant breakthrough. The development of in-depth knowledge is hardly possible with quasi-experiments. Instead, researchers need to break away from the crippling limitations of stress and coping models discussed throughout this book and focus on the dynamics of systemic processes.

The following explains this more specifically. Validation of experimental research or *ex-post-facto* correlational group comparisons after events such as catastrophes or major job layoffs depends on the control of alternative hypotheses (Murphy, 1991). In stress and coping frameworks, control refers to three groups of variables: preexisting variables, stress appraisal, and other mediating variables. On the level of the individuum, preexisting variables are demographics, personal traits, and personal coping mechanisms (Lazarus & Folkman, 1984b). Preexisting variables in the community address unemployment quotas, business climate, crime rates, social programs, and many more. Stress appraisal has been extensively discussed by Lazarus and Folkman (1984b) and refers to perceptions that determine whether a situation is perceived to be harmful or challenging. Finally, mediating factors comprise all other variables that have an effect on the coping process. Examples are resources and social support (Norbeck, 1988). The control of these groups of variables, especially if family and community levels of systems are included, is cumbersome if not impossible. Random sampling, often considered the panacea by researchers who strive toward generalizations, washes out the effects of any one of these interfering variables on the system. Findings do not reveal the operations of systemic processes or the variations in systemic processes among subjects.

Other methods of control, such as strict inclusion criteria or stratification of the sample, permit the elimination of certain known interferences, for example, single parenthood or certain attitudes or beliefs, and facilitate the equalization of comparison groups along the remaining preexisting or mediating variables. Strictly defined samples, however, do not allow the generalization to other population groups and may reduce the systemic process to a skeleton of operations seen as being separate from the whole. Because the whole is different from its parts (von Bertalanffy, 1968), such findings have little clinical relevance.

Finally, instead of eliminating interfering variables, stress and coping researchers have attempted to define and measure them as components of causal models. Although this approach is the most useful, it does not do justice to systemic complexity. Systems are in constant motion in that countless interfering variables interact with each other circularly and nonrecursively rather than independently. Therefore, variations among systems seem to become considerably greater than the commonalities, and the processes leading to variations are poorly understood. Ironically, the information clinicians and policymakers need is precisely the kind not provided by conventional research, namely, knowledge about these variations and their processes.

In sum, quasi-experiments yield valid results only in a controlled environment, but the real world presents confusing patterns of inter-acting and interrelated forces that mutually contribute to systemic outcomes. Manipulating or eliminating one or more of these variables will change the system, but the change is not linear and therefore difficult to estimate. Due to the great variability of systemic processes, the statistical determination of common interaction or direct effects of the variables is problematic. In short, the approach to conceptuali-zation and research defines the knowledge that can be generated when, in fact, the knowledge in need of being generated, that is, sys-temic processes and their variability, should define the approach to conceptualization and research.

Research on Family and Community Reactions to Environmental Crises

In contrast to stress and coping theory, the framework of systemic organization requires a conceptualization of phenomena that reaches beyond the linear effect of a stimulus. The systemic researcher thinks of intervening variables as constituents of the total life process. Thus, the systemic process represents *the* major variable in determining out-come of disasters. If the researcher is to control for life process rather than a myriad of independent mediators, the primary problem refers to the measurement of the systemic process.

All three questions posed at the beginning of this chapter refer to systems processes; the first one addresses the community as a whole. Process at the community level is most difficult to describe (Murphy, 1991). The definition of community is the first challenge. In the example in Chapter 16, Alice was involved with various communities that all contributed to her crisis and recovery. The assault happened in the city. The city also provided the services needed for Alice's medical emergency and the pursuit of justice with the aim of promoting safety for all citizens. Alice also interfaced with the rural community of her family. That community had originally shaped its inhabitants' attitudes toward work and education, similar to Alice's father's, but more recently reflected a conflict of ideologies that separated the generations and was played out in Alice's family. Finally, Alice became part of the medical community, a subcommunity within the city that also served rural areas. Based on this, it becomes clear that to find answers about community processes, researchers need to focus on functional communities rather than on geographic or political systems.

Communities were studied descriptively as they responded to disasters by measuring the economic impact, the interruption of services, and ultimately the processes of restoration. Models for disaster response have been developed (e.g., Kreps, 1978; Wenger, 1978), whereby community structure, history, resources, and preparedness have been linked with the type and impact of the disaster. Likewise, many types of functional community assessments are constantly being made to determine the efficiency and effectiveness of various physical and mental health services and their accessibility. This includes an abundance of federal, state, and local surveys about consumer status, resource availability, and use. Such data banks are very useful for researchers, but are not always disseminated and made available. Furthermore, variables and their measurement differ from study to study, which makes comparisons difficult.

In working with the framework of systemic organization, such assessments take on a more in-depth perspective. An assessment of community process refers to both the health of the community as a system and the community's ability to promote health of its people. In Alice's case, one could study the city emergency system, the medical system, or the mental health system. Their health is determined by the four process dimensions. Therefore, a researcher would want to know how the system is maintained through policies and procedures, decision making, assignment of jobs and workloads, financial resources, materials, and supplies. In terms of coherence, the commitment of workers, job satisfaction, channels of communication, and the relationship between administration and staff are of the essence. Individuation is apparent if the system is open to new ideas, if individuals' growth is promoted and encouraged, and if education and training are made available. The second criterion for health is the satisfaction of the constituents, and the final evidence is the fit with the larger environment. The latter requests a look at problems the system is to address and the function it is to perform to determine the system's legitimacy. For example, a medical system is legitimate if its services are in demand, if the people's actual needs are met by the services, and if it allows access to all people in need of the services.

In nursing, in addition to available aggregate community data, a client-focused community assessment may be most relevant. Such an assessment relates to the other two questions mentioned at the beginning of this chapter: the interface of the individual with the community and with family and community. For example, a case study focusing on Alice's situation would examine how Alice was served by her community: all systems that became activated or failed to activate in response to her emergency. This includes her own family. The systemic process in focus is Alice's very own at the point of crisis as it interfaces with the services meant to sustain Alice until the time of full recovery. Beyond the immediate medical care, Alice needed to restore a sense of safety through diligent action by the police in investigating the case and arresting the assailant. Optimally, Alice hoped that the judicial system would remove the assailant from the streets and the penitentiary system would rehabilitate him. Furthermore, to feel safe, Alice needed to believe that further incidents were preventable. The community and a relative provided Alice with housing in a safer neighborhood brightly lighted at night and with gadgets that decreased the likelihood of break-ins, such as a burglar alarm and safety locks. In terms of Alice's coherence, mental health counseling and empathetic talks with her parents were needed to help Alice regain self-respect and a sense of control over her life. Therapy for her family helped the parents and siblings in supporting Alice's coherence. Finally, individuation needed to take place in terms of finding a meaning for the incident and a change of the family's worldview. Alice needed help in thinking through the issues either during counseling sessions or with her parents. She also wanted to continue her education and personal development with her parents' full support.

In case management and family therapy, assessments of the larger systems that examine the responses to the needs of victims as listed earlier are of essence. For example, Imber-Black (1988) provides detailed procedural instructions to clinicians. It seems that such clinical assessments could be conducted with the consultation of a researcher to include sufficient rigor and thus qualify as scientific research. A series of well-planned case studies of this nature could lead to more informed interventions and suitable referrals of clients. In addition, such studies have a high potential to influence policy making and the political process for the sake of all individuals and families in similar crises.

If the study of community services and their interface with the processes of the family and the individuals directly affected by their environment is applied to multiple families in similar situations, the designs can be descriptive, qualitative, quantitative, or, most advantageous, triangulated by methods.

The community process can be assessed with an evaluation study as described in Chapter 15. This time, the viewpoints of individuals and families about the services are of primary importance. Included in the evaluation are accessibility and effectiveness of the services as well as the outcomes of the interventions relative to the recovery process measured at the individual and family levels.

This framework guides the researcher in choosing the phenomena of study of family community interface. Here, they include the individuals' perceptions of their own needs and the effectiveness of family support and community services. After a disastrous event, the families gain depth by being pulled into this process with questions about their own interpretations of the event and the needs of the affected member(s). They are also questioned about related family issues and interactional patterns of the family with the affected member(s). In addition, key professionals may be interviewed about their view of the situation. All these viewpoints are then compared and contrasted.

Research on Work Issues

A focus on systemic processes and their interface is equally important if the study concerns work issues. Researchers are beginning to acknowledge the need to look at the totality of all interacting stresses as an explanation for coping (Bolger, DeLongis, Kessler, & Wethington, 1989). In family-work research, two theoretical positions are discussed. The first is role theory and the proposition that role overload is created by excessive demands, especially of women. Distress builds and affects coping at work and in the family. Consequently, spillover can occur from family to work or from work to family.

The second position, role expansion theory, seems to be contrary to the first. It relates to findings that multiple roles can have positive effects on the individuals (Marks, 1977). Multiple roles are believed to provide access to additional resources that counteract the effect of role overload and promote satisfaction (Kibria, Barnett, Baruch, Marshall, & Pleck, 1990).

Both positions may have validity if they constitute predominant mechanisms in the life process. Researchers have argued that a person's life process, specifically the person's emotional constitution (coherence) (Kandel & Davies, 1986) or learned values about work roles (system maintenance), will determine what roles and how many the person will assume and how work conflicts and crises are avoided (Moen, Kain, & Elder, 1983). Such propositions, even though not widespread in the literature, concur with the framework of systemic organization.

For example, if according to this framework all women learn their roles through individuation starting early in childhood, their life process expresses these role behaviors as well as their attitudes and beliefs. Their systemic process, therefore, determines their desire to engage in work roles and their capability to do so. There would be no problem if each woman had a free choice. This is, however, seldom the case. Pressure to assume or not to assume work roles may be derived from economic need, the partner's expectation, or social pressure in terms of fitting in with friends or the neighborhood. All of these lead to incongruence if the work-related behaviors assumed clash with values in the woman's system maintenance. For example, incongruence occurs when the individual is forced to work but has strong beliefs, such as "a good mother stays home with the child." Likewise, problems occur if a woman believes that engagement in the world of work is needed for self-growth but is forced to stay home and tend to the children.

Research with this framework is therefore research about incongruence. The example of Herb and Margaret's family is typical in that the basic incongruence lies within the values that support the individuals' system maintenance. These are values about the roles at work and in the family. As the actual situation threatens these values and the individuals resist system change, the conflict is carried into the family process. The researcher's challenge is a design for a study that addresses the main components (the key individuals' system maintenance, specifically values about work and family roles; the actual work situation and the individuals' response to it; family system maintenance and coherence, specifically the conflict played out in interpersonal relationships; and the outcomes in terms of family and individual health variables) and provides in-depth knowledge about the process.

What was stated in previous chapters about designs that research the family life process is also valid here. Designs that address work-family incongruence need to be longitudinal and focus on change. How the change occurs is more important than its outcome, and change needs to be evaluated on both the individual and family levels. The optimal design uses methods triangulation to take advantage of the ease of administration and analysis of standardized tools and the power of qualitative data to explain individuals' viewpoints and family processes. For example, a study of families in Herb and Margaret's situation may involve an instrument exploring work attitudes of both partners; a tool measuring family role perceptions of both partners; and a family functioning tool that provides scores for family system maintenance, coherence, individuation, and family conflict filled out by as many members as possible. Instruments measuring satisfaction with the family and the mental and physical health of all family members could be used to determine the outcome. The tools could be administered at the height of a family crisis and at regular intervals thereafter.

Qualitative data are indispensable for understanding the life process as it strives to find new health. Each person's perceptions about his or her own work and family roles and those of other family members need to be recorded. Changes, as they occur over time, are described by all family members. Some families may engage in a course of therapy, and its effect may need to be assessed with mental or physical health outcome measures. However, for a complete understanding of treatment effects, the researcher wants to know how values about work and family have shifted, how relationships have changed, and how the family has renewed its general process. The framework of systemic organization will guide the questions to be asked. For example, if the regeneration of the family life process signifies better coherence of the family and learning from the experience, questions that elicit informative responses would address such family dynamics in very general terms with the caution that subjects are not to be directed toward the desired answers.

Quantitative analyses need to respect constancy of the unit of measurement. There may be a need for various regression models, one for each family member's perceptions about the self and the family, or a family model, if family scores make conceptual sense. In addition to determining main and interactive effects in predicting outcomes, the researcher needs to assess the nature of change. For that purpose, data from each participating family must be used to describe family process from one point of measurement to the next. The convergence or divergence of the various types of data is then analyzed in the search for explanations. If the explanations are strictly guided by the propositions of this framework, they will qualify as theory testing.

Another type of conflict is workplace incongruence. According to the framework of systemic organization, individuals learn basic life patterns, such as patterns of relating, achievement, control-dependency, and problem solving, that they tend to pursue not only in the family but in all other systems in which they assume roles (DeMarco, 1994). Workplace congruence is possible if expectations at work concur with the individuals' basic patterns. If there is incongruence due to a mismatch of family and work patterns, the individual is likely to perceive tension and anxiety about the work situation. Today's economic conditions may make it difficult for individuals to change positions and find others more in tune with their own system. For example, nurses who have a strong need for stability are likely to become increasingly insecure and threatened within today's health care environment, which is marked by phenomenal changes and has high expectations of professionals in terms of flexibility, willingness to work in teams, individuation, and abilities to make changes.

The expansion of the framework of systemic organization, therefore, has applicability in a new and highly relevant area of research as of yet untapped. The survival of health care institutions depends on the hard work and cooperation of their constituents. If patterns of family life of nurses are reflected in the interactive patterns of these nurses in the teams in their unit, the question arises as to how unit staff or teams could better accommodate a diversity of patterns or how one could screen nurses and assign them to units that match their own life process to enhance productivity. DeMarco (1994) has begun this kind of work with the development of a work questionnaire based on the dimensions of the framework of systemic organization, and efforts to validate it qualitatively are on the way. Much more needs to be done in the future.

Family and work patterns should be measured and their level of congruence determined in relation to the well-being of individuals and the health of the workplace. For example, studies on the individual level might examine activity-rest rhythms at home and at work, patterns of relatedness, decision making, assertiveness, or self-development, and workplace studies could focus on the systemic functioning of a team in relation to the life processes of its members.

Research on Unemployment and Economic Hardship

Chapters 18 and 19, which refer to economic stress, unemployment, and severe poverty, include an overview of the research exploring effects of unemployment and poverty on families and children. Again, the conceptual models used have been linear. Although the exploration of processes is talked about and a phenomenological approach to the problem is suggested by Barling (1990), little has been done. A beginning is marked by the interpersonal model of Elder, Conger, Foster, and Ardelt (1992), which suggests that an unfavorable income-need ratio, adverse income change, and unstable work conditions create a situation of economic pressure that tends to encourage hostilities between the partners. The researchers proceeded to expand the model horizontally to other family relationships to show that the father's hostility elicited reciprocal hostility from the children, which suggests circular reinforcement but remains to be researched in the future.

Friedemann and Webb's (1995) study on family effects of economic stress constitutes one of few studies with a longitudinal perspective. Although the study was originally based on a stress and coping framework, its follow-up 6 years later had implications relative to the framework of systemic organization. First, the proposition that family incongruence leads to incongruence in individuals and is experienced as anxiety or related emotions was supported in that family health (the perception of family effectiveness within the four dimensions measured with the Assessment of Strategies in Families [ASF] instrument) predicted one third of the variance of anxiety and two thirds of depression. In addition, the results indicated perceptional differences between men and women. The women's mental health was clearly related to internal processes of the family, namely, role functions related to system maintenance and coherence, but the husbands expected families to accommodate to their needs for individuation. Interestingly, both genders felt that the family ultimately benefited from their economic crisis, but the women saw the benefit as improved coherence and the men as better individuation. Finally, the exploratory study suggested that economic stress compounded by a troublesome marital relationship and ongoing family hardship over 6 years could lead to chronic incongruence through a process that maintained anxiety. These findings encourage the use of expanded systemic models for further study of family phenomena with triangular designs described earlier.

In the study of economic hardship and poverty, processes in need of exploration are internal family operations attempting to adjust to economic hardship and/or reverse it. They address system maintenance in terms of making do with less, individuation through learning new ways of procuring resources or learning from the situation, and system change in relation to assuming new attitudes and values about the family and the environment. Other processes of importance are those of the family's macrosystem. Economic bleakness, unavailability of jobs, transportation to jobs, educational opportunities, discrimination, and the like have serious repercussions on the personal and family levels. Researchers of families who confront harsh and dangerous conditions in their immediate environment can build knowledge only if they examine the family life process in its totality. This includes seemingly unrelated problems and changes that threaten family health concurrently. A focus on perceptions is of extreme importance because family health is subjective and each member's perceptions of the family process, its members' contributions to the process, and the family interchange with its environment determine the level of congruence.

A study of old men in the Bowery is an example of an anthropological field project that has provided an in-depth description of the life processes of homeless men. The study contributes to a new understanding of the men's situation by describing them as personal casualties or victims of the larger system. The study includes personal stories and interviews about the men's history, daily activities, relationships, and their meaning of life. Concurrently, the researchers describe the men's environment in great detail, deriving data from multiple and diverse sources (Cohen & Sokolovsky, 1989). Such broad-based studies are perhaps the best in providing the information needed by health care, mental health, and social organizations. They can be applied to families as well as individuals. Nevertheless, disadvantages exist in that these studies are extensive in effort, have a high cost, and take a long time to complete. Smaller studies may be more feasible and also valuable as long as the design addresses family processes and their interface with the macrosystem. Researchers using the framework of systemic organization may draw on many creative ways of exploring these processes as long as they do not violate research principles and tests of validity.

Concluding Remarks

This book has taken the readers on a journey through nursing with the framework of systemic organization. Initially, they were familiarized with the basic concepts and the dynamic process of systems: individual, family, and larger groups and organizations as well as the process of nursing. The theoretical section was followed by practical applications in a variety of nursing situations. On their journey, readers were exposed to healthy processes of individuals and families attempting to continuously regain congruence through the adjustment of values and behaviors working toward the desired systemic targets of stability, growth, control, and spirituality. These healthy processes were then contrasted with crises that stifled the growth of family systems and the development of the individuals within. Numerous examples guided the readers through the nursing process aimed at crisis resolution through supporting families in system change.

I believe that a focus on systems larger than the individual is absolutely necessary in all types of nursing. Because physical disease is often intertwined with a difficult life situation, seemingly simple cases often turn out to be immensely complex. I hope that nurses in clinical settings who observe incongruence and crisis of individuals and families have found in this book the necessary tools to work on sharpening their skills of assessing situations, asking the right questions, finding existing strengths and resources, and supporting clients in pursuing a course toward better health. Experts in nursing have the opportunity to expand their understanding of the clients' life process to include all areas of family life as well as the environment, its culture, resources, dangers, and temptations. The framework of systemic organization provides the necessary structure to organize assessment data of complex situations, determine on what level to enter the system, set goals with the clients, and find ways to pursue them.

Studying the case examples may have surprised many readers about seemingly unconventional approaches undertaken with families. Ever so often, behaviors that appear problematic on the surface turn out to be assets for families when their motivations and effects are examined in greater depth. Perhaps the most valuable merit of the framework of systemic organization is its guidance in examining values, beliefs, and motivations. Values and beliefs serve as the foundation out of which the life process evolves and as a backdrop for behavior patterns. Working with the framework of systemic organization, nurses avoid judging behaviors at face value without seeing them in the context of the dynamic overall life process. Thus, the framework promotes true cultural sensitivity, not through the knowledge about peculiarities of ethnic patterns pertaining to certain groups of people, but through the revelation of the role these patterns play in attaining the systemic targets of families in maintaining stability while adjusting to an environment that poses continuously changing demands. Cultural sensitivity reaches beyond ethnicity and race to a sensitivity to the many variations of human existence. The first step toward such sensitivity is the knowledge and appreciation of one's own peculiarities that can then reach out to the clients'. On the basis of the process of individuation, nurses working with the framework of systemic organization slowly transform their own culture in that they accept and value differences and experience growth through interactions with families and communities.

This explains why nursing with the framework of systemic organization challenges neophytes and develops experts. It defies "cookbook" approaches to nursing as well as ready-made and good-for-all interventions. The framework individualizes care, not in terms of superficial demographic differences, but according to the clients' view of their world. The clients' world can open up to every nurse and reveal the secrets of humanity, the very essence that promotes growth within the nursing profession.

Like the clinician, the researcher is driven by the same fascination for human nature and social interactions. The task of the researcher is the exploration of process, and knowledge is generated from the understanding of humans, families, clients, and nurses as complex, evolving, and constantly moving systems. That understanding drives the methods, all limited in many ways. If methods are used in combination, however, researchers can minimize shortcomings and optimize explanatory power. Therefore, through methods triangulation, a variety of creative methods is encouraged to generate in-depth knowledge. In research, truth is relative to the subjects' understanding of their world and the researcher attempts to capture that understanding. Common to all research designs is the necessity for subjects to play an integral part in the exploration process, because it is through the subjects that truth evolves.

In short, the framework of systemic organization leads to innovative clinical approaches and research designs with families and family members, and it can be expanded to the environment of individuals, groups, and families. The broad systemic understanding of phenomena played out in families and organizations has the potential to assist nurses in assuming visionary leadership and guiding policymakers away from surface solutions to health and social problems, such as promoting the return to an antiquated family ideal unsuitable for many, and to turn them toward those policies that benefit both wealthy and poor individuals, traditional and nontraditional families, and people in urban and rural settings. Based on the tenets of this framework and the conviction that all nursing, by necessity, has to be family nursing, it is my sincere hope that nurses increasingly become ardent advocates of their patients' families and that researchers reveal to the world the essence of family life, human interaction, and the social process of groups and organizations.

References

Aaronson, L. S., & Burman, M. E. (1994). Focus on psychometrics. Use of health records in research: Reliability and validity issues. *Research in Nursing & Health, 17,* 67-73.

Abbott, D. D., & Brody, G. H. (1985). The relation of child age, gender, and number of children to the marital adjustment of wives. *Journal of Marriage and the Family, 47*(1), 77-84.

Ablon, J., & Ames, G. M. (1989). Culture and family. In C. L. Gilliss, B. L. Highley, B. M. Roberts, & I. M. Martinson (Eds.), *Toward a science of family nursing* (pp. 124-145). Reading, MA: Addison-Wesley.

Ackoff, R. L. (1974). *Redesigning the future: A systems approach to societal problems.* New York: John Wiley.

Adams, G. R., & Jones, R. M. (1983). Female adolescents' identity development: Age comparisons and perceived child-rearing experience. *Developmental Psychology, 19,* 249-256.

Agar, M. H. (1986). *Speaking of ethnography.* Beverly Hills, CA: Sage.

Ajzen, I., & Fishbein, M. (1980). *Understanding attitudes and predicting social behavior.* Englewood Cliffs, NJ: Prentice Hall.

Allen, K. R. (1993). The dispassionate discourse of children's adjustment to divorce. *Journal of Marriage and the Family, 55*(1), 46-49.

Alston, L. T., & Aguire, B. (1987). Elderly Mexican Americans: Nativity and health access. *International Migration Review, 21,* 626-642.

Amato, P. R. (1993). Children's adjustment to divorce: Theories, hypotheses, and empirical support. *Journal of Marriage and the Family, 55*(1), 23-38.

American Nurses Association. (1980). *Nursing: A social policy statement* (ANA Pub. No. NP-63 35M). Kansas City, MO: Author.

American Psychiatric Association. (1980). *Diagnostic and statistical manual of psychiatric disorders* (3rd ed.). Washington, DC: Author.

Anderson, E. (1989). Sex codes and family life among poor inner-city youths. In W. J. Wilson (Ed.), *The ghetto underclass: Social science perspectives* (pp. 59-78). Newbury Park, CA: Sage.

Andrews, G., Tennant, C., Hewson, D. M., & Vaillant, G. E. (1978). Life event stress—Social support, coping style, and risk of psychological impairment. *Journal of Nervous and Mental Diseases, 166*(5), 307-316.

Andrews, S., Williams, A. B., & Neil, K. (1993). The mother-child relationship in the HIV-1 positive family. *Image, 25*(3), 193-198.

Antonovsky, A. (1979). *Health, stress, and coping.* San Francisco: Jossey-Bass.

Aries, P. (1962). *Centuries of childhood—Social history of family life.* New York: Knopf.

Aroian, K. J., & Patsdaughter, C. A. (1989). Multiple-method, cross-cultural assessment of psychological distress. *Image, 21*(2), 90-93.

Asen, K., Berkowitz, R., Cooklin, A., Leff, J., Loader, P., Piper, R., & Rein, L. (1991). Family therapy outcome research: A trial for families, therapists, and researchers. *Family Process, 30*(1), 3-30.

Atchley, R. C. (1980). *The social forces in later life: An introduction to social gerontology.* Belmont, CA: Wadsworth.

Atchley, R. C. (1982). Retirement: Leaving the world of work. *The Annals of the American Academy of Political and Social Science, 464,* 120-131.

Atkinson, T., Liem, R., & Liem, J. (1986). The social costs of unemployment: Implications for social support. *Journal of Health and Social Behavior, 27,* 317-331.

Auerswald, E. H. (1987). Epistemological confusion in family therapy and research. *Family Process, 26,* 317-330.

Avery, R., Goldscheider, F., & Speare, A. (1992). Feathered nest/gilded cage: Parental income and leaving home in the transition to adulthood. *Demography, 29,* 375-388.

Baker, A. F. (1989). How families cope. *Journal of Psychosocial Nursing, 27*(1), 31-36.

Baker, O. V., Druckman, J. M., & Flagle, J. E. (1980). *Helping youth and families of separation, divorce and remarriage.* Palo Alto, CA: American Institutes for Research.

Bandura, A. (1969). *Principles of behavior modification.* New York: Holt, Rinehart & Winston.

Bandura, A. (1979). The social learning perspective: Mechanism of aggression. In H. Toch (Ed.), *Psychology of crime and criminal justice* (pp. 191-225). New York: Holt, Rinehart & Winston.

Bane, M. J. (1986). Household compositions and poverty. In S. Danziger & D. Weinberg (Eds.), *Fighting poverty* (pp. 209-232). Cambridge, MA: Harvard University Press.

Bane, M. J., & Ellwood, D. T. (1986). Slipping into and out of poverty: The dynamics of spells. *Journal of Human Resources, 21,* 1-23.

Barkauskas, V. H. (1986). Community health nursing. In B. B. Logan & C. E. Dawkins (Eds.), *Family-centered nursing in the community* (pp. 4-30). Reading, MA: Addison-Wesley.

Barling, J. (1990). *Employment, stress and family functioning.* New York: John Wiley.

Barnett, R. C., & Baruch, G. K. (1987). Social roles, gender and psychological distress. In R. C. Barnett, L. Biener, & G. K. Baruch (Eds.), *Gender and stress* (pp. 122-143). New York: Free Press.

Baron, R. M., & Kenney, D. A. (1986). The moderator-mediator variable distinction in social psychological research: Conceptual, strategic, and statistical considerations. *Journal of Personality and Social Psychology, 51,* 1173-1182.

Bateson, G. (1961). The biosocial integration of behavior in the schizophrenic family. In N. W. Ackerman, F. L. Beatman, & S. N. Sherman (Eds.), *Exploring the base for family therapy* (pp. 116-122). New York: Family Service Association.

Bateson, G., & Jackson, D. D. (1964). Some varieties of pathogenic organization. In D. M. Rioch & E. A. Weinstein (Eds.). *Disorders of communication, Vol. XLII: Research Publications* (pp. 270-283). Baltimore: Williams & Wilkins.

Beavers, W. R. (1981). A systems model of family for family therapists. *Journal of Marital and Family Therapy, 7*, 299-308.

Beck, C. J. (1989). *Everyday Zen: Love & work*. San Francisco: HarperCollins.

Bedsworth, J. A., & Molen, M. T. (1982). Psychological stress in spouses of patients with myocardial infarctions. *Heart and Lung, 11*, 450-456.

Belenky, M. F., Clinchy, B. M., Goldberger, N. R., & Turule, J. M. (1986). *Women's ways of knowing: The development of self, voice, and mind*. New York: Basic Books.

Bennett, L. A., & Ames, G. M. (1985). *The American experience with alcohol: Contrasting cultural perspectives*. New York: Plenum.

Benoliel, J. Q. (1987). Health care providers and dying patients: Critical issues in terminal care. *Omega, 18*(4), 341-363.

Bepko, C., & Krestan, J. (1985). *The responsibility trap: A blueprint for treating the alcoholic family*. New York: Free Press.

Berardo, F. M. (1990). Trends and directions in family research in the 1980's. *Journal of Marriage and the Family, 52*(11), 809-817.

Berg, D., & Smith, K. (1988). *The self in social inquiry: Researching methods*. Newbury Park, CA: Sage.

Bergier, J.-F. (1971). *The industrial bourgeoisie and the rise of the working class, 1700-1914*. London: Cambridge University Press.

Berkey, K. M., & Harmon-Hanson, S. M. (1991). *Pocket guide to family assessment and intervention*. St. Louis, MO: C. V. Mosby.

Bernheim, K. (1989). Psychologists and families of the severely mentally ill: The role of family consultation. *American Psychologist, 44*, 562-564.

Billingsley, A. (1968). *Black families in white America*. Englewood Cliffs, NJ: Prentice Hall.

Bleathman, C. (1987). The practical management of the Alzheimer's disease patient in the hospital setting. *Journal of Advanced Nursing, 12*(4), 531-534.

Blood, R. O., & Wolfe, D. M. (1960). *Husbands and wives: The dynamics of married living*. New York: Free Press.

Boatright, C. J. (1985). Children as victims of disaster. In J. Laube & S. A. Murphy (Eds.), *Perspectives on disaster recovery* (pp. 131-149). Norwalk, CT: Appleton-Century-Crofts.

Bolger, N., DeLongis, A., Kessler, R. C., & Wethington, E. (1989). The contagion of stress across multiple roles. *Journal of Marriage and the Family, 51*, 175-183.

Bomar, P. J. (Ed.). (1989). *Nurses and family health promotion: Concepts, assessment, and interventions*. Baltimore, MD: Williams & Wilkins.

Borysenko, J. (1984). Stress, coping and the immune system. In J. D. Matarazzo, S. M. Weiss, J. A. Herd, N. E. Miller, & S. M. Weiss (Eds.), *Behavioral health: A handbook of health enhancement and disease prevention* (pp. 248-260). New York: John Wiley.

Boss, P., Caron, W., Horbal, J., & Mortimer, J. (1990). Predictors of depression in caregivers of dementia patients: Boundary ambiguity and mastery. *Family Process, 29*(3), 245-254.

Boumann, C. C. (1984). Identifying priority concerns of families of ICU patients. *Dimension of Critical Care Nursing, 3,* 313-319.

Bournaki, M. C., & Germain, C. P. (1993). Esthetic knowledge in family-centered nursing care of hospitalized children. *Advances in Nursing Science, 16*(2), 81-89.

Bowen, M. (1976). Theory in the practice of psychotherapy. In P. J. Guerin (Ed.), *Family therapy: Theory and practice* (pp. 42-90). New York: Gardner.

Bowers, B. J. (1988). Family perceptions of care in a nursing home. *The Gerontologist, 28,* 361-368.

Bowker, L. H. (1993). A battered woman's problems are social, not psychological. In R. J. Gelles & D. R. Loseke (Eds.), *Current controversies on family violence* (pp. 154-165). Newbury Park, CA: Sage.

Bowman, P. J. (1993). The impact of economic marginality among African American husbands and fathers. In H. P. McAdoo (Ed.), *Family ethnicity: Strength in diversity* (pp. 120-137). Newbury Park, CA: Sage.

Boyd-Franklin, N. (1989). *Black families in therapy: A multisystems approach.* New York: Guilford.

Bozett, F. W., & Gibbons, R. (1983). The nursing management of families in the critical care setting. *Critical Care Update, 10,* 22-27.

Breitmayer, B. J., Ayres, L., & Knafl, K. A. (1993). Triangulation in qualitative research: Evaluation of completeness and confirmation purposes. *Image, 25*(3), 237-243.

Brenner, M. H. (1987). Economic change, alcohol consumption and heart disease mortality in nine industrialized countries. *Social Science and Medicine, 25*(2), 119-132.

Breunlin, D. C. (1988). Oscillation theory and family development. In C. J. Falicov (Ed.), *Family transitions: Continuity and change over the life cycle* (pp. 133-155). New York: Guilford.

Brody, E. M. (1985). Parent caring as a normative family stress. *The Gerontologist, 25,* 19-25.

Brown, M. A., & Powell-Cope, G. (1993). Themes of loss and dying in caring for a family member with AIDS. *Research in Nursing & Health, 16,* 179-191.

Buckley, W. (1967). *Sociology and modern systems theory.* Englewood Cliffs, NJ: Prentice Hall.

Bullough, V., & Bullough, B. (1981). *Health care for the other Americans.* Norwalk, CT: Appleton-Century-Crofts.

Burns, N., & Grove, S. K. (1993). *The practice of nursing research: Conduct, critique, and utilization* (2nd ed.). Philadelphia: Saunders.

Burr, W. R. (1970). Satisfaction with various aspects of marriage over the life cycle: A random middle class sample. *Journal of Marriage and the Family, 32,* 29-37.

Burr, W. R. (1972). Role transitions: A reformulation of theory. *Journal of Marriage and the Family, 34,* 407-416.

Buss, T., & Redburn, F. S. (1983). *Mass unemployment: Plant closings and mental health* (Sage Studies in Community Mental Health, Vol. 6). Beverly Hills, CA: Sage.

Caine, R. M. (1991). Incorporating CARE into caring for families in crisis. *AACN Clinical Issues, 2*(2), 236-241.

Calam, R., Waller, G., Slade, P., & Newton, T. (1990). Eating disorders and perceived relationships with parents. *International Journal of Eating Disorders, 9,* 479-485.

Campbell, D. T., & Fiske, D. W. (1959). Convergent and discriminant validation by the multitrait multimethod matrix. *Psychological Bulletin, 56*(2), 81-105.

Campbell, R. T., Mutran, E., & Parker, R. N. (1987). Longitudinal design and longitudinal analysis. *Research on Aging, 8*(4), 480-504.

Cantor, M. H. (1979). Neighbors and friends: An overlooked resource in the informal support system. *Research on Aging, 1,* 434-463.

Caper, B. (1978). Fundamental patterns of knowing in nursing. *Advances in Nursing Science, 1*(1), 13-23.

Caplan, G. (1964). *Principles of preventive psychiatry.* New York: Basic Books.

Caplan, G. (1982). *The family as support system.* In H. McCubbin, A. Cauble, & J. Patterson (Eds.), *Family stress, coping, and social support* (pp. 200-220). Springfield, IL: Charles C Thomas.

Carpenito, L. J. (1989). *Handbook of nursing diagnoses* (3rd ed.). Philadelphia: J. B. Lippincott.

Carter, E. A., & McGoldrick, M. (Eds.). (1980). *The family life cycle: A framework for family therapy.* New York: Gardner.

Carter, E. A., & McGoldrick, M. (Eds.). (1988). *The family life cycle: A framework for family therapy* (2nd ed.). New York: Gardner.

Chandler, L. A. (1982). *Children under stress: Understanding emotional adjustment reactions.* Springfield, IL: Charles C Thomas.

Chekryn-Reimer, J., Davies, B., & Martens, N. (1991). Palliative care: The nurse's role in helping families through the transition of "fading away." *Cancer Nursing, 14*(6), 321-327.

Chesla, C., Martinson, I., & Muwaswes, M. (1994). Continuities and discontinuities in family members' relationships with Alzheimer's patients. *Family Relations, 43*(1), 3-9.

Chinn, P. L. (1985). Debunking myths in nursing theory and research. *Image, 17,* 45-49.

Cicirelli, V. G. (1992). *Family caregiving: Autonomous and paternalistic decision making.* Newbury Park, CA: Sage.

Clark, M. D. (1985, January 2). Loss of job status. *Nursing Times,* pp. 53-54.

Clements, I. W., & Roberts, F. B. (1983). *Family health: A theoretical approach to nursing care.* New York: John Wiley.

Cobb, S., & Kasl, S. (1977). *Termination: The consequences of job loss.* Cincinnati, OH: National Institute of Occupational Safety and Health.

Cochran, M., Larner, M., Riley, D., Gunnarsson, L., & Henderson, C. R. (1990). *Extending families: The social networks of parents and their children.* Cambridge, NY: Cambridge University Press.

Cohen, C. I., & Sokolovsky, J. (1989). *Old men of the Bowery: Strategies for survival among the homeless.* New York: Guilford.

Cohen, F. (1984). Coping. In J. D. Matarazzo, S. M. Weiss, J. A. Herd, N. E. Miller, & S. M. Weiss (Eds.), *Behavioral health: A handbook of health enhancement and disease prevention* (pp. 217-254). New York: John Wiley.

Cohn, M. O., & Jay, G. M. (1988). Families in long-term-care settings. In M. A. Smyer, M. D. Cohn, & D. Brannon (Eds.), *Mental health consultation in nursing homes* (pp. 142-191). New York: New York University Press.

Collins, C., Given, B., & Berry, D. (1989). Longitudinal studies as intervention. *Nursing Research, 38*(4), 251-253.

Constantine, L. L. (1986). *Family paradigms: The practice and theory in family therapy.* New York: Guilford.

Conway, K. (1985). Coping with the stress of medical problems among black and white elderly. *International Journal of Aging and Human Development, 21*(1), 39-47.

Cook, J. A. (1988). Who mothers the chronically mentally ill? *Family Relations, 37,* 42-49.

Cook, T. D., & Campbell, D. T. (1979). *Quasi-experimentation: Design and analysis issues for field settings.* Boston: Houghton Mifflin.

Corner, J. (1991). In search of more complete answers to research questions. Quantitative versus qualitative research methods: Is there a way forward? *Journal of Advanced Nursing, 16,* 718-727.

Couch, A. (1970). The psychological determinants of interpersonal behavior. In K. Gergen & D. Marlowe (Eds.), *Personality and social behavior* (pp. 77-89). Reading, MA: Addison-Wesley.

Coward, D. D. (1990). Critical multiplism: A research strategy for nursing science. *Image, 22*(3), 163-167.

Cox Dzurec, L. (1994). Schizophrenic clients' experiences of power: Using hermeneutic analysis. *Image, 26*(2), 155-159.

Cromwell, R. L., Butterfield, E. C., Brayfield, F. M., & Curry, J. J. (1977). *Acute myocardial infarction: Reaction and recovery.* St. Louis, MO: C. V. Mosby.

Cromwell, V. L., & Cromwell, R. E. (1978). Perceived dominance in decision making and conflict resolution among Anglo, black, and Chicano couples. *Journal of Marriage and the Family, 40,* 749-759.

Cronbach, L. J. (1975). Beyond the two disciplines of scientific psychology. *American Psychological Journal, 30,* 123-134.

Crotty, P., & Kulys, R. (1986). Are schizophrenics a burden to their families? Significant others' views. *Health and Social Work, 3,* 173-188.

Crouter, A. C., & Manke, B. (1994). The changing American workplace: Implications for individuals and families. *Family Relations, 43*(2), 117-124.

Crouter, A. C., & McHale, S. M. (1993). The long arm of the job: Influence of parental work on childrearing. In T. Luster & L. Okagaki (Eds.), *Parenting: An ecological perspective* (pp. 179-202). Hillsdale, NJ: Lawrence Erlbaum.

Curran, D. (1985). *Stress and the healthy family.* Minneapolis, MN: Winston.

Dainton, M. (1993). The myths and misconceptions of the stepmother identity: Descriptions and prescriptions for identity management. *Family Relations, 42*(1), 93-98.

Daniels, M., & Irwin, M. (1989). Caregiver stress and well-being. In E. Light & B. D. Lebowitz (Eds.), *Alzheimer's disease and family stress: Direction for research* (pp. 292-309). Rockville, MD: U.S. Department of Health and Human Services, Alcohol, Drug Abuse, and Mental Health Administration, National Institutes of Health.

Davies, B., Chekryn-Reimer, J., & Martens, N. (1990). Families in supportive care. Part 1: The transition of fading away: The nature of the transition. *Journal of Palliative Care, 6,* 12-20.

De Chesney, M. (1986). Promoting healthy family functioning in acute care units. *Journal of Pediatric Nursing 1*(2), 96-101.

Delgado, M. (1987). Puerto Ricans. In A. Minahan (Ed.), *Encyclopedia of social work* (Vol. 2, pp. 427-432). Silver Springs, MD: National Association of Social Workers.

DeMarco, R. (1994). *Within and between method triangulation: Developing a summative rating scale using qualitative and quantitative paradigms* (Predoctoral field study). Detroit: Wayne State University.

Demo, D. H. (1993). The relentless search for effects of divorce: Forging new trails or tumbling down the beaten path? *Journal of Marriage and the Family, 55*(1), 42-45.

Denzin, N. K. (1989). *The research act: A theoretical introduction to sociological methods* (3rd ed.). New York: McGraw-Hill.

Devore, W., & Schlesinger, E. G. (1987). *Ethnic sensitive social work practice* (2nd ed.). Columbus, OH: Merrill.

Dew, M. A., Bromet, E. J., & Schulberg, H. C. (1987). A comparative analysis of two community stressors' long-term mental health effects. *American Journal of Community Psychology, 15,* 167-184.

Dew, M. A., Penkower, L., & Bromet, E. J. (1991). Effects of unemployment on mental health in the contemporary family. *Behavior Modification, 15*(4), 501-544.

Diekelmann, N., Allen, D., & Tanner, C. (1989). *The NLN criteria for appraisal of baccalaureate programs: A critical hermeneutic analysis* (Pub. No. 15-2253). New York: The National League for Nursing Press.

Doherty, W. J. (1985). Family interventions in health care. *Family Relations, 34,* 129-137.

Dohrenwend, B. S. (1973). Social status and stressful life events. *Journal of Personality and Social Psychology, 28,* 225-235.

Dooley, I. D., & Catalano, R. (1980). Economic change as a cause of behavioral disorder. *Psychological Bulletin, 87,* 450-468.

Dornbush, S., Carlsmith, J. M., Bushwall, S. J., Ritter, P. L., Leiderman, H., Hastorf, A. H., & Gross, R. T. (1985). Single parents, extended households, and the control of adolescents. *Child Development, 56,* 326-341.

Douglas, A. (1977). *The feminization of American culture.* New York: Avon.

Draper, T. W., & Marcos, A. C. (Eds.). (1990). *Family variables: Conceptualization, measurement, and use.* Newbury Park, CA: Sage.

Duffy, M. E. (1987). Methodological triangulation: A vehicle for merging quantitative and qualitative research methods. *Image, 19*(3), 130-133.

Dunst, C. J., Trivette, C. M., & Deal, A. G. (1988). *Enabling and empowering families: Principles and guidelines for practice.* Cambridge, MA: Brookline.

Duvall, E. M. (1977). *Marriage and family development* (5th ed.). Philadelphia: J. B. Lippincott.

Duxbury, L., Lee, C., Higgins, C. A., & Mills, S. (1992). Time spent in paid employment. *Optimum, 23,* 38-45.

Dzurec, L. C., & Abraham, I. L. (1993). The nature of inquiry: Linking quantitative and qualitative research. *Advances in Nursing Science, 16*(1), 73-79.

Eisenberg, L. (1977). Disease and illness: Distinctions between professional and popular ideas of sickness. *Culture, Medicine and Psychiatry, 1,* 9-23.

Elder, G. H. (1974). *Children of the Great Depression: Social change in life experience.* Chicago: University of Chicago Press.

Elder, G. H., Conger, R. D., Foster, E. M., & Ardelt, M. (1992). Families under economic pressure. *Journal of Family Issues, 13*(1), 5-37.

Engel, G. L. (1980). The clinical application of the biopsychosocial model. *American Journal of Psychiatry, 137,* 535-544.

Engel, G. L. (1982). The biopsychosocial model and medical education: Who are to be the teachers? *New England Journal of Medicine, 306,* 802-805.

Erickson, R. J. (1993). Reconceptualizing family work: The effect of emotion work on perceptions of marital quality. *Journal of Marriage and the Family, 55*(4), 888-900.

Erikson, E. H. (1950). *Childhood and society.* New York: Norton.

Erikson, E. H. (1968). *Identity, youth and crisis.* New York: Norton.

Etzioni, A. (1974). Marriage and maternity as endangered species seen in perspective. *Human Behavior, 3,* 10-11.

Fawcett, J. (1975). The family as a living open system: An emerging conceptual framework for nursing. *International Nursing Review, 22,* 113-116.

Feetham, S. L., Meister, S. B., Bell, J. M., & Gilliss, C. L. (Eds.). (1993). *The nursing of families: Theory/research/education/practice.* Newbury Park, CA: Sage.

Feldman, H. (1971). The effects of children on the family. In A. Michel (Ed.), *Family issues of employed women in Europe and America* (pp. 107-125). Leiden, the Netherlands: E. J. Brill.

Ferree, M. M. (1988, November). *Negotiating household roles and responsibilities: Resistance, conflict, and change.* Paper presented at the annual meeting of the National Council on Family Relations, Philadelphia.

Ferree, M. M. (1990). Beyond separate spheres: Feminism and family research. *Journal of Marriage and the Family, 52,* 866-884.

Fielding, N., & Fielding, J. (1986). *Linking data.* Beverly Hills, CA: Sage.

Fiese, B. H. (1993). Family rituals in alcoholic and nonalcoholic households: Relations to adolescent health symptomatology and problem drinking. *Family Relations, 42*(2), 187-192.

Fisher, L., Ransom, D. C., Terry, H. E., Lipkin, M., & Weiss, R. (1992). The California Family Health Project: Introduction and a description of adult health. *Family Process, 31*(3), 231-250.

Flanzer, J. P. (1993). Alcohol and other drugs are key causal agents of violence. In R. J. Gelles & D. R. Loseke (Eds.), *Current controversies on family violence* (pp. 171-181). Newbury Park, CA: Sage.

Florin, I., Nostadt, A., Reck, C., Franzen, U., & Jenkins, M. (1992). Expressed emotion in depressed patients and their partners. *Family Process, 31*(2), 163-171.

Floyd, J. (1993). The use of across-method triangulation in the study of sleep concerns in healthy older adults. *Advances in Nursing Science, 16*(2), 70-80.

Friedemann, M. L. (1986). Family economic stress and unemployment: Child's peer behavior and parent's depression. *Child Study Journal, 16*(2), 125-141.

Friedemann, M. L. (1987). Families of the unemployed worker: Need for nursing intervention and prevention. *Archives of Psychiatric Nursing, 1*(2), 81-87.

Friedemann, M. L. (1989a). Closing the gap between grand theory and mental health practice with families. Part 1: The framework of systemic organization for nursing of families and family members. *Archives of Psychiatric Nursing, 3*(1), 10-19.

Friedemann, M. L. (1989b). Closing the gap between grand theory and mental health practice with families. Part 2: The Control-Congruence Model for mental health nursing of families. *Archives of Psychiatric Nursing, 3*(1), 20-28.

Friedemann, M. L. (1991a). An instrument to evaluate effectiveness in family functioning. *Western Journal of Nursing Research, 13*(2), 220-236.

Friedemann, M. L. (1991b). Closing the gap between grand-theory and mental health practice. The framework of systemic organization and the Control-Congruence Model for mental health nursing of families. In J. Fawcett & A. Whall (Eds.), *Family theory development in nursing: State of the science and art* (pp. 317-342). Philadelphia: F. A. Davis.

Friedemann, M. L. (1992). *Enhancing families with the Congruence Model: A counseling/education model.* Detroit: Wayne State University, College of Nursing.

Friedemann, M. L. (1994). Evaluation of the Congruence Model with rehabilitating substance abusers. *International Journal of Nursing Studies, 31*(1), 97-108.

Friedemann, M. L., & Andrews, M. (1990). Family support and child adjustment in single-parent families. *Issues in Comprehensive Pediatric Nursing, 13*(4), 289-301.

Friedemann, M. L., & Musgrove, J. (1994). Perceptions of inner-city substance abusers about their families. *Archives of Psychiatric Nursing, 8*(2), 115-123.

Friedemann, M. L., & Webb, A. A. (1995). Family health and mental health six years after economic stress and unemployment. *Issues in Mental Health Nursing, 16,* 51-66.

Friedemann, M. L., & Youngblood, M. (1992). Applying the Congruence Model to an alcoholic family in a multiproblem context [Case study]. *Families in Societies, 73*(7), 432-438.

Friedman, M. M. (1992). *Family nursing: Theory and practice* (3rd ed.). Norwalk, CT: Appleton & Lange.

Fritz, B., & Williams, J. (1988). Issues of adolescent development for survivors of childhood cancer. *Journal of the American Academy of Child and Adolescent Psychiatry, 27,* 712-715.

Fullinwider-Bush, N., & Jacobvitz, D. B. (1993). The transition to young adulthood: Generational boundary dissolution and female identity development. *Family Process, 32*(1), 87-103.

Furstenberg, F. F., Jr. (1990). Coming of age in a changing family system. In S. Feldman & G. Elliott (Eds.), *At the threshold: The developing adolescent* (pp. 147-170). Cambridge, MA: Harvard University Press.

Gacic, B. (1986). An ecosystemic approach to alcoholism: Theory and practice. *Contemporary Family Therapy, 8*(4), 264-278.

Gelfand, D. Z., & Fandetti, D. V. (1980). Suburban and urban white ethnics: Attitudes toward care of the aged. *The Gerontologist, 20,* 588-595.

Gelles, R. J., & Loseke, D. R. (Eds.). (1993). *Current controversies on family violence.* Newbury Park, CA: Sage.

Gentry, W., Shows, W., & Thomas, M. (1974). Chronic low back pain: A psychological profile. *Psychosomatics, 15,* 174-177.

Gershwin, M. W., & Nilsen, J. M. (1989). Healthy families: Forms and processes. In C. L. Gilliss, B. L. Highley, B. M. Roberts, & I. M. Martinson (Eds.), *Toward a science of family nursing* (pp. 77-91). Reading, MA: Addison-Wesley.

Gerson, J. M., & Peiss, K. (1985). Boundaries, negotiation, consciousness: Reconceptualizing gender relations. *Social Problems, 32,* 317-331.

Gil, D. G. (1970). *Violence against children: Physical abuse in the United States.* Cambridge, MA: Harvard University Press.

Gillian, D. (1990, June 7). On slang, prosecution's guilty. *Washington Post,* p. D3.

Gilligan, C. (1987). Adolescent development reconsidered. In C. E. Irwin, Jr. (Ed.), *New directions for child development: Adolescent social behavior and health* (Vol. 37). San Francisco: Jossey-Bass.

Gilliss, C. L., Highley, B. L., Roberts, B. M., & Martinson, I. M. (1989). (Eds.). *Toward a science in family nursing.* Reading, MA: Addison-Wesley.

Giordano, J., & Giordano, G. (1977). *The ethno-cultural factor in mental health.* New York: Institute on Pluralism and Group Identity of the American Jewish Community.

Glaser, B. G., & Strauss, A. L. (1965). *Awareness of dying.* Hawthorne, NY: Aldine.

Glazier, N., & Moynihan, D. P. (1975). *Beyond the melting pot* (3rd ed.). Cambridge: MIT Press.

Glenn, N. (1975). The contribution of marriage to the psychological well-being of males and females. *Journal of Marriage and the Family, 37,* 594-599.

Glick, P. C. (1947). The family cycle. *American Sociological Review, 12,* 164-174.

Glick, P. C. (1983). Prospective changes in marriage, divorce, and living arrangement. *Journal of Family Issues, 33*(5), 7-26.

Glick, P. C. (1988). Fifty years of family demography: A record of social change. *Journal of Marriage and the Family, 50*(4), 861-873.

Glick, P. C. (1989). Remarried families, stepfamilies and stepchildren: A brief demographic profile. *Family Relations, 38,* 24-27.

Golan, N. (1981). *Passing through transitions.* New York: Free Press.

Goldscheider, F., & Da Vanzo, J. (1989). Pathways to independent living in early adulthood: Marriage, semiautonomy, and premarital residential independence. *Demography, 26,* 597-614.

Gorenberg, B. (1983). The research tradition of nursing: An emerging issue. *Nursing Research, 32*(6), 347-349.

Grafstrom, M., Norberg, A., & Hagberg, B. (1993). Relationships between demented elderly people and their families: A follow-up study of caregivers who had previously reported abuse when caring for their spouses and parents. *Journal of Advanced Nursing, 18,* 1747-1757.

Grayson, J. P. (1985). The closure of a factory and its impact on health. *International Journal of Health Sciences, 15,* 69-93.

Green, R. J. (1990). Family communication and children's learning disabilities: Evidence for Coles' theory of interactivity. *Journal of Learning Disabilities, 23,* 145-148.

Greenberg, D., Kazak, A., & Meadows, A. (1989). Psychologic functioning in 8- to 16-year-old cancer survivors and their parents. *Journal of Pediatrics, 114,* 488-493.

Greenhaus, J., & Beutell, N. (1985). Sources of conflict between work and family roles. *Academy of Management Review, 10,* 76-88.

Griffith, J. L., Griffith, M. E., & Slovik, L. S. (1989). Mind-body patterns of symptom generation. *Family Process, 28,* 137-152.

Grynch, J. H., & Fincham, F. D. (1990). Marital conflict and children's adjustment: A cognitive-contextual framework. *Psychological Bulletin, 108,* 267-290.

Gutek, B., Searle, S., & Kelpa, I. (1991). Rational versus gender role explanations for work family conflict. *Journal of Applied Psychology, 76,* 560-568.

Haase, J. E., & Myers, S. T. (1988). Reconciling paradigm assumptions of qualitative and quantitative research. *Western Journal of Nursing Research, 10*(2), 128-137.

Hackett, T. P., & Cassem, N. T. (1982). Coping with cardiac disease. *Advanced Cardiology, 31,* 212-217.

Hahlweg, K., Goldstein, M. J., Nuechterlein, K. H., Magana, A., Mintz, J., Doane, J. A., Miklowitz, D. J., & Snyder, K. S. (1989). Expressed emotion and patient-relative interaction in families of recent onset schizophrenics. *Journal of Consulting and Clinical Psychology, 57,* 11-18.

Haley, J. (1959). The family of the schizophrenic: A model system. *Journal of Nervous and Mental Diseases, 129,* 357-374.

Haley, J. (1976). *Problem-solving therapy.* San Francisco: Jossey-Bass.

Hall, G. R. (1988). Care of the patient with Alzheimer's disease living at home. *Nursing Clinics of North America, 23*(1), 31-46.

Hanson, S. M. (1987). Family nursing and chronic illness. In L. M. Wright & M. Leahy (Eds.), *Families and chronic illness* (pp. 3-32). Springhouse, PA: Springhouse Corp.

Hardgrove, C., & Roberts, B. M. (1989). The family with a hospitalized child. In C. L. Gilliss, B. L. Highley, B. M. Roberts, & I. M. Martinson (Eds.), *Toward a science of family nursing* (pp. 248-261). Reading, MA: Addison-Wesley.

Hareven, T. K. (1987). American families in transition: Historical perspectives on change. In F. Walsh (Ed.), *Normal family processes* (pp. 446-465). New York: Guilford.

Hartley, J. (1987). Managerial unemployment: The wive's perspective role. In S. Fineman (Ed.), *Unemployment: Personal and social consequences*. Philadelphia: Open University Press.

Hartog, J., & Hartog, E. (1983). Cultural aspects of health and illness behavior in hospitals. *Western Journal of Medicine, 139,* 910-916.

Hatch, L. R. (1991). Informal support patterns of older African-American and white women. *Research on Aging, 13*(2), 144-170.

Hatfield, A. B. (1978). Psychological costs of schizophrenia to the family. *Social Work, 23,* 355-359.

Hatfield, A. B. (1990). *Family education in mental illness.* New York: Guilford.

Hayghe, H. (1986). Rise in mothers' labor force activity includes those with infants. *Monthly Labor Review, 109,* 43-45.

Healy, J. M., Malley, J. E., & Stewart, A. J. (1990). Children and their fathers after parental separation. *American Journal of Orthopsychiatry, 60,* 531-543.

Hepworth, S. J. (1980). Moderating factors of the psychological impact of unemployment. *Journal of Occupational Psychology, 53,* 139-145.

Herndon, A. (1982, August). Do we know enough about the predominant family form of the 21st century? *Wake Forest,* pp. 36-37.

Heron, J. M., & Leheup, R. (1984). Happy families? *British Journal of Psychiatry, 145,* 136-138.

Hetherington, E. M., Cox, M., & Cox, R. (1981). The aftermath of divorce. In E. M. Hetherington & R. D. Parke (Eds.), *Contemporary readings in child psychology* (2nd ed., pp. 99-109). New York: McGraw-Hill.

Hetherington, E. M., Cox, M., & Cox, R. (1982). Effects of divorce on parents and children. In M. Lamb (Ed.), *Nontraditional families: Parenting and child development* (pp. 233-288). Hillsdale, NJ: Lawrence Erlbaum.

Hinds, P. S. (1989). Method triangulation to index change in clinical phenomena. *Western Journal of Nursing Research, 11*(4), 440-447.

Hirschfeld, M. (1983). Homecare versus institutionalization: Family caregiving and senile brain disease. *International Journal of Nursing Studies, 20,* 23-32.

Hobbs, D. (1968). Transition to parenthood: A replication and extension. *Journal of Marriage and the Family, 30,* 413-417.

Hobbs, N., Dokecki, P., Hoover-Dempsey, K., Moroney, R., Shayne, M., & Weeks, K. (1984). *Strengthening families.* San Francisco: Jossey-Bass.

Hobbs, P. R., Ballinger, C. B., McClure, A., Martin, B., & Greenwood, C. (1985). Factors associated with psychiatric morbidity in men—a general practice survey. *Acta Psychiatrica Scandinavica, 71,* 281-286.

Hochschild, A. (1989). *The second shift.* New York: Viking.

Hodovanic, B. H., Reardon, D., Reese, W., & Wedges, B. (1984). Family crisis intervention program in the medical intensive care unit. *Heart and Lung, 13,* 243-249.

Hoffman, I. W. (1988). Foreword. In A. E. Gottfried & A. W. Gottfried (Eds.), *Maternal employment and children's development—longitudinal research* (pp. ix-xii). New York: Plenum.

Hofland, B. F. (1988). Autonomy in long term care: Background issues and a programmatic response. *The Gerontologist, 28*(Suppl.), 3-9.

Hood, J. C. (1983). *Becoming a two-job family.* New York: Praeger.

Horwitz, A., Tessler, R., Fisher, G., & Gamache, G. (1992). The role of adult siblings in providing social support to the severely mentally ill. *Journal of Marriage and the Family, 54,* 233-241.

Hough, E. E., Lewis, F. M., & Woods, N. F. (1991). Family response to mother's chronic illness: Case studies of well- and poorly adjusted families. *Western Journal of Nursing Research, 13*(5), 568-596.

Howard, A., & Bray, D. W. (1988). *Managerial lives in transition: Advancing age and changing times.* New York: Guilford.

Howard, P. B. (1994). Lifelong maternal caregiving for children with schizophrenia. *Archives of Psychiatric Nursing, 8*(2), 107-114.

Howze, D. C., & Kotch, J. B. (1984). Disentangling life events, stress and social support: Implications for the primary prevention of child abuse and neglect. *Child Abuse & Neglect, 8,* 401-409.

Hugentobler, M. K., Israel, B. A., & Schurman, S. J. (1992). An action research approach to workplace health: Integrating methods. *Health Education Quarterly, 19*(1), 55-76.

Hull, M. M. (1989). Family needs and supportive nursing behaviors during terminal cancer: A review. *Oncology Nursing Forum, 16,* 787-792.

Hull, M. M. (1991). Hospice nurses: Caring support for caregiving families. *Cancer Nursing, 14*(2), 63-70.

Humphrey, L. L. (1986). Family dynamics in bulimia. In S. C. Feinstein, A. H. Esman, J. G. Looney, A. Z. Schwartzberg, A. D. Sorosky, & M. Sugar (Eds.), *Annals of adolescent psychiatry: Vol. 13. Developmental and clinical studies* (pp. 315-332). Chicago: University of Chicago Press.

Imber-Black, E. (1988). *Families and larger systems.* New York: Guilford.

Ironson, G. (1992). Work, job stress, and health. In S. Zedeck (Ed.), *Work, families and organizations* (pp. 33-69). San Francisco, CA: Jossey-Bass.

Jackson, D. D. (1957). The question of family homeostasis. *Psychiatric Quarterly, 31*(Suppl. 1), 79-90.

Jackson, P. R., & Warr, P. B. (1984). Unemployment and psychological ill-health: The moderating role of duration and age. *Psychological Medicine, 14,* 605-614.

Jacobson, G. F. (1974). Programs and techniques of crisis intervention. In S. Arieti (Ed.), *American handbook of psychiatry* (Vol. 2, pp. 810-823). New York: Basic Books.

Jahoda, M. (1988). Economic recession and mental health: Some conceptual issues. *Journal of Social Issues, 44*(4), 13-23.

Jahoda, M., Lazarsfeld, P. F., & Zeisel, H. (1971). *Marienthal: The sociography of an unemployed community.* Hawthorne, NY: Aldine.

Jicks, T. D. (1979). Mixing qualitative and quantitative methods: Triangulation in action. *Administration Science Quarterly, 24,* 602-611.

Joelson, L., & Wahlquist, L. (1987). The psychological meaning of job insecurity and job loss: Results of a longitudinal study. *Social Science Medicine, 25*(2), 179-182.

Johnson, H. C. (1987). Biologically based deficit in the identified patient: Indications for psychoeducational strategies. *Journal of Marital and Family Therapy, 13,* 337-348.

Johnson-Saylor, M. T. (1984). *Unemployment and health: Issues in a primary care practice.* Cambridge, MA: Blackwell Scientific Publishing.

Jones, L. (1990). Unemployment and child abuse. *Families in Society: Journal of Contemporary Human Services, 71*(10), 578-586.

Jones, L. (1991). Unemployed fathers and their children: Implications for policy and practice. *Child and Adolescent Social Work, 8*(2), 101-125.

Jones, P. S., & Martinson, I. M. (1992). The experience of bereavement in caregivers of family members with Alzheimer's disease. *Image, 24*(3), 172-175.

Joselevich, E. (1988). Family transitions, cumulative stress, and crises. In C. J. Falicov (Ed.), *Family transitions: Continuity and change over the life cycle* (pp. 273-291). New York: Guilford.

Josselson, R. (1987). *Finding herself: Pathways to identity development in women.* San Francisco: Jossey-Bass.

Jung, C. G. (1953). *Collected works.* New York: Pantheon.

Kandel, D., & Davies, M. (1986). Adult sequelae of adolescent depressive symptoms. *Archives of General Psychiatry, 43,* 255-262.

Kantor, D., & Lehr, W. (1975). *Inside the family.* San Francisco: Jossey-Bass.

Kantrowitz, B., & Wingert, P. (1990, Winter/Spring). Step by step. *Newsweek—Special Issue,* pp. 24-37.

Kaplan, S., & Kaplan, R. (1981). *Cognition and environment.* Ann Arbor, MI: Ulrich.

Karasek, R. (1979). Job demands, job decision latitude and mental strain: Implications for job redesign. *Administrative Science Quarterly, 24,* 285-307.

Kasl, S., & Cobb, S. (1967). Effects of parental status + incongruence and discrepancy on physical and mental health of adult offspring. *Journal of Personality and Social Psychology Monograph, 7*(2, Pt. 2), 1-15.

Kaufman, J., & Zigler, E. (1987). Do abused children become abusive parents? *American Journal of Orthopsychiatry, 57,* 186-192.

Kelly, R. F., & Voydanoff, P. (1985). Work/family role strain among employed parents. *Family Relations, 34*(3), 367-374.

Kelvin, P., & Jarret, J. E. (1985). *Unemployment: Its social psychological effects.* Cambridge, UK: Cambridge University Press.

Kent, J. S., & Clopton, J. R. (1992). Bulimic women's perception of their family relationships. *Journal of Clinical Psychology, 48,* 281-292.

Kessler, R. C., McLeod, J. D., & Wethington, E. (1985). The costs of caring: A perspective on the relationship between sex and psychological distress. In I. G. Sarason & B. R. Sarason (Eds.), *Social support: Theory, research, and application.* The Hague, the Netherlands: Marinus Nijhof.

Kessler, R. C., Turner, J. B., & House, J. S. (1987). Intervening processes in the relationship between unemployment and health. *Psychological Medicine, 17,* 949-961.

Kibria, N., Barnett, R. C., Baruch, G. K., Marshall, N. L., & Pleck, J. H. (1990). Homemaking-role quality and the psychological well-being and distress of employed women. *Sex Roles, 22,* 327-347.

Kidd, P., & Morrison, E. F. (1988). The progression of knowledge in nursing: A search for meaning. *Image, 20*(4), 222-224.

Kidwell, J., Fischer, J. L., Dunham, R. M., & Baranowski, M. (1983). Parents and adolescents: Push and pull of change. In H. I. McCubbin & C. R. Figley (Eds.), *Stress and the family. Vol. 1: Coping with normative transitions* (pp. 74-89). New York: Brunner/Mazel.

Kikumura, A., & Kitano, H. (1973). Interracial marriage: A picture of the Japanese Americans. *Journal of Social Issues, 29,* 67-81.

Killian, K. D. (1994). Fearing fat: A literature review of family systems understandings and treatments of anorexia and bulimia. *Family Relations, 43*(3), 311-318.

Kimchi, J., Polivka, B., & Stevenson, J. S. (1991). Triangulation: Operational definitions. *Nursing Research, 40*(6), 364-366.

King, I. M. (1981). *A theory for nursing: Systems, concepts and process.* New York: John Wiley.

Kirby, H. D., & Luker, K. A. (1986). The experience of unemployment and its effects on family life. *Health Visitor, 59*, 312-314.

Kiresuk, T., & Sherman, R. (1975). Process and outcome measurement using goal attainment scaling. In J. Zusman & C. R. Wurster (Eds.), *Program evaluation: Alcohol, drug abuse, and mental health services* (pp. 213-228). Lexington, MA: D. C. Health and Company.

Knafl, K. A., Pettengill, M. M., Bevis, M. E., & Kirchhoff, K. T. (1988, January/February). Blending qualitative and quantitative approaches to instrument development and data collection. *Journal of Professional Nursing,* pp. 30-37.

Knoll, J. (1994). Key concepts in family support policy. *Inclusive Communities (Developmental Disability Institute, Wayne State University), 2*(2), 4-5, 8.

Kog, E., & Vandereycken, W. (1985). Family characteristics of anorexia and bulimia: A review of the research literature. *Clinical Psychology Review, 5*, 159-180.

Kog, E., & Vandereycken, W. (1989). Family interaction in eating disorder patients and normal controls. *International Journal of Eating Disorders, 8*, 11-23.

Komarovsky, M. (1940). *The unemployed man and his family.* New York: Dryden.

Kotarba, J. (1983). The social control function of holistic health in bureaucratic settings: The case of space medicine. *Journal of Health and Social Behavior, 24*, 275-288.

Krahn, G. L. (1993). Conceptualizing social support in families of children with special health needs. *Family Process, 32*(2), 235-248.

Krause, N. (1988). Gender and ethnicity differences in psychological well-being. *Annual Review of Gerontology and Geriatrics, 8*, 156-188.

Kreps, G. A. (1978). The organization of disaster response: Some fundamental theoretical issues. In E. L. Quarantelli (Ed.), *Disasters: Theory and research* (pp. 65-85). Beverly Hills, CA: Sage.

Kübler-Ross, E. (1969). *On death and dying.* New York: Macmillan.

Kuhlman, G. J., Wilson, H. S., Hutchinson, S. A., & Wallhagen, M. (1991). Alzheimer's disease and family caregiving: Critical synthesis of the literature and research agenda. *Nursing Research, 40*(6), 331-337.

Kuhnert, K., Sims, R. R., & Lahey, M. A. (1989). The relationship between job security and employee health. *Group and Organization Studies, 14*, 399-410.

Kumabe, K. T., Nishida, C., & Hepworth, D. H. (1985). *Bridging ethnocultural diversity in social work and health.* Honolulu: University of Hawaii, School of Social Work.

Kupferschmid, B. J., Briones, T. L., Dawson, C., & Drongowski, C. (1991). Families: A link of a liability? *AACN Clinical Issues, 2*(2), 252-257.

Kurdek, L. A. (1993). Issues in proposing a general model of the effects of divorce on children. *Journal of Marriage and the Family, 55*(1), 39-41.

Lang, A. R. (1981, October). *Drinking and disinhibition: Contributions from psychological research.* Paper presented at the Social Research Group of the University of California at Berkeley School of Public Health and the National Institute of Alcohol Abuse and Alcoholism, Berkeley, CA.

Larson, J. H. (1984). The effect of husband's unemployment on marital and family relations in blue collar families. *Family Relations, 33*, 503-511.

Larson, J. H., Wilson, S. M., & Beley, R. A. (1988, November). *Job insecurity at a university: Its impact upon the marital and family relations of married faculty and staff members.* Paper presented at the annual meeting of the National Council on Family Relations, Atlanta, GA.

Lawler, E. E. (1990). Achieving competitiveness by creating new organization cultures and structures. In D. B. Fishman & C. Cherniss (Eds.), *The human side of corporate competitiveness* (pp. 69-101). Newbury Park, CA: Sage.

Lawton, M. P., Brody, E. M., & Saperstein, A. R. (1989). A controlled study of respite service for caregivers of Alzheimer's patients. *The Gerontologist, 29*(1), 8-16.

Lazarus, R. S., & Alfert, E. (1964). Short-circuiting of threat by experimentally altering cognitive appraisal. *Journal of Abnormal and Social Psychology, 69,* 195-205.

Lazarus, R. S., & Folkman, S. (1984a). *Stress appraisal and coping.* New York: Springer.

Lazarus, R. S., & Folkman, S. (1984b). The coping process: An alternative to traditional formulations. In R. S. Lazarus & S. Folkman (Eds.), *Stress appraisal and coping* (pp. 141-180). New York: Springer.

Lazear, L. D. (1991). *Seven ways of teaching: The artistry of teaching with multiple intelligences.* Chicago: Skylight.

Lefley, H. P. (1987). Aging parents as caregivers of mentally ill adult children: An emerging social problem. *Hospital and Community Psychiatry, 38,* 1063-1070.

Lego, S. (1994). AIDS-related anxiety and coping methods in a support group for caregivers. *Archives of Psychiatric Nursing, 8*(3), 200-207.

Leininger, M. (1985). Nature, rationale, and the importance of qualitative research methods in nursing. In M. Leininger (Ed.), *Qualitative research methods in nursing* (pp. 1-25). Philadelphia: Saunders.

Leininger, M. (1992). Current issues, problems, and trends to advance qualitative paradigmatic research methods for the future. *Qualitative Health Research, 2*(4), 392-415.

Levine, S. (1989). *A gradual awakening.* Garden City, NY: Doubleday.

Lewis, F. M., & Bloom, J. R. (1979). Psychosocial adjustment to breast cancer: A review of selected literature. *International Journal of Psychiatric Medicine, 9*(1), 1-17.

Lewis, J. M., Beavers, W. R., Gossett, J. T., & Phillips, V. A. (Eds.). (1976). *No single thread: Psychological health in family systems.* New York: Brunner/Mazel.

Lewis, O. (1965). *La vida.* New York: Random House.

Liem, G. R., & Liem, J. H. (1988). The psychological effects of unemployment on workers and their families. *Journal of Social Issues, 44*(4), 87-106.

Liem, J. H., & Liem, G. R. (1990). Understanding the individual and family effects of unemployment. In J. Eckenrode & S. Gore (Eds.), *Stress between work and family* (pp. 175-204). New York: Plenum.

Liepman, M. R., Silva, L. V., & Nirenberg, T. D. (1989). The use of family behavior loop mapping for substance abuse. *Family Relations, 38*(3), 282-287.

Lillard, J., & Marietta, L. (1989). Palliative care nursing: Promoting family integrity. In C. L. Gilliss, B. L. Highley, B. M. Roberts, & I. M. Martinson (Eds.), *Toward a science of family nursing.* Reading, MA: Addison-Wesley.

Lillie-Blanton, M., Anthony, J. C., & Schuster, C. R. (1993). Probing the meaning of racial/ethnic group comparisons in crack cocaine smoking. *Jama, 269*(8), 993-997.

Lin, C., & Liu, W. T. (1993). Intergenerational relationships among Chinese immigrant families from Taiwan. In H. P. McAdoo (Ed.), *Family ethnicity: Strength in diversity* (pp. 271-286). Newbury Park, CA: Sage.

Lindemann, E. (1944). Symptomatology and management of acute grief. *American Journal of Psychiatry, 101,* 141-148.

Locke, L. A. (1969). What is job satisfaction? *Organizational Behaviour and Human Performance, 4,* 3-23.

Lowenberg, J. S. (1993). Interpretive research methodology: Broadening the dialogue. *Advances in Nursing Science, 16*(2), 57-69.

Lynn-McHale, D. J., & Bellinger, A. (1988). Need satisfaction levels of family members of critical care patients and accuracy of nurses' perceptions. *Heart and Lung, 17,* 447-453.

Lynn-McHale, D. J., & Smith, A. (1991). Comprehensive assessment of families of the critically ill. *AACN Clinical Issues, 2*(2), 195-209.

MacEwen, K. E., & Barling, J. (1991). Effects of maternal employment experiences on children's behavior via mood, cognitive difficulties, and parenting behavior. *Journal of Marriage and the Family, 53*(3), 635-644.

Malone, J. A. (1990). Schizophrenia research update: Implications for nursing. *Journal of Psychosocial Nursing and Mental Health Services, 28*(8), 4-9.

Malveaux, J. (1989). The economic statuses of black families. In H. P. McAdoo (Ed.), *Black families* (2nd ed.). Newbury Park, CA: Sage.

Margolis, L. H., & Farran, D. C. (1984). Unemployment and children. *International Journal of Mental Health, 13,* 107-124.

Marks, S. (1977). Multiple roles and role strain: Some notes on human energy, time, and commitment. *American Sociological Review, 42,* 921-936.

Marlatt, G. A., & Gordon, J. R. (Eds.). (1985). *Relapse prevention.* New York: Guilford.

Marlatt, G. A., & Rohsenow, D. J. (1980). Cognitive processes in alcohol use: Expectancy and the balanced placebo design. In N. K. Mello (Ed.), *Advances in substance abuse* (Vol. 1). Greenwich, CT: JAI.

Marsden, C., & Dracup, K. (1991). Different perspectives: The effect of heart disease on patients and spouses. *AACN Clinical Issues, 2*(2), 285-292.

Marsden, D. (1982). *Workless.* London: Croom Hill.

Masters, J., Cerreto, M., & Mendlowitz, D. (1983). The role of the family in coping with childhood chronic illness. In T. Burish & L. Bradley (Eds.), *Coping with chronic disease* (pp. 381-407). San Diego: Academic Press.

May, R. (1977). *The meaning of anxiety* (Rev. ed.). New York: Norton.

McAdoo, H. P. (1993). Ethnic families: Strengths that are found in diversity. In H. P. McAdoo (Ed.), *Family ethnicity: Strength in diversity* (pp. 3-14). Newbury Park, CA: Sage.

McCubbin, H. I., & Patterson, J. M. (1983). Family transitions: Adaptation to stress. In H. I. McCubbin & C. R. Figley (Eds.), *Stress and the family. Vol. 1: Coping with normative transitions* (pp. 5-25). New York: Brunner/Mazel.

McCubbin, M. A., & McCubbin, H. I. (1987). Family stress theory and assessment. The T-Double ABCX Model of family adjustment and adaptation. In H. I. McCubbin, & A. I. Thompson (Eds.), *Family assessment inventories for research and practice* (pp. 1-25). Madison: The University of Wisconsin—Madison.

McGinnis, S. (1986). How can nurses improve the quality of life of hospice client and family? An exploratory study. *Hospice Journal, 2*(1), 23-36.

McGoldrick, M., & Carter, E. A. (1982). The family life cycle. In F. Walsh (Ed.), *Normal family processes* (pp. 167-195). New York: Guilford.

McHale, S. M., & Crouter, A. C. (1992). You can't always get what you want: Incongruence between sex-role attitudes and family work roles and its implications for marriage. *Journal of Marriage and the Family, 54*(3), 537-547.

McLoyd, V. C. (1989). Socialization and development in a changing economy: The effects of paternal job and income loss on children. *American Psychologist, 44,* 293-302.

McShane, R. E. (1991). Family theoretical perspectives and implication for nursing practice. *AACN Clinical Issues, 2*(2), 210-219.

Mechanic, D. (1987). Correcting misconceptions in mental health policy: Strategies for improved care of the seriously mentally ill. *Milbank Quarterly, 65*(2), 203-230.

Mederer, H., & Hill, R. (1983). Critical transitions over the family life span: Theory and research. In H. I. McCubbin, M. B. Sussman, & J. M. Patterson (Eds.), *Social stress and the family: Advances in family stress theory and research* (pp. 39-60). New York: Haworth.

Mederer, H. J. (1993). Division of labor in two-earner homes: Task accomplishment versus household management as critical variables in perceptions about family work. *Journal of Marriage and the Family, 55*(1), 133-145.

Mednick, M. T. (1987). Single mothers: A review and critique of current research. *Applied Social Psychology Annual, 7,* 184-201.

Melick, M. E. (1985). The health of postdisaster populations: A review of the literature. In J. Laube & S. A. Murphy (Eds.), *Perspectives on disaster recovery* (pp. 179-209). Norwalk, CT: Appleton-Century-Crofts.

Miller, B. C., & Myers-Walls, J. A. (1983). Parenthood: Stresses and coping strategies. In H. I. McCubbin & C. R. Figley (Eds.), *Stress and the family. Vol. 1: Coping with normative transitions* (pp. 54-73). New York: Brunner/Mazel.

Miller, D., & Jang, M. (1977). Children of alcoholics: A 20-year longitudinal study. *Social Work Research, 13,* 23-29.

Miller Ham, L., & Chamings, P. A. (1983). Family nursing: Historical perspectives. In I. W. Clements & F. B. Roberts (Eds.), *Family health: A theoretical approach to nursing care* (pp. 33-43). New York: John Wiley.

Minuchin, S. (1974). *Families and family therapy.* Cambridge, MA: Harvard University.

Minuchin, S., Baker, L., Rosman, B. L., Liebman, R., Milman, L., & Todd, T. C. (1975). A conceptual model of psychosomatic illness in children: Family organization and family therapy. *Archives of General Psychiatry, 32,* 1031-1038.

Mirowsky, J., & Ross, C. (1989). *Social causes of psychological distress.* New York: Aldine de Gruyter.

Mirr, M. P. (1991). Decisions made by family members of patients with severe head injury. *AACN Clinical Issues, 2*(2), 242-251.

Mischke-Berkey, K., Warner, P., & Hanson, S. (1989). Family health assessment and intervention. In P. Bomar (Ed.), *Nursing and family health promotion* (pp. 115-154). Baltimore, MD: Williams & Wilkins.

Mitchell, E. S. (1986). Multiple triangulation: A methodology for nursing science. *Advances in Nursing Science, 8*(3), 18-26.

Moen, P., Kain, E. L., & Elder, G. H. (1983). Economic condition and family life: Contemporary and historical perspectives. In R. R. Nelson & F. Skidmore (Eds.), *American families and the economy: The high costs of living* (pp. 213-259). Washington, DC: National Academy Press.

Mohamed, S., Weisz, E., & Waring, E. (1978). The relationship of chronic pain to depression, marital adjustment and family dynamics. *Pain, 5,* 285-292.

Molter, N. (1979). Needs of relatives of critically ill patients: A descriptive study. *Heart and Lung, 8,* 332-339.

Molter, N. C., & Leske, J. S. (1983). *Critical care family needs inventory.* Milwaukee: University of Wisconsin—Milwaukee, School of Nursing. [Instrument available from authors.]

Moltz, D. A. (1993). Bipolar disorder and the family: An integrative model. *Family Process, 32*(4), 409-423.

Montgomery, R. J. (1987). Social service utilization. In G. Maddox (Ed.), *Encyclopedia of aging* (pp. 630-632). New York: Springer.

Montgomery, R. J., & Borgatta, E. F. (1985). *Family support project* (Final report to the Administration on Aging). Seattle: University of Washington, Institute on Aging/Long-Term Care Center.

Montgomery, R. J., & Kosloski, K. (1994). A longitudinal analysis of nursing home placement for dependent elders cared for by spouses vs. adult children. *Journal of Gerontology, 49*(2), S62-S74.

Moorman, J. E., & Hernandez, D. J. (1989). Married couple families with step, adopted, and biological children. *Demography, 26,* 267-277.

Moos, R. H. (1974). Systems for the assessment and classification of human environments: An overview. In R. Moos & P. Insel (Eds.), *Issues in social ecology* (pp. 5-28). Palo Alto, CA: National.

Moos, R. H. (1986). *Family Environment Scale: Manual* (2nd ed.). Palo Alto, CA: Consulting Psychologists.

Morse, J. M. (1991). Approaches to qualitative-quantitative methodological triangulation. *Nursing Research, 40*(1), 120-123.

Moss, M., & Kurland, P. (1979). Family visiting with institutionalized mentally impaired aged. *Journal of Gerontological Social Work, 1,* 271-278.

Motenko, A. K. (1989). The frustrations, gratifications, and well-being of dementia caregivers. *The Gerontologist, 29,* 166-172.

Moynihan, D. (1986). The tangle of pathology. In R. Staples (Ed.), *The black family: Essays and studies* (3rd ed., pp. 5-14). Belmont, CA: Wadsworth.

Murphy, S. (1986). Family study and nursing research. *Image, 18*(4), 170-174.

Murphy, S. A. (1989). Multiple triangulation: Applications in programs of nursing research. *Nursing Research, 38*(5), 294-297.

Murphy, S. A. (1991). Human responses to catastrophe. In J. J. Fitzpatrick, R. L. Taunton, & A. K. Jacox (Eds.), *Annual review of nursing research* (Vol. 9, pp. 57-76). New York: Springer.

Myers, J., Lindenthal, J., & Pepper, M. (1974). Social class, life events and psychiatric symptoms: A longitudinal study. In B. S. Dohrenwend & B. P. Dohrenwend (Eds.), *Stressful life events: Their nature and effects* (pp. 191-205). New York: John Wiley.

Naisbett, J. (1982). *Megatrends—Ten new directions transforming our lives.* New York: Warner.

Nanji, A. A. (1993). The Muslim family in North America: Continuity and change. In H. P. McAdoo (Ed.), *Family ethnicity: Strength in diversity* (pp. 229-242). Newbury Park, CA: Sage.

Nelson, M. A. (1993). Race, gender, and the effect of social supports on the use of health services by elderly individuals. *International Journal of Aging and Human Development, 37*(3), 227-246.

Neugarten, B. L. (1979). Time, age and the life cycle. *American Journal of Psychiatry, 136,* 887-894.

Neuman, B. (1982). *The Neuman systems model: Application to nursing education and practice.* Norwalk, CT: Appleton-Century-Crofts.

Newman, M. (1979). *Theory development in nursing.* Philadelphia: F. A. Davis.

Newman, M. (1983). Newman's health theory. In I. W. Clements & F. B. Roberts (Eds.), *Family health: A theoretical approach to nursing care* (pp. 161-175). New York: John Wiley.

Newman, M. (1990). Newman's theory of health. *Nursing Science Quarterly, 3*(1), 37-41.

Newman, M. (1992). Prevailing paradigms in nursing. *Nursing Outlook, 40*(1), 10-13, 32.

Nobles, W. (1978). Toward an empirical and theoretical framework for defining black families. *Journal of Marriage and the Family, 40,* 679-698.

Norbeck, J. S. (1988). Social support. In J. J. Fitzpatrick, R. L. Taunton, & J. Q. Benoliel (Eds.), *Annual review of nursing research* (Vol. 6, pp. 85-109). New York: Springer.

Norris, L. O., & Grove, S. K. (1986). Investigation of selected psychosocial needs of family members of critically ill adult patients. *Heart and Lung, 15,* 194-199.

Norton, A., & Glick, P. (1986). One parent families: A social and economic profile. *Family Relations, 35*(1), 9-17.

Oberst, M. T., & James, R. H. (1985). Going home: Patient and spouse adjustment following cancer surgery. *Topics of Clinical Nursing, 7,* 46-57.

Oden, B. (1986). The family yesterday and today—an historical perspective. *Socialmedicininsk Tidskrift, 5*(6), 200-207.

Oiler Boyd, C. (1993). Toward a nursing practice research method. *Advances in Nursing Science, 16*(2), 9-25.

Olshansky, S. (1962). Chronic sorrow: A response to having a mentally defective child. *Social Case Work, 43,* 190-193.

Olson, D. H., McCubbin, H. I., Barnes, H. L., Larsen, A. S., Muxen, M. J., & Wilson, M. A. (1984). *Families: What makes them work?* Beverly Hills, CA: Sage.

Olson, D. H., Portner, J., & Lavee, Y. (1985). *FACES III.* St. Paul, MN: University of Minnesota, Family Social Science.

Orem, D. E. (1985). *Nursing: Concepts of practice* (3rd ed.). New York: McGraw-Hill.

Orona, C. J. (1990). Temporality and identity loss due to Alzheimer's disease. *Social Science in Medicine, 30,* 1247-1256.

Osterman, P. (1993). Why don't "they" work? Employment patterns in a high pressure economy. *Social Science Research, 22,* 115-130.

Pagalow, M. D. (1981). *Women-battering: Victims and their experiences.* Beverly Hills, CA: Sage.

Parks, C. M. (1975). The emotional impact of cancer on patients and their families. *Journal of Laryngology and Ontology, 89,* 1271-1279.

Patterson, G. R., & Capaldi, D. (1991). Antisocial parents: Unskilled and vulnerable. In P. Cowan & E. M. Hetherington (Eds.), *Family transitions* (pp. 195-218). Hillsdale, NJ: Lawrence Erlbaum.

Patterson, J. M., Budd, J., Goetz, D., & Warwick, W. J. (1993). Family correlates of a 10-year pulmonary health trend in cystic fibrosis. *Pediatrics, 91*(2), 383-389.

Patton, M. Q. (1987). *How to use qualitative methods in evaluation.* Newbury Park, CA: Sage.

Payne, R. L., & Hartley, J. (1987). A test of a model for explaining the affective experience of unemployed men. *Journal of Occupational Psychology, 60,* 31-47.

Pearlin, L. I. (1983). Role strains and personal stress. In H. B. Kaplan (Ed.), *Psychological stress: Trends in theory and research* (pp. 3-32). San Diego: Academic Press.

Pearlin, L. I. (1990). The sociological study of stress. *Journal of Health and Social Behavior, 30,* 241-256.

Pearlin, L. I., Lieberman, M. A., Menaghan, E. G., & Mullan, J. T. (1981). The stress process. *Journal of Health and Social Behavior, 22,* 337-356.

Peele, S., & Brodsky, A. (1975). *Love and addiction.* Los Angeles: Taplinger.

Pender, N. J. (1987). *Health promotion in nursing practice* (2nd ed.). Norwalk, CT: Appleton & Lange.

Perry-Jenkins, M., & Crouter, A. C. (1990). Implications of men's provider role attitudes for household work and marital satisfaction. *Journal of Family Issues, 11,* 136-156.

Peters, M., & deFord, C. (1986). The solo mother. In R. Staples (Ed.), *The black family: Essays and studies* (3rd ed., pp. 164-172). Belmont, CA: Wadsworth.

Pettingale, K. W., Morris, T., Greer, S., & Haybittle, J. L. (1985, Winter). Mental attitudes to cancer: An additional prognostic factor. *Lancett,* p. 750.

Phillips, J. R. (1988). Research issues: Research blenders. *Nursing Science Quarterly, 1*(1), 4-5.

Phillips, L. R., & Rempusheski, V. F. (1986). Caring for the frail elderly at home: Toward a theoretical explanation of the dynamics of poor quality family caregiving. *Advances in Nursing Science, 8,* 62-84.

Pilisuk, M., & Acredolo, C. (1988). Fear of technological hazards: One concern of many? *Social Behavior, 3,* 17-24.

Pill, C. J. (1990). Stepfamilies: Redefining the family. *Family Relations, 39,* 186-193.

Pittman, F. S. (1987). *Turning points: Treating families in transition and crisis.* New York: Norton.

Pittman, F. S. (1988). Family crises: Expectable and unexpectable. In C. J. Falicov (Ed.), *Family transitions: Continuity and change over the life cycle* (pp. 255-271). New York: Guilford.

Polit, D., & Hungler, B. (1991). *Nursing research: Principles and methods* (4th ed.). Philadelphia: J. B. Lippincott.

Polit, D. F., & Hungler, B. P. (1989). *Essentials of nursing research: Methods, appraisal, and utilization* (2nd ed.). Philadelphia: J. B. Lippincott.

Potuchek, J. L. (1992). Employed wives' orientations to breadwinning: A gender theory analysis. *Journal of Marriage and the Family, 54*(3), 548-558.

Price, R. H. (1990). Strategies for managing plant closings and downsizing. In D. B. Fishman & C. Cherniss (Eds.), *The human side of corporate competitiveness* (pp. 127-151). Newbury Park, CA: Sage.

Pruchno, R., & Kleban, M. H. (1993). Caring for an institutionalized parent: The role of coping strategies. *Psychology and Aging, 8*(1), 18-25.

Pruchno, R. A., & Resch, N. L. (1989). Mental health of caregiving spouses: Coping as mediator, moderator, or main effect? *Psychology and Aging, 4,* 454-463.

Ragiel, C. A. (1984). The impact of critical injury on patient, family and clinical systems. *Critical Care Quarterly, 7,* 73-78.

Ragsdale, D., Kotarba, J. A., & Morrow, J. R. (1992). Quality of life of hospitalized persons with AIDS. *Image, 24*(4), 259-265.

Rait, D., & Lederberg, M. (1989). The family of the cancer patient. In J. Holland & J. Rowland (Eds.), *Handbook of psychooncology: Psychological care of the patient with cancer.* New York: Oxford University Press.

Rando, T. A. (1984). *Grief, dying and death: Clinical interventions for caregivers.* Champaign, IL: Research Press.

Rankin, S. H. (1989). Family transitions expected and unexpected. In C. L. Gilliss, B. L. Highley, B. M. Roberts, & I. M. Martinson (Eds.), *Toward a science of family nursing* (pp. 173-186). Reading, MA: Addison-Wesley.

Ransom, D. C., Fisher, L., & Terry, H. E. (1992). The California Family Health Project: II. Family world view and adult health. *Family Process, 31*(3), 251-267.

Rapoport, R. (1963). Normal crisis, family structure and mental health. *Family Process, 2,* 68-80.

Rappaport, J. (1987). Terms of empowerment/exemplars of prevention: Toward a theory for community psychology. *American Journal of Community Psychology, 15,* 121-148.

Ravitch, D. (1974). *The great school wars.* New York: Basic Books.

Ray, S., & McLoyd, V. (1986). Fathers in hard times: The impact of unemployment and poverty on paternal and maternal relationships. In M. Lamb (Ed.), *The father's role: Applied perspectives* (pp. 339-383). New York: John Wiley.

Reback, M. (1994, October 2). Disabled student often swept away by mainstream. *The Detroit News,* p. 3B.

Reigel, B., Omery, A., Calvillo, E., Elsayed, G., Lee, P., Shuler, P., & Siegal, B. E. (1992). Moving beyond: A generative philosophy of science. *Image, 24*(2), 115-120.

Reinhard, S. C. (1994). Perspectives on the family's caregiving experience in mental illness. *Image, 26*(1), 70-74.

Retzer, A., Simon, F. B., Weber, G., Stierlin, H., & Schmidt, G. (1991). A follow-up study of manic-depressive and schizoaffective psychoses after systemic family therapy. *Family Process, 30*(2), 139-153.

Riehl, J. P., & Roy, S. C. (1980). *Conceptual models for nursing practice.* Norwalk, CT: Appleton-Century-Crofts.

Roberts, C. S., & Feetham, S. L. (1982). Assessing family functioning across three areas of relationships. *Nursing Research, 81*(4), 231-235.

Rodgers, C. D. (1983). Needs of relatives of cardiac surgery patients during the critical care phase. *Focus on Critical Care, 10,* 50-55.

Rogers, M. (1970). *An introduction to the theoretical basis of nursing.* Philadelphia: F. A. Davis.

Rogers, M. E. (1980). Nursing: A science of unitary man. In J. P. Riehl & C. Roy, *Conceptual models for nursing practice* (2nd ed., pp. 329-337). Norwalk, CT: Appleton-Century-Crofts.

Ronco, W. R., & Peattie, I. (1988). Making work: A perspective from social science. In R. Pahl (Ed.), *On work: Historical, comparative, and theoretical approaches* (pp. 709-721). Cambridge, MA: Blackwell.

Rook, K., Dooley, D., & Catalano, R. (1991). Stress transmission: The effects of husbands' job stressors on the emotional health of their wives. *Journal of Marriage and the Family, 53*(1), 165-177.

Rosen, K. H., & Stith, S. M. (1993). Intervention strategies for treating women in violent dating relationships. *Family Relations, 42*(4), 427-433.

Rosman, B. (1988). Family development and the impact of a child's chronic illness. In C. J. Falicov (Ed.), *Family transitions: Continuity and change over the life cycle* (pp. 293-309). New York: Guilford.

Ross, C. E., Mirowski, J., & Goldstein, K. (1990). The impact of the family on health: The decade in review. *Journal of Marriage and the Family, 52*(4), 1059-1078.

Roth, P. (1989a). Family health promotion during transitions. In P. J. Bomar (Ed.), *Nurses and family health promotion: Concepts, assessment, and interventions* (pp. 320-347). Baltimore, MD: Williams & Wilkins.

Roth, P. (1989b). Family social support. In P. J. Bomar (Ed.), *Nurses and family health promotion: Concepts, assessment, and interventions* (pp. 90-102). Baltimore, MD: Williams & Wilkins.

Rousseau, D. M. (1978). Relations of work to nonwork. *Journal of Applied Psychology, 33,* 513-517.

Rowley, K. M., & Feather, N. T. (1987). The impact of unemployment in relation to age and length of unemployment. *Journal of Occupational Psychology, 60,* 323-332.

Rubin, R. H. (1983). Epilogue: Families and alternative lifestyles in an age of technological revolution. In E. D. Macklin & R. H. Rubin (Eds.), *Contemporary families and alternative life styles* (pp. 400-409). Beverly Hills, CA: Sage.

Ryder, R. G. (1973). Longitudinal data relating marriage satisfaction and having a child. *Journal of Marriage and the Family, 35,* 604-606.

Sacks, O. (1987). *The man who mistook his wife for a hat and other clinical tales.* New York: Harper Perennial.

Sadler, J. Z., & Hulgus, Y. F. (1991). Clinical controversy and the domains of scientific evidence. *Family Process, 30*(1), 21-26.

Sandelowski, M. (1993). Rigor or rigor mortis: The problem of rigor in qualitative research revisited. *Advances in Nursing Science, 16*(2), 1-18.

Santi, L. L. (1987). Changes in the structure and size of American households: 1970 to 1985. *Journal of Marriage and the Family, 49*(4), 833-837.

Santrock, J. W., & Warshak, R. A. (1979). Father custody and social development in boys and girls. *Journal of Social Issues, 35,* 112-125.

Sarter, B. J. (1990). Philosophical foundations of nursing theory. In N. Chaska (Ed.), *The nursing profession: Turning points* (pp. 223-229). St. Louis, MO: C. V. Mosby.

Sawhill, I. (1988). Poverty in the U.S.: Why is it so persistent? *Journal of Economic Literature, 26*(3), 1073-1119.

Sayles-Cross, S. (1993). Perceptions of familial caregivers of elder adults. *Image, 25*(2), 88-92.

Schaefer, M. T., & Olson, D. H. (1981). Assessing intimacy: The PAIR inventory. *Journal of Marital and Family Therapy, 7,* 47-60.

Seligman, M. (1975). *Helplessness: On depression, development, and death.* San Francisco: Freeman.

Seligman, M., & Darling, R. B. (1989). *Ordinary families, special children: A systems approach to childhood disability.* New York: Guilford.

Selvini-Palazzoli, M., Cirillo, S., Selvini, M., & Sorrentino, A. M. (1989). *Family games: General models of psychotic processes in the family.* New York: Norton.

Serra, P. (1993). Physical violence in the couple relationship: A contribution toward the analysis of the context. *Family Process, 32*(1), 21-33.

Shamir, B. (1986). Unemployment and the household division of labor. *Journal of Marriage and the Family, 48*(1), 195-206.

Shapiro, J. (1983). Family reactions and coping strategies in response to the physically ill or handicapped child: A review. *Social Science Medicine, 17,* 913-931.

Shorter, E. (1975). *The making of the modern family.* New York: Basic Books.

Silva, M. C., & Rothbart, D. (1984). Analysis of changing trends in philosophies of science on nursing theory development and testing. *Advances in Nursing Science, 6*(1), 1-13.

Silva, M. C., & Sorrel, J. M. (1992). Testing of nursing theory: Critique and philosophical expansion. *Advances in Nursing Science, 14*(4), 12-23.

Silver, R. L., & Wortman, C. B. (1980). Coping with undesirable life events. In J. Garber & M. E. Seligman (Eds.), *Human helplessness* (pp. 279-341). New York: Academic Press.

Simpson, T. (1991). The family as a source of support for the critically ill adult. *AACN Clinical Issues, 2*(2), 229-235.

Sloman, L., & Konstantareas, M. M. (1990). Why families of children with biological deficits require a systems approach. *Family Process, 29*(4), 417-429.

Small, S. A., & Riley, D. (1990). Toward a multidimensional assessment of work spillover into family life. *Journal of Marriage and the Family, 52*(1), 51-62.

Smilkstein, G. (1978). The family APGAR: A proposal for a family function test and its use by physicians. *Journal of Family Practice, 6,* 1231-1239.

Smith, G. C., Smith, M. F., & Toseland, R. W. (1991). Problems identified by family caregivers in counseling. *The Gerontologist, 31,* 15-22.

Smith, K., & Bengston, V. (1979). Positive consequences of institutionalization: Solidarity between elderly parents and their middle-aged children. *The Gerontologist, 19,* 438-443.

Smith, K., Kupferschmid, B. J., Dawson, C., & Briones, T. L. (1991). A family-centered critical care unit. *AACN Clinical Issues, 2*(2), 258-266.

Snell, J. E., Rosenwald, R. J., & Robey, A. (1964). The wifebeater's wife: A study of family interaction. *Archives of General Psychiatry, 11,* 107-112.

Sohier, R. (1988). Multiple triangulation and contemporary nursing research. *Western Journal of Nursing Research, 10*(6), 732-742.

Spanier, G. B., & Lewis, R. A. (1980). Marital quality: A review of the seventies. *Journal of Marriage and the Family, 42,* 825-839.

Spector, R. (1979). *Cultural diversity in health and illness.* Norwalk, CT: Appleton-Century-Crofts.

Speer, D. C. (1970). Family systems: Morphostasis and morphogenesis, or "is homeostasis enough?" *Family Process, 9,* 259-278.

Stack, C. (1986). Sex roles and survival strategies in an urban black community. In R. Staples (Ed.), *The black family: Essays and studies* (3rd ed., pp. 88-98). Belmont, CA: Wadsworth.

Stack, C. (1990). Different voices, different visions: Gender, culture, and moral reasoning. In F. Ginsburg & A. L. Tsing (Eds.), *Uncertain terms: Negotiating gender in American culture* (pp. 19-27). Boston: Beacon Press.

Staines, G., & O'Connor, P. (1980). Conflicts among work, leisure, and family roles. *Monthly Labor Review, 103,* 35-39.

Staples, R. (1974). The black family revisited: A review and a preview. *Journal of Social and Behavioral Sciences, 20,* 65-78.

Staples, R. (1986). Changes in black family structure: The conflict between family ideology and structural conditions. In R. Staples (Ed.), *The black family: Essays and studies* (3rd ed., pp. 20-28). Belmont, CA: Wadsworth.

Staples, R. (1989). Family life in the 21st century: An analysis of old forms, current trends, and future scenarios. In C. L. Gilliss, B. L. Highley, B. M. Roberts, & I. M. Martinson (Eds.), *Toward a science of family nursing* (pp. 156-170). Reading, MA: Addison-Wesley.

Staples, R., & Mirande, A. (1980). Racial and cultural variations among American families: A decennial review of the literature on minority families. *Journal of Marriage and the Family, 42*(4), 887-903.

Stattin, H., & Klackenberg, G. (1992). Discordant family relations in intact families: Developmental tendencies over 18 years. *Journal of Marriage and the Family, 54*(4), 940-956.

Steinberg, L. (1990). Autonomy, conflict, and harmony in the family relationship. In S. S. Feldman & G. R. Elliott (Eds.), *At the threshold: The developing adolescent* (pp. 255-276). Cambridge, MA: Harvard University Press.

Steinberg, L. D., Catalano, R., & Dooley, D. (1981). Economic antecedents of child abuse and neglect. *Child Development, 52,* 975-983.

Steinglass, P., Bennett, L. A., Wolin, S. J., & Reiss, D. (1987). *The alcoholic family.* New York: Basic Books.

Stevens, B. J. (1979). *Nursing theory: Analysis, application, evaluation.* Boston: Little, Brown.

Stevens, G. L., Walsh, R. A., & Baldwin, B. A. (1993). Family caregivers of institutionalized elderly individuals. *Nursing Clinics of North America, 28*(2), 349-362.

Stoll, R. I. (1989). The essence of spirituality. In V. B. Carson (Ed.), *Spiritual dimensions of nursing practice* (pp. 4-23). Philadelphia: Saunders.

Stoller, E., & Earl, L. (1983). Help with activities of everyday life: Sources of support for the noninstitutionalized elderly. *The Gerontologist, 23,* 64-70.

Strober, M., Lampert, C., Morrell, W., Burroughs, J., & Jacobs, C. (1990). A controlled family study of anorexia nervosa: Evidence of familial aggregation and lack of shared transmission with affective disorders. *International Journal of Eating Disorders, 9,* 239-253.

Suarez, Z. E. (1993). Cuban Americans: From golden exiles to social undesirables. In H. P. McAdoo (Ed.), *Family ethnicity: Strength in diversity* (pp. 164-176). Newbury Park, CA: Sage.

Sullivan, H. S. (1953). *Interpersonal theory of psychiatry.* New York: Norton.

Sullivan, M. L. (1989). Absent fathers in the inner city. In W. J. Wilson (Ed.), *The ghetto underclass: Social science perspectives* (pp. 48-58). Newbury Park, CA: Sage.

Suppe, F., & Jacox, A. K. (1985). Philosophy of science and the development of nursing theory. In H. H. Werly & J. J. Fitzpatrick (Eds.), *Annual review of nursing research* (pp. 241-267). New York: Springer.

Symons, D. K., & McLeod, P. J. (1993). Maternal employment plans and outcomes after the birth of an infant in a Canadian sample. *Family Relations, 42*(4), 442-446.

Taitz, L. S., King, J. M., Nicholson, J., & Kessel, M. (1987). Unemployment and child abuse. *British Medical Journal, 294,* 1074-1076.

Teachman, J. D., Polonko, K. A., & Scanzoni, J. (1987). Demography of the family. In M. B. Sussman & S. Steinmetz (Eds.), *Handbook of marriage and the family* (pp. 3-36). New York: Plenum.

Tennstedt, S. L., Crawford, S. L., & McKinlay, J. B. (1993). Is family care on the decline? A longitudinal investigation of the substitution of formal long-term care services for informal care. *The Milbank Quarterly, 71*(4), 601-624.

Tennstedt, S. L., & McKinlay, J. B. (1989). Informal care for frail older persons. In M. G. Ory & K. Band (Eds.), *Aging and health care* (pp. 145-165). New York: Routledge.

Thomas, L., McCabe, E., & Berry, J. (1980). Unemployment and family stress: A reassessment. *Family Relations, 29,* 517-524.

Thompson, L. (1991). Family work: Women's sense of fairness. *Journal of Family Issues, 12,* 181-196.

Thornton, A., Young-DeMarco, L., & Goldscheider, F. (1993). Leaving the parental nest: The experience of a young white cohort in the 1980s. *Journal of Marriage and the Family, 55*(1), 216-229.

Tilly, L., & Scott, J. (1978). *Women, work, and family.* New York: Holt, Rinehart & Winston.

Tinbergen, E. A., & Tinbergen, N. (1972). *Early childhood autism: An ethological approach. Advances in ethology* (Vol. 10). Berlin: Paul Parey.

Tripp-Reimer, T., & Lauer, G. M. (1987). Ethnicity and families with chronic illness. In L. M. Wright & M. Leahy (Eds.), *Families and chronic illness* (pp. 77-100). Springhouse, PA: Springhouse Corp.

Trygar-Artinian, N. (1991). Strengthening nurse-family relationships in critical care. *AACN Clinical Issues, 2*(2), 269-275.

Turner, R. J. (1983). Direct, indirect, and moderating effects of social support on psychological distress and associated conditions. In H. B. Kaplan (Ed.), *Psychosocial stress* (pp. 105-155). San Diego: Academic Press.

Udelman, H., & Udelman, L. D. (1980). The family and chronic illness. *Arizona Medicine, 37,* 491-494.

U.S. Congress, House Committee on Ways and Means. (1986, March 18). *Hearing before subcommittee on public assistance and unemployment compensation, 99th Congress, 2d Sess.* Washington, DC: Author.

Valle, R. (1989). U.S. ethnic minority group access to long-term care. In T. Schwab (Ed.), *Caring for an aging world: International models for long-term care, financing, and delivery* (pp. 339-363). New York: McGraw-Hill.

Vanicelli, M. (1987). Treatment of alcoholic couples in outpatient group therapy. *Group, 11*(4), 247-257.

Vaughan, F. (1986). *The inward arc: Healing and wholeness in psychotherapy and spirituality.* Boston: New Science Library.

Vaughn, C. E., & Leff, J. P. (1976). The influence of family and social factors on the course of psychiatric illness: A comparison of schizophrenic and depressed neurotic patients. *British Journal of Psychiatry, 129,* 125-137.

Verbosky, S. J., & Ryan, D. A. (1988). Female partners of Vietnam veterans: Stress by proximity. *Issues in Mental Health Nursing, 9,* 95-104.

Violon, A., & Guirgea, D. (1984). Familial models for chronic pain. *Pain, 18,* 199-203.

Visher, E., & Visher, J. (1988). *Old loyalties, new ties: Therapeutic strategies with stepfamilies.* New York: Brunner/Mazel.

Visher, E. B., & Visher, J. S. (1978). Major areas of difficulty for stepparent couples. *International Journal of Family Counseling, 6,* 70-80.

Visher, E. B., & Visher, J. S. (1982). Stepfamilies and stepparenting. In F. Walsh (Ed.), *Normal family processes* (pp. 331-353). New York: Guilford.

von Bertalanffy, L. (1968). *General systems theory.* New York: George Braziller.

Voydanoff, P. (1984). Economic distress and families: Policy issues. *Journal of Family Issues, 5,* 273-288.

Voydanoff, P. (1988). Work role characteristics, family structure demands and work/family conflict. *Journal of Marriage and the Family, 50*(3), 749-761.

Voydanoff, P. (1990). Economic distress and family relations: A review of the eighties. *Journal of Marriage and the Family, 52*(4), 1099-1115.

Voydanoff, P., & Donnelly, B. W. (1988). Economic distress, family coping, and quality of family life. In P. Voydanoff & I. C. Majka (Eds.), *Families and economic distress* (pp. 97-116). Newbury Park, CA: Sage.

Walker, L. E. (1979). *The battered woman.* New York: Harper & Row.

Walker, L. E. (1984). *The battered woman syndrome.* New York: Springer.

Walker, L. E. (1993). The battered woman syndrome is a psychological consequence of abuse. In R. J. Gelles & D. R. Loseke (Eds.), *Current controversies on family violence* (pp. 133-153). Newbury Park, CA: Sage.

Wasserman, I. M. (1984). A longitudinal analysis of the linkage between suicide, unemployment, and marital dissolution. *Journal of Marriage and the Family, 46*(4), 853-859.

Watson, J. (1985). *Nursing: Human science and human care.* Norwalk, CT: Appleton-Century-Crofts.

Watzlawick, P., Beavin, J. H., & Jackson, D. D. (1967). *Pragmatics of human communication: A study of interactional patterns, pathologies and paradoxes.* New York: Norton.

Watzlawick, P., Weakland, C. E., & Fisch, R. (1974). *Change: Principles of problem formation and problem resolution.* New York: Norton.

Webb, A. A., & Friedemann, M. L. (1991). Six years after an economic crisis: Child's anxiety and quality of peer relationships. *Journal of Community Health Nursing, 8*(4), 233-243.

Wegscheider, S. (1981). *Another chance: Hope and health for the alcoholic family.* Palo Alto, CA: Science and Behavior Books.

Weigel, R. R. (1988). Coping with economic stress: Implications for helping professionals. *Lifestyles: Family and Economic Issues, 9*(4), 367-382.

Weinberg, G. M. (1975). *Introduction to general systems thinking.* New York: Wiley Interscience.

Wenger, D. E. (1978). Community response to disaster: Functional and structural alterations. In E. L. Quarantelli (Ed.), *Disasters: Theory and research* (pp. 17-47). Beverly Hills, CA: Sage.

Werner, E. E. (1986). Resilient offspring of alcoholics: A longitudinal study from birth to age 18. *Journal of Studies on Alcohol, 47,* 34-40.

Whall, A. L. (1986). *Family therapy theory for nursing.* Norwalk, CT: Appleton-Century-Crofts.

Whall, A. L. (1993). Disciplinary issues related to family theory development in nursing. In S. L. Feetham, S. B. Meister, J. M. Bell, & C. L. Gilliss (Eds.), *The nursing of families* (pp. 13-17). Newbury Park, CA: Sage.

Whall, A. L., & Fawcett, J. (1991). The family as a focal phenomenon in nursing. In A. L. Whall & J. Fawcett (Eds.), *Family theory development in nursing: State of the science and art* (pp. 7-29). Philadelphia: F. A. Davis.

Whelan, C. T. (1992). The role of income, life-style deprivation and financial strain in mediating the impact of unemployment on psychological distress: Evidence from the Republic of Ireland. *Journal of Occupational and Organizational Psychology, 65,* 331-344.

Widom, C. S. (1989). Does violence beget violence? A critical examination of the literature. *Psychological Bulletin, 106,* 3-28.

Wilk, J. (1988). Family environments and the young chronically mentally ill. *Journal of Psychosocial Nursing, 26*(10), 15-20.

Willie, C. (1988). *A new look at black families* (3rd ed.). Dix Hills, NY: General Hall.

Wilson, H. S. (1993). Family caregiving for a relative with Alzheimer's dementia: Coping with negative choices. In G. D. Wegner & R. J. Alexander (Eds.), *Readings in family nursing* (pp. 197-207). Philadelphia: J. B. Lippincott.

Wilson, H. S., & Hutchinson, S. A. (1991). Triangulation of qualitative methods: Heideggerian hermeneutics and grounded theory. *Qualitative Health Research, 1*(2), 263-276.

Wilson, J. W. (1987). *The truly disadvantaged: The inner city, the underclass, and public policy.* Chicago: University of Chicago Press.

Wilson, S. M., Larson, J. H., & Stone, K. I. (1993). Stress among job insecure workers and their spouses. *Family Relations, 42*(1), 74-80.

Wolfer, J. (1993). Aspects of "reality" and ways of knowing in nursing: In search of an integrating paradigm. *Image, 25*(2), 141-145.

Wolfson, C., Handfield-Jones, R., Glass, K. C., McClaran, J., & Keyserlingk, E. (1993). Adult children's perceptions of their responsibility to provide care for dependent elderly parents. *The Gerontologist, 33*(3), 315-323.

Wolin, S. J., & Bennett, L. A. (1984). Family rituals. *Family Process, 23,* 401-420.

Woods, N. F., & Catanzaro, M. (1988). *Nursing research: Theory and practice.* St. Louis, MO: C. V. Mosby.

Woolfolk, R., Sass, L., & Messer, S. (1988). Introduction to hermeneutics. In S. Messer, L. Sass, & R. Woolfolk (Eds.), *Hermeneutics and psychological theory: Interpretive perspectives on personality, psychotherapy, and psychopathology* (pp. 2-26). New Brunswick, NJ: Rutgers University Press.

Wright, B. (1986, January 15). A doleful existence. *Nursing Times,* pp. 46-47.

Wright, L. M., & Leahy, M. (1984). *Nurses and families: A guide to family assessment and intervention.* Philadelphia: F. A. Davis.

Wright, L. M., & Leahy, M. (1988, May). *Family nursing trends in academic and clinical settings.* Proceedings of the International Family Nursing Conference, Calgary, Alberta, Canada.

Wynne, L. C. (1988). An epigenetic model of family processes. In C. J. Falicov (Ed.), *Family transitions: Continuity and change over the life cycle* (pp. 81-106). New York: Guilford.

Wynne, L. C., Shields, C. G., & Sirkin, M. I. (1992). Illness, family theory, and family therapy: I. Conceptual issues. *Family Process, 31*(1), 3-18.

Young, R. (1983). The family-illness intermesh: Theoretical aspects and their application. *Social Science Medicine, 17,* 395-398.

Zarit, S. H., & Anthony, C. R. (1986). Interventions with dementia patients and their families. In M. L. Gilhooly, S. H. Zarit, & J. E. Birren (Eds.), *The dementias: Policy and management* (pp. 66-92). Englewood Cliffs, NJ: Prentice Hall.

Zimmerman, C. C. (1947). *Family and civilization.* New York: Harper Brothers.

Zimmerman, S. L. (1988). *Understanding family policy: Theoretical approaches.* Newbury Park, CA: Sage.

Zlotnick, C., & Cassanego, M. (1992). Unemployment and health. *Nursing & Health Care, 13*(2), 78-82.

Zvonkovic, A. M., Schmiege, C. J., & Hall, L. D. (1994). Influence strategies used when couples make work-family decisions and their importance for marital satisfaction. *Family Relations, 43*(2), 182-188.

Index

Aaronson, L. S., 288
Abbott, D. D., 82
Ablon, J., 86, 87
Abraham, I. L., 101, 183
Acculturation, 88
Ackoff, R. L., 4
Acredolo, C., 300
Adams, G. R., 81
Addiction:
  as misguided spirituality, 154
  cognitive model of, 154
  cyclical patterns of, 169-170
  disease model of, 154
  etiology of, 170-171
  experimental psychology model of,
    154
  framework of systemic organization
    model of, 170
  life process with, 171-172
  medical model of, 170-171
  morality model of, 154
  social learning model of, 154
  See also Addictions; Addictive family
    roles/life processes
Addictions, 154
  alcoholism, 155
  domestic violence, 155

good habits becoming, 154
obsession and, 155
seesaw coupling and, 169
See also Addiction; Addictive family
  roles/life processes
Addictive family roles/life processes, 156
  alcohol and power, 156-159
  examples of, 156-169
  jealousy, love, and violence, 159-164
  success, control, and drugs, 164-169
  to stabilize family system, 156
African American families:
  cultural schizophrenia of, 97
  kinship networks of, 96
  lifestyle deviances of, 97
  patterns, 96, 97
  predominant matriarchal structure of,
    95
  role of church in, 96
  See also African American family
    system
African American family system:
  as resilient system, 331
  female heads of household in, 331
  survival of amid poverty, 331
  See also African American families
Africanity model, 96-97

377

About the Author

Marie-Luise Friedemann is Associate Professor and Assistant Dean for the Area of Family, Community, and Mental Health Nursing at Wayne State University, College of Nursing, in Detroit. She has a master's degree in psychiatric nursing and a clinical background in community health nursing. Her specialty area is nursing and the health of families. Dr. Friedemann has researched the functioning of families—specifically, families with substance abusers, elders in nursing homes, and unemployed members—and has developed an assessment tool of family effectiveness. The theory of systemic organization has evolved since 1987 and forms the basis of all of Dr. Friedemann's teaching, research, and clinical work. Based on the theory is the Congruence Model, a structured approach to substance-abusing families that she has tested, taught to nurses and other professionals, and is currently using in her clinical work as an ANA-certified nurse family therapist.